Horizons in Medicine

number **12**

Edited by

Peter Weissberg MD FRCP FMedSci

*BHF Professor of Cardiovascular Medicine
Addenbrooke's Centre for Clinical Investigation,
Addenbrooke's Hospital, Cambridge*

**Royal College of
Physicians of London**

Cover illustrations

Front cover: A barium swallow showing lower oesophaeal narrowing due to myopathy. From: Swain, P. Endoscopic ultrasound.

Back cover (top): Interface hepatitis: lymphocytes and plasma cells surround periportal hepatocytes (H & E). From: Bassendine, MF. Autoimmune hepatitis.

Back cover (bottom): A 'remodelled' asthmatic small airway. From: Holgate, ST. Gene-environment interactions in the pathogenesis of asthma.

Royal College of Physicians of London
11 St Andrews Place, London NW1 4LE

Registered Charity No. 210508

Copyright © 2000 Royal College of Physicians of London
ISBN 1 86016 135 9

Typeset by Dan-Set Graphics, Telford, Shropshire
Printed in Great Britain by The Lavenham Press Ltd, Sudbury, Suffolk

British Library Cataloguing in Publication Data
A catalogue record of this book is available from the British Library

Editor's Introduction

You are familiar with the scene: a colleague contacts you, out of the blue, to ask a 'small favour'. 'We would like you to organise the RCP Advanced Medicine Conference. All you have to do is determine the programme and identify the speakers. We do the rest'. What an honour; what can you say? Of course, you agree. However, the initial sense of ego-boosting flattery rapidly gives way to anxiety when you discover that not only must the speakers be asked to deliver a carefully planned lecture aimed at the clinical non-specialist, but they are also to prepare a manuscript for this publication. Those of us whose day-to-day lives include frequent 'off the shelf'-type talks have no problem with yet another; but a talk that requires thought and preparation is something else, and a manuscript requires serious time and commitment, resources that are universally being stretched to the limit. Anxiety gives way to despair when you realise that all your bright ideas for a sensational programme have been used in previous years by your predecessors.

Thankfully, my fears proved unfounded since, first, the reputation and stature of the RCP Advanced Medicine Conference is such that speakers are as keen to speak as delegates are to listen. Almost all the speakers I approached agreed enthusiastically to participate without hesitation. Secondly, staff in the College conference and publications offices really did do all the rest, for which I am eternally grateful. I can therefore reassure future organisers that, not only is organising the conference and editing *Horizons in Medicine* a valuable educational experience, it is a pleasure.

Emphasis is placed on the fact that this volume represents proceedings of the Advanced Medicine Conference, rather than its sister, Science in Medicine. However, science and clinical medicine cannot be dissociated since yesterday's scientific discovery underpins today's medicine. It is not the science but its communication that is difficult. It is a tribute to the speakers and authors of this book that they have seemingly effortlessly communicated the science of their medicine through its application to patient care. At a time when there is increasing pressure on doctors to deliver protocol-driven health care, it is essential that we do not lose sight of the fact that medicine is all about manipulation of basic pathophysiological processes and can only evolve through science. This year we also recognised the contribution of science, in its broadest sense, to the practice of medicine by inclusion of a highly successful session devoted to new technologies in medicine.

The practice of medicine is increasingly dominated by the use of 'high tech' investigational and interventional procedures, and these are well represented in *Horizons in Medicine 12*. However, it is also greatly influenced by its social context, hence the equally important inclusion of chapters on so-called recreational drug abuse, food poisoning and allergies, and the growing burden of obesity. As a specialist who finds it increasingly difficult to keep up with advances in all fields of medicine, I have tried to cover some of the most important aspects of today's 'advanced medicine'. I hope that, like its predecessors, *Horizons in Medicine 12* provides something for everyone, and I sincerely hope that readers will gain as much from reading it as I have from editing it.

PETER WEISSBERG
November 2000

Contributors

JOSEPH BARBENEL *Professor, Bioengineering Unit, University of Strathclyde, Wolfson Centre, 106 Rottenrow, Glasgow G4 0NW*

MARGARET F BASSENDINE *Professor of Hepatology, The Medical School, University of Newcastle and Honorary Consultant Physician, Newcastle upon Tyne United Hospitals Trust*

PAUL BEATTY *Senior Lecturer, Division of Imaging Science and Bio-medical Engineering, The Stopford Building, University of Manchester, Oxford Road, Manchester M13 9PT*

ADRIAN B BOMFORD *Reader in Medicine & Honorary Consultant Physician, Institute of Liver Studies, GKT School of Medicine, King's Denmark Hill Campus, Bessemer Road, London SE5 9JP*

LESZEK K BORYSIEWICZ *Professor of Medicine, Department of Medicine, University of Wales College of Medicine, Heath Park, Cardiff CF4 4XX*

MARTIN M BROWN *Professor of Stroke Medicine, Institute of Neurology, University College London, National Hospital for Neurology & Neurosurgery, Queen Square, London WC1N 3BG*

CHRISTOPHER D BYRNE *Professor of Endocrinology & Metabolism, Director Wellcome Clinical Research Facility & Honorary Consultant Physician, South Academic Block, Level D (MP 811), Southampton General Hospital, Southampton SO16 6YD*

SARAH C CLARKE *Specialist Registrar in Cardiology, Papworth Hospital, Papworth Everard, Cambridge CB3 8RE*

JULIET COMPSTON *Reader in Metabolic Bone Disease and Honorary Consultant Physician, Department of Medicine, University of Cambridge School of Clinical Medicine, Addenbrooke's Hospital, Cambridge CB2 2QQ*

MERERID EVANS *MRC Clinical Training Fellow, Department of Medicine, University of Wales College of Medicine, Heath Park, Cardiff CF4 4XX*

PAMELA W EWAN *Consultant in Allergy & Clinical Immunology, Addenbrooke's Hospital, Cambridge CB2 2QQ*

NICK FINER *Consultant Physician and Endocrinologist, Luton & Dunstable Hopsital NHS Trust, Visiting Specialist, Addenbrooke's Hospital, Cambridge and Visiting Professor, Luton University*

JOHN D FIRTH *Consultant Physician and Nephrologist, Addenbrooke's Hospital, Cambridge CB2 2QQ*

JANE FLINT *Consultant Cardiologist, Department of Cardiology, Wordsley Hospital, Stream Road, Wordsley, Stourbridge, West Midlands DY8 5QX*

TIM FRYER *Senior Research Associate, Wolfson Brain Imaging Centre, University of Cambridge Clinical School, Addenbrooke's Hospital, Cambridge CB2 2QQ*

JOHN D S GAYLOR *Reader, Bioengineering Unit, University of Strathclyde, Wolfson Centre, 106 Rottenrow, Glasgow G4 0NW*

J SIMON R GIBBS *Senior Lecturer in Cardiology, National Heart & Lung Institute at Imperial College of Science, Technology and Medicine, London.*

CHRISTOPHER E M GRIFFITHS *Professor of Dermatology, University of Manchester, Dermatology Centre, Hope Hospital, Salford M6 8HD*

CHRISTOPHER J HAWKEY *Professor of Gastroenterology, Division of Gastroenterology, University Hospital Nottingham, Queen's Medical Centre, Nottingham NG7 2UH*

JOHN HENRY *Professor of Accident and Emergency Medicine, Imperial College School of Medicine, St Mary's Hospital, Praed Street, London W2 1NY*

STEPHEN T HOLGATE *MRC Clinical Professor of Immunopharmacology, Respiratory Cell and Molecular Biology Research Division, Medical Specialties, Southampton General Hospital, Southampton SO16 6YD*

PHILIP W IND *Senior Lecturer and Honorary Consultant Physician, Respiratory Medicine, NHLI, Hammersmith Hospital, Imperial College, London W12 0NN*

ADITYA KAPOOR *Research Fellow, Department of Cardiological Sciences, St George's Hospital Medical School, London SW17 0RE*

RICHARD F A LOGAN *Professor of Clinical Epidemiology, Division of Public Health and Epidemiology, University of Nottingham Medical School, Queens Medical Centre, Nottingham NG7 2UH*

STEPHEN MAN *Royal Society Research Fellow, Department of Medicine, University of Wales College of Medicine, Heath Park, Cardiff CF4 4XX*

ROBERT MARCUS *Consultant Haematologist, Department of Haematology, Addenbrooke's Hospital, Cambridge CB2 2QQ*

JOHN J V MCMURRAY *Professor of Medical Cardiology, CRI in Heart Failure, Wolfson Building, University of Glasgow, Glasgow G12 8QQ*

GRAEME MOYLE *Associate Director of HIV Research, Chelsea and Westminster Hospital, London SW10 9NH*

PETER ORMEROD *Consultant Chest Physician, Blackburn Royal Infirmary, Blackburn and Professor of Respiratory Medicine, Lancashire Postgraduate School of Medicine and Health, University of Central Lancashire, Preston, Lancashire.*

HUGH PENNINGTON *Professor of Bacteriology, Department of Medical Microbiology, University of Aberdeen, Medical School, Foresterhill, Aberdeen AB25 2ZD*

ALED O PHILLIPS *Senior Lecturer and Consultant Nephrologist, Institute of Nephrology, University of Wales College of Medicine, Heath Park, Cardiff CF14 4XN*

RICHARD J PYE *Consultant Dermatologist, Addenbrooke's Hospital, Cambridge CB2 2QQ*

NIALL QUINN *Professor of Clinical Neurology, Department of Clinical Neurology, Institute of Neurology, Queen Square, London WC1N 3BG*

STUART H RALSTON *Department of Medicine and Therapeutics, University of Aberdeen Medical School, Foresterhill, Aberdeen AB25 2ZD*

EDWARD ROWLAND *Consultant Cardiologist, Department of Cardiological Sciences, St George's Hospital Medical School, London SW17 0RE*

PETER M SCHOFIELD *Consultant Cardiologist, Papworth Hospital, Papworth Everard, Cambridge CB3 8RE*

ANETTE SCHRAG *Honorary Lecturer, Department of Clinical Neurology, Institute of Neurology, Queen Square, London WC1N 3BG*

ALISON SEED *Clinical Research Fellow, CRI in Heart Failure, Wolfson Building, University of Glasgow, Glasgow G12 8QQ*

ROBERT STOCKLEY *Professor of Medicine, Department of Medicine, Queen Elizabeth Hospital, Edgbaston, Birmingham B15 2TH*

PAUL SWAIN *Professor of Gastrointestinal Endoscopy, Endoscopy Unit, Royal London Hospital, Whitechapel Road, London E1 1BB*

ANTHONY P WEETMAN *Professor of Medicine, University of Sheffield, Clinical Sciences Centre, Northern General Hospital, Sheffield S5 7AU*

MARK WILES *Professor of Neurology, Department of Medicine (Neurology), University of Wales College of Medicine, Heath Park, Cardiff CF14 4XN*

ADRIAN WILSON *Professor of Medical Physics, Department of Physics, University of Warwick, Coventry CV4 7AL and Director of Clinical Physics & Biomedical Engineering, Walsgrave Hospital, Coventry CV2 2DX. (Chapter written whilst at Department of Medical Physics and Clinical Engineering, The Royal Hallamshire Hospital, Glossop Road, Sheffield S10 2JF)*

DAVID A WOOD *Professor of Cardiology, National Heart & Lung Institute, Imperial College School of Medicine, Dovehouse Street, London SW3 6LY*

Contents

Editor's introduction iii

List of contributors v

CARDIOLOGY AND CARDIOVASCULAR RISK MANAGEMENT

Developments in percutaneous and surgical myocardial
revascularisation 1
Sarah C Clarke and Peter M Schofield

Management of heart failure 15
Alison Seed & John J V McMurray

Cardiac arrhythmias – when to intervene 27
Edward Rowland & Aditya Kapoor

Reducing risk of atherosclerotic vascular disease in the diabetic
population 39
Christopher D Byrne

Strategies for reducing cardiovascular risk in the NHS 57
Jane Flint & David A Wood

RESPIRATORY MEDICINE AND IMMUNOLOGY

The treatment of asthma in adults 73
Philip W Ind

The clinical management of pulmonary hypertension 87
J Simon R Gibbs

Drug resistant tuberculosis 97
Peter Ormerod

Peanut and other food allergies 105
Pamela W Ewan

Bronchial disease 115
Robert A Stockley

The Lumleian Lecture
Gene-environment interactions in the pathogenesis of asthma 127
Stephen T Holgate

NEUROLOGY AND RHEUMATOLOGY

Advances in treatment for acute stroke 145
Martin M Brown

Disorders of the basal ganglia and their modern management 163
Anette Schrag & Niall Quinn

Physiotherapy in neurological disease: evidence-based medicine 175
Mark Wiles

What's new in metabolic bone disease? 185
Stuart H Ralston

Osteoporosis: how and who to treat 193
Juliet Compston

HEPATOLOGY AND GASTROENTEROLOGY

Autoimmune hepatitis 203
Margaret F Bassendine

Haemochromatosis 213
Adrian Bomford

Endoscopic ultrasound 223
Paul Swain

Screening for colorectal cancer – time to start? 233
Richard F A Logan

Impact of coxibs 243
Christopher J Hawkey

DIABETES, ENDOCRINOLOGY AND ONCOLOGY

Medical management of obesity 253
Nick Finer

New developments in thyroid disease 267
Anthony P Weetman

Monoclonal antibodies in the treatment of cancer   281
Robert Marcus

Vaccine strategies for cancer   289
Mererid Evans, Stephen Man & Leszek K Borysiewicz

RENAL AND DERMATOLOGY

Diabetic nephropathy: significance, treatment options and future
prospects   301
Aled O Phillips

Acute renal failure   315
John D Firth

Psoriasis   327
Christopher E M Griffiths

The hidden epidemic of basal cell carcinoma   339
Richard J Pye

INFECTION AND TOXICOLOGY

Refining the management of HIV: the impact of recent therapies, drugs
in development and new diagnostics   347
Graeme Moyle

Food poisoning   357
Hugh Pennington

The current drug scene   367
John Henry

NEW TECHNOLOGIES IN MEDICINE

New imaging techniques: positron emission tomography   379
Tim Fryer

Advances in patient monitoring   395
Paul Beatty

Decision support systems in medicine   409
Adrian Wilson

Artificial organs for renal therapy   421
Joseph P Barbenel & John D S Gaylor

Developments in percutaneous and surgical myocardial revascularisation

Sarah C Clarke and Peter M Schofield

□ INTRODUCTION

Angina pectoris due to underlying coronary artery disease remains a common clinical problem in the western world. In many patients symptoms can be adequately controlled by medication, but percutaneous coronary intervention is required in some. Recent developments in balloon coronary angioplasty and coronary stenting will be described here. Coronary artery bypass surgery remains an effective treatment for the relief of symptoms and in certain situations for an improvement in prognosis. The long-term results of saphenous vein bypass grafts and the results of arterial conduits for this type of surgery will be examined. There have been developments in the recent past towards less invasive coronary artery surgery in respect of a mini-thoracotomy and no cardiopulmonary bypass (MIDCAB procedure) as well as a standard sternotomy but no cardiopulmonary bypass ('off-pump' coronary artery bypass (OPCAB) procedure). In a small proportion of patients, angina proves refractory to medical treatment, and percutaneous coronary intervention and coronary artery bypass surgery are not possible due to the diffuse and distal nature of the coronary artery disease. In this group of patients, laser revascularisation has been used in the recent past, initially using a surgical approach (anterolateral thoracotomy), and more recently a percutaneous catheter-based approach. These new developments will also be described.

□ PERCUTANEOUS CORONARY INTERVENTION

Percutaneous transluminal coronary angioplasty

Coronary angioplasty using balloon dilatation has been carried out for over 20 years. It provides symptomatic improvement in patients with angina, and involves a short in-hospital stay. It is now frequently undertaken as a day-case procedure or with a 'one night' stay. Patients are able to return to work within a few days and the procedure carries a low morbidity and mortality. The disadvantages of percutaneous transluminal coronary angioplasty (PTCA) include re-stenosis at the site of balloon dilatation and the fact that some lesions are not suitable for the technique (eg long-standing total occlusions which cannot be crossed with a guidewire).

The procedure involves crossing the lesion with a fine guidewire, passing the deflated balloon catheter over the guidewire to the lesion and then inflating the balloon at the site of stenosis (Fig. 1). The long-term observational data for PTCA are encouraging. In 5,000 patients followed up for five years, there was an in-hospital mortality of 0.5%, a one-year survival of 98% and a five-year survival of 91% [1]. There was, however, an event-free survival of only 70% at three years due to the requirement for re-investigation or repeat intervention in the first six months after PTCA.

If re-stenosis occurs following PTCA, it tends to occur within the first six months. Angiographic re-stenosis occurs in up to 35% of patients, and in about 25% the return of symptoms requires repeat intervention. This difference arises because some patients with an original lesion causing 95% stenosis may have a 50% residual stenosis on a routine six-month angiogram but remain free of angina. They are classified as angiographic re-stenosis but not clinical re-stenosis.

Various features are involved in the development of re-stenosis. First, it is caused by the formation of new tissue by the vessel wall in response to injury. The trauma caused by balloon dilatation results in the local release of growth factors which lead to new scar tissue forming inside the artery at the site of the procedure. Secondly, there may be some elastic 'recoil' of the vessel following PTCA which contributes to restenosis. Thirdly, intravascular ultrasound studies have demonstrated a process termed 'negative remodelling'. This is the opposite to that which normally occurs in

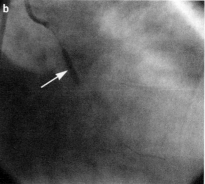

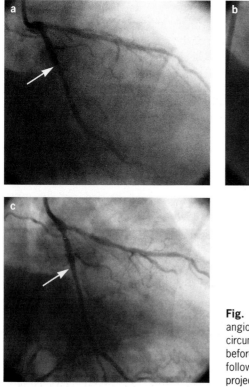

Fig. 1 Percutaneous transluminal coronary angioplasty procedure. A stenosis in the circumflex branch of the left coronary artery **(a)** before, **(b)** during balloon inflation, and **(c)** following dilatation (right anterior oblique projection).

atheromatous arteries. When an artery becomes narrowed by atheromatous tissue, it grows in size to 'accommodate' the progressive narrowing. Following PTCA however, negative remodelling can occur with the artery actually getting smaller.

The Angioplasty Compared with Medicine (ACME) trial compared angioplasty with medical therapy for patients with single-vessel disease and exercise-induced myocardial ischaemia [2]. PTCA resulted in an improvement in angina symptoms as well as increased exercise capacity as compared with medical treatment. The Randomised Intervention Treatment of Angina (RITA)-1 trial compared the outcome in patients with single or multi-vessel disease who, being considered suitable for angioplasty or coronary surgery, were randomised to one or other treatment [3]. There was no difference in early mortality between the two groups. At six months, more patients had angina or required repeat revascularisation in the PTCA group. By two years, these differences were less marked and, despite the greater requirement for re-intervention, the overall two-year cost for PTCA was substantially less than for coronary artery surgery. The results from several other trials (CABRI, EAST and BARI) [4–7] have shown the same trends – the longer-term results favour non-surgical intervention.

Coronary artery stenting

The introduction of coronary artery stents has had a major impact on percutaneous coronary intervention. During balloon inflation, there is disruption of the atheromatous plaque. In some cases, extensive dissection of the vessel wall results, and this may lead to occlusion of the vessel requiring emergency coronary artery bypass grafting (CABG). In this situation, stents restore flow by acting as a scaffold to prevent intimal flap occlusion and therefore obviate the need for emergency surgery. They are also useful when there is an inadequate angiographic result following PTCA. The clinical evidence indicates that the earlier a stent is deployed after a poor initial angiographic result following PTCA, the better the eventual outcome. Coronary artery stents come mounted on a balloon catheter. They are advanced over the angioplasty guidewire to the site of stenosis or dissection. The balloon is then inflated to high pressure (typically 12–16 atm), which pushes the stent into the wall of the artery (Fig. 2).

Coronary stents are therefore useful in the acute phase of intervention if there is a poor angiographic result after PTCA or significant dissection. They also have longer-term benefits. Stents produce greater luminal gain at the time of the procedure, so there is less angiographic and clinical re-stenosis. As a result, there is a longer event-free survival. In the Benestent study, there was an angiographic re-stenosis rate of 32% following PTCA and 22% following coronary stenting [8]. Other studies have also demonstrated a reduced angiographic re-stenosis rate following coronary artery stenting as compared with PTCA.

Indications for coronary artery stenting include an inadequate angiographic result after PTCA, extensive dissection following PTCA, the treatment of re-stenotic lesions, when treating lesions in saphenous vein grafts and when dealing with totally occluded vessels. For these last two indications, the angiographic and clinical

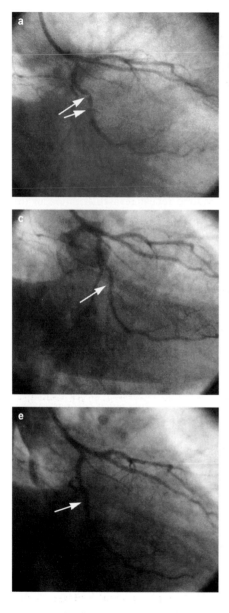
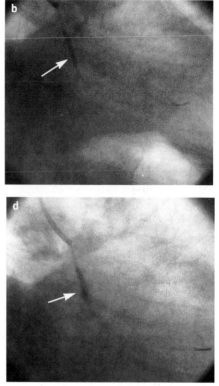

Fig. 2 Coronary artery stenting procedure. A stenosis in the first obtuse marginal branch of the circumflex artery **(a)** before, and **(b)** after balloon dilatation. **(c)** There was a residual stenosis, so a coronary stent was deployed **(d)**, with a good angiographic result **(e)** (right anterior oblique projection).

re-stenosis rates are substantially higher than expected when using balloon angioplasty alone. The use of coronary stents has increased steadily in recent years (Fig. 3). However, problems can be encountered following coronary artery stenting. There is a reported incidence of subacute thrombosis of up to 4%. This may occur up to two weeks after the procedure when the patient has returned home and lead to myocardial infarction (MI). The incidence of subacute thrombosis has been substantially reduced by the widespread use of high pressure stent deployment (to prevent there being dead spaces between the stent and the vessel wall where a clot could form) and the routine use of antiplatelet agents (aspirin plus ticlopidine or

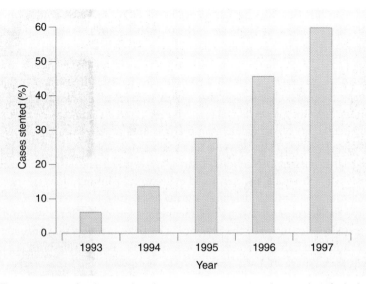

Fig. 3 The percentage of patients undergoing percutaneous coronary intervention who had coronary stents (UK data, 1993–1997).

aspirin plus clopidogrel) following stenting. It has also become clear that if re-stenosis occurs within a coronary stent, treatment is difficult. If the tissue ingrowth extends for more than 75% of the length of the stent, balloon angioplasty results in a re-restenosis rate of around 60% [9]. More recently, radiation therapy has come to the fore as a potential way of preventing in-stent re-stenosis or treating it once it has developed. Brachytherapy has been demonstrated to arrest tissue growth and is currently under evaluation. The stent itself may be made radioactive using beta-emitting activity (^{32}P).

There has been considerable interest in the role of PTCA or coronary stenting in acute MI. Some studies have demonstrated a benefit of 'primary angioplasty/ stenting' over thrombolysis [10]. There may be an improved coronary vessel patency rate, a lower re-infarction rate and a lower mortality rate. Such findings have not been demonstrated consistently, however, and the results of percutaneous intervention depend on the adequacy of the angiographic result, which in turn depends on the experience of the operator. A second problem is that most acute infarct patients present to hospitals that do not have interventional facilities. There would have to be a high investment to develop the infrastructure to support primary angioplasty for acute MI to enable rapid treatment by experienced operators. In the UK, therefore, it is likely to be used in a minority of cases for the foreseeable future.

☐ CORONARY ARTERY BYPASS GRAFTING

Saphenous vein grafts/arterial conduits

CABG is an established technique which has been shown to provide effective relief of angina and in certain situations to prolong life. Saphenous vein has been the standard conduit for the bypass procedures (Fig. 4). However, vein grafts demonstrate a proliferative response in their walls as soon as they are connected to the arterial circulation. Any trauma during procurement exaggerates this response and may serve as a nidus for atherosclerosis. Whereas arterial smooth muscle is adapted to pulsatile flow, smooth muscle in transplanted veins exhibits a proliferative response. Veins are also poorly suited to inhibiting the platelet-mediated thrombotic events that characterise the arterial circulation.

The patency rate of saphenous vein grafts is 80% at one year, 75% at five years and 50% at 10 years (Fig. 5). Vein graft disease is composed of three patho-physiological processes: thrombosis, intimal hyperplasia and atherosclerosis. The early patency of vein grafts is determined by technical considerations (ie the quality of the anastomoses), endothelial injury during harvesting, the arterial run-off (ie the state of the native coronary artery) and the use of aspirin. The longer-term patency of vein grafts is determined by the presence of diabetes mellitus, the continuation of cigarette smoking and the level of cholesterol. The Cholesterol Lowering Atherosclerosis Study (CLAS) showed that lipid lowering drugs may reduce progressive vein graft atherosclerosis. More recently, the Post-Coronary Artery Bypass Graft (P-CABG) trial showed benefit from lipid-lowering with a statin [11].

Following coronary artery bypass surgery, an important predictor of late outcome is the type of bypass conduit used for grafting. The left internal thoracic artery grafted to the left anterior descending artery is an important predictor of both survival and event-free survival (Fig. 6). The internal thoracic artery has a media which receives its entire oxygen requirement from the lumen. It is a metabolically active conduit which releases endothelium-derived nitric oxide and prostacyclin. These properties inhibit mitogenesis and smooth muscle proliferation, which protects against thrombosis and atherosclerosis. The endothelial release of these biochemical mediators enhances graft survival. Patency rates of the left internal thoracic artery grafts to the left anterior descending artery are 85–90% after 10 years.

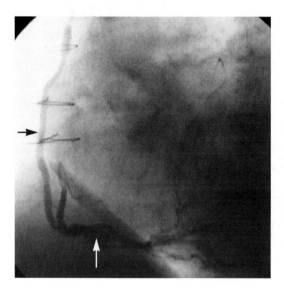

Fig. 4 A saphenous vein graft (small arrow) anastomosed to the ascending aorta proximally and the right coronary artery distally (large arrow) eight years following surgery. The bypass graft is unobstructed and fills the native vessel well (right anterior oblique projection).

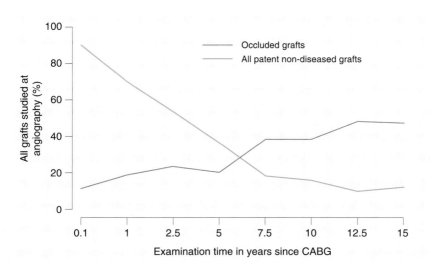

Fig. 5 Serial angiographic follow-up of saphenous vein grafts showing those which were occluded or patent and non-diseased (those patent but diseased are not shown) (CABG = coronary artery bypass graft).

As a result, patients have reduced re-operation rates and improved survival. If both internal thoracic arteries are used for grafting, the re-operation rate falls even further. The potential problem with bilateral internal thoracic artery grafting is sternal healing and the occurrence of mediastinitis [12]. This seems to be more common in obese patients and those with diabetes mellitus.

The radial artery was initially used as a conduit in the early 1970s, but was abandoned due to low early patency rates. In the late 1980s radial artery grafting was

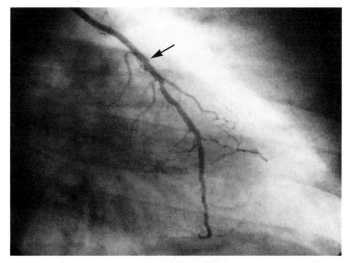

Fig. 6 A left internal mammary artery graft anastomosed (arrow) to the left anterior descending artery (right anterior projection).

re-introduced with patency rates of 93–95% at 18 months. Why was there this improvement? Like all the other arterial conduits, the radial artery develops spasm during harvesting. Since the media of the radial artery is much thicker than the media of the other conduits, the spasm is more intense and more difficult to reverse. Surgeons used to treat spasm by hydrostatically dilating the radial artery or by passing probes, both of which damaged the endothelium. It is likely that the current success of grafting radial artery is related to reduced trauma during harvesting and avoidance of mechanical and hydrostatic dilatation of the conduit (Fig. 7). In many cardiothoracic centres, calcium channel blockers are used peri-operatively and then continued for 3–12 months following surgery to reduce the problem of spasm. The use of radial artery conduits for coronary artery bypass continues to increase. One unresolved issue is whether the preferred proximal anastomosis is to the aorta directly or to the internal thoracic artery.

The gastroepiploic artery was introduced in the late 1980s and also has high patency rates. The procedure usually involves using the conduit *in situ*, when patency rates of 92% at two years have been reported [13]. Occasionally, it is used as a free conduit from the aorta. However, the graft is difficult to harvest in the obese patient and is vulnerable to twisting and technical error. The gastoepiploic artery is also prone to spasm and tends to be smaller at the point of anastomosis than other arteries used for coronary artery grafting. Surgery involves an additional abdominal procedure and, although complications are infrequent, an increased incidence of pancreatitis has been reported. The literature suggests that the best long-term results of coronary artery surgery occur when both internal thoracic arteries are used, supplemented by radial or gastroepiploic grafts. Consideration needs to be given, however, to the patient's age and general medical state, the presence of diabetes mellitus and whether the patient is obese.

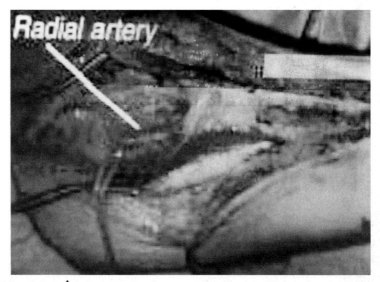

Fig. 7 A radial artery during harvesting for a coronary artery bypass procedure.

Less invasive coronary artery surgery

There have been many developments in recent years in the field of less invasive coronary artery surgery. A number of different incisions have been advocated for less invasive access, although some of these may have been simply for 'cosmetic' reasons. Coronary artery surgery has been so successful to date because of good myocardial protection, good exposure and clear vision of the vessels in a dry motionless field. Currently, the two approaches being used more widely are off-pump surgery, first, via a MIDCAB and, secondly, via a standard sternotomy OPCAB. Clearly, both techniques are performed without the need for cardiopulmonary bypass. At the end of the day, the quality of the anastomosis has a major impact on the long-term outcome following coronary artery grafting.

The access for the MIDCAB procedure is via a mini-thoracotomy which is usually placed transversely in the 5th intercostal space (Fig. 8). The surgery requires the dissection of a good and undamaged length of internal thoracic artery and clear access to the relevant coronary artery, usually the left anterior descending vessel. In this operation, only one graft is deployed (occasionally a 'jump' to the diagonal with two distal anastomoses is used) and the surgery depends on a good quality internal thoracic artery. The early experience with MIDCAB procedures did not involve the use of stabilisers. A number of stabilisers are now available which facilitate the anastomosis to the coronary artery and make it much easier to

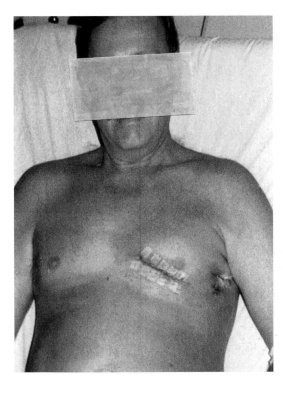

Fig. 8 A patient who has recently undergone a mini-thoracotomy with no cardiopulmonary bypass (MIDCAB) procedure, showing the mini-thoracotomy.

operate on a beating heart. Since temporary occlusion of the native coronary vessel is required to perform the anastomosis, there is local myocardial ischaemia. This can cause arrhythmia and reduced myocardial contractility. If the vessel to be grafted is already occluded, less ischaemia occurs during surgery since more effective collateral channels have usually developed. In about 5% of cases, it is necessary to convert to a standard sternotomy for technical reasons. Since the introduction of stabilisers, the combined occlusion and stenosis rate has been reported to be 5% [14].

For the OPCAB procedure, a full sternotomy is usually performed. Whilst this may not be 'minimally invasive', it allows multiple CAGB to be carried out without the need for cardiopulmonary bypass. Once again, the introduction of stabilisers has greatly facilitated the technique. During the anastomosis, there is local ischaemia due to transient occlusion of the vessel. Although this is rarely of clinical significance, it can be a problem if the vessel is dominant and the proximal lesion of only moderate severity. In this situation, it is unlikely that any collateral channels are well developed. Methods used to combat temporary ischaemia include pharmacological slowing of the heart, pre-conditioning, and the use of intracoronary shunts. Although shunts are effective in preventing ischaemia, their placement is cumbersome and may damage the endothelium of the native vessel. The conversion rate with OPCAB procedures to a standard cardiopulmonary bypass technique is around 5%. The results of OPCAB surgery have demonstrated an early graft occlusion or stenosis rate of 5–6%. The overall success of both MIDCAB and OPCAB surgery since the introduction of stabilisers encourages the further use of these minimally invasive procedures.

☐ MYOCARDIAL LASER REVASCULARISATION

Transmyocardial revascularisation

Most patients with angina due to underlying coronary artery disease can be successfully treated by medication, coronary angioplasty/stenting or CAGB surgery. Some patients, however, have angina which cannot be controlled by medication and have diffuse and distal coronary artery disease which is not suitable for angioplasty or CABG. These patients have usually already undergone several conventional revascularisation procedures. Transmyocardial revascularisation (TMR) is a laser technique which has been evaluated in recent years for the treatment of such patients. TMR is usually performed through a left anterolateral thoracotomy and uses laser energy to create transmural channels in the ischaemic myocardium (Fig. 9). At first, a high-energy carbon dioxide laser was used. There have now been several reports of the efficacy of TMR, including uncontrolled trials, registry data and more recently randomised controlled studies. Reports indicate that TMR improves the symptomatic status of patients (CCS angina score) and their exercise capacity (usually on serial exercise tests). However, the data on improvement in myocardial perfusion using nuclear techniques or positron emission tomography

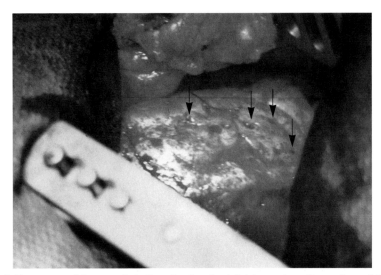

Fig. 9 Transmyocardial revascularisation showing the 'pits' (arrows) on the surface of the left ventricle after delivery of laser energy.

scanning have been inconsistent. The mechanism of action of TMR remains uncertain. It appears that direct perfusion of the myocardium through the laser channels does not occur; the channels tend to close post-operatively. There is increasing evidence to support new vessel formation (angiogenesis) as a possible mechanism, and denervation, as well as a placebo effect, may also contribute. The technique of TMR carries a peri-operative mortality rate of almost 5% and also has a significant procedural morbidity. This may include infection (respiratory or wound), arrhythmia (typically transient atrial fibrillation) and left ventricular failure.

Because of developments in fibreoptic technology, and using a Holmium-YAG laser energy source, it is now possible to produce tissue ablation from the endocardial surface of the left ventricle via a catheter-based approach. This is known as percutaneous myocardial laser revascularisation (PMR) (Fig. 10). The technique involves introducing an aligning ('guiding') catheter, a laser delivery catheter and an extendable laser fibre via the femoral artery (Fig. 11). The results of a randomised prospective trial involving over 200 patients, the PACIFIC trial [15], have recently been reported. PMR provides good symptomatic improvement, with a 25% increase in treadmill exercise times (from around 400 sec at baseline). Importantly, there were no peri-operative deaths and the procedural morbidity was very low: 1% of patients required percutaneous drainage of pericardial effusion for cardiac tamponade. The risk:benefit ratio for PMR is much more favourable than for TMR which, however, may still have a role as an adjunct to coronary artery grafting when complete revascularisation cannot be achieved [16]. It is likely that PMR will be used more widely in such patients, and in the future may be combined with the intra-myocardial delivery of angiogenic peptides further to induce new blood vessel formation.

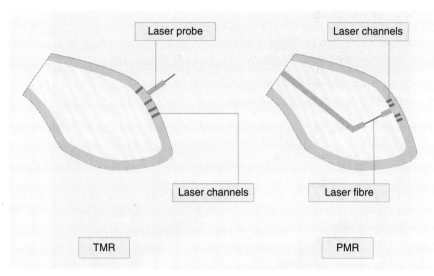

Fig. 10 Laser revascularisation with transmyocardial revascularisation (TMR). The laser probe is placed on the epicardial surface of the left ventricle and transmural channels are created. With percutaneous myocardial laser revascularisation (PMR), the laser fibre is placed on the endocardial surface of the left ventricle and channels created which are not transmural but which penetrate to a depth of about 6 mm.

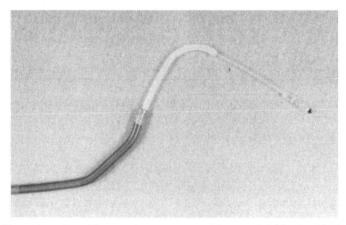

Fig. 11 The equipment used for percutaneous myocardial revascularisation: an aligning ('guiding') catheter (2.5 mm in diameter), a laser delivery catheter and an extendable laser fibre.

REFERENCES

1   Mick M, Piedmonte M, Arnold AM, *et al*. Risk stratification for long-term outcome after elective coronary angioplasty: a multivariate analysis of 5,000 patients. *J Am Coll Cardiol* 1994; **24**: 74–80.

2   Parisi AF, Folland ED, Hartigan P. A comparison of angioplasty with medical therapy in the treatment of single vessel coronary disease. *N Engl J Med* 1992; **326**: 10–6.

3   Coronary angioplasty versus coronary artery bypass surgery: the Randomized Intervention Treatment of Angina (RITA) trial. *Lancet* 1993; **341**: 573–80.

4 Weintraub WS, Mauldin PD, Becker E, *et al*. A comparison of the costs of and quality of life after coronary angioplasty or coronary surgery for multivessel coronary artery disease. Results from the Emory Angioplasty Versus Surgery Trial (EAST). *Circulation* 1995; **92**: 2831–40.

5 Anonymous. Influence of diabetes on 5-year mortality and morbidity in a randomised trial comparing CABG and PTCA in patients with multivessel disease. The Bypass Angioplasty Revascularisation Investigation (BARI). *Circulation* 1997; **96**: 1761–9.

6 Pocock SJ, Henderson RA, Rickards AF, *et al*. Meta-analysis of randomised trials comparing coronary angioplasty with bypass surgery. *Lancet* 1995; **346**: 1184–9.

7 Rickards AF, Davies SW. Coronary angioplasty versus coronary surgery in the management of angina. *Curr Opin Cardiol* 1995; **10**: 399–403.

8 Serruys PW, De Jaegere P, Kiemeneij F, *et al*. A comparison of balloon-expandable-stent inplantation with balloon angioplasty in patients with coronary artery disease. Benestent Study Group. *N Engl J Med* 1993; **328**: 673–9.

9 Eltchaninoff H, Koning R, Tron C, *et al*. Balloon angioplasty for the treatment of coronary in-stent re-stenosis: immediate results and 6 month angiographic recurrent stenosis rate. *J Am Coll Cardiol* 1998; **32**: 980–4.

10 Grines CL, Browne KF, Marco J, *et al*. A comparison of immediate angioplasty with thrombolytic therapy for acute myocardial infarction. The Primary Angioplasty in Myocardial Infarction Study Group. *N Engl J Med* 1993; **328**: 673–9.

11 The Post-Coronary Artery Bypass Graft Trial Investigators. The effect of aggressive lowering of low-density lipoprotein cholesterol levels and low-dose anticoagulation on obstructive changes in saphenous vein coronary artery bypass grafts. *N Engl J Med* 1997; **336**: 153–62.

12 Loop FD. Coronary artery surgery: the end of the beginning. *Eur J Cardiothorac Surg* 1998; **14**: 554–71.

13 Barner HB. The continuing evolution of arterial conduits. *Ann Thorac Surg* 1999; **68**: S1–8.

14 Stanbridge R, Hadjinikolaou LK. Technical adjuncts in beating heart surgery. Comparison of MIDCAB to off-pump sternotomy: a meta-analysis. *Eur J Cardiothorac Surg* 1999; **16**: S24–33.

15 Oesterle SN, Ali N, Sanborn TA, *et al*. Percutaneous transmyocardial laser revascularisation (PMR). Final results from the PACIFIC trial. *Circulation* 1999; **100**: 1592 (abstract).

16 Clarke SC, Schofield PM. Myocardial laser revascularization. *Eur Heart J* 1999; **20**: 1213–4.

☐ SELF ASSESSMENT QUESTIONS

1 Percutaneous balloon coronary angioplasty:
   (a) Is associated with an in-hospital mortality of 2%
   (b) Is associated with an angiographic re-stenosis rate of 35%
   (c) Is ideal for treating chronic total occlusions
   (d) Is associated with improvement in angina symptoms when compared to medical treatment
   (e) Improves the prognosis of patients with coronary artery disease

2 Coronary artery stenting:
   (a) Is useful to correct dissection of the vessel wall during angioplasty
   (b) Is associated with a lower re-stenosis rate than balloon angioplasty
   (c) Is contraindicated in diseased saphenous vein grafts
   (d) Prevents subacute intravascular thrombosis
   (e) Requires treatment with antiplatelet agents

3 With coronary artery bypass surgery:
   (a) The patency rate of saphenous vein grafts at five years is 75%

(b) The patency rate for internal thoracic artery grafts at 5 years is 75%
(c) Prognosis is improved in all patients
(d) Lipid lowering drugs may reduce progressive vein graft atherosclerosis
(e) The gastroepiploic artery can be used as a conduit

4 With coronary artery bypass grafting:
(a) Bilateral internal thoracic artery grafting is associated with impaired healing of the sternum
(b) The patency rate of radial artery grafts is 93% at 18 months
(c) Cardiopulmonary bypass is always required
(d) Using a 'mini-thoracotomy', typically three grafts are placed
(e) Patients are usually off work for at least six months

5 Myocardial laser revascularisation:
(a) Improves prognosis in patients with advanced coronary artery disease
(b) Can be performed percutaneously using a carbon dioxide laser
(c) Is preferred to 're-do' coronary artery bypass grafting
(d) Improves angina symptoms in patients with advanced coronary artery disease
(e) Carries less risk when performed using a percutaneous approach

ANSWERS

1a False	2a True	3a True	4a True	5a False
b True	b True	b False	b True	b False
c False	c False	c False	c False	c False
d True	d False	d True	d False	d True
e False	e True	e True	e False	e True

Management of heart failure

Alison Seed and John J V McMurray

□ INTRODUCTION

This review discusses the pharmacological management of chronic heart failure (CHF) caused by left ventricular (LV) systolic dysfunction. There is an excellent evidence base, enabling firm recommendations to be made for the treatment of this type of CHF [1–3]. Unfortunately, this is not so for other types of CHF, for example CHF associated with preserved LV systolic function.

□ A FRAMEWORK FOR UNDERSTANDING THERAPY

Although CHF is, at least initially, a primary mechanical and haemodynamic problem, it is now also recognised as a syndrome characterised by neurohumoral activation (Fig. 1) [4,5]. Chronic activation of certain neurohumoral systems, for

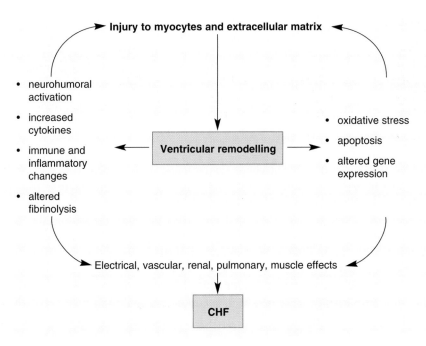

Fig. 1 The neurohumoral model of heart failure (CHF = chronic heart failure).

example the renin angiotensin aldosterone system (RAAS), seems to be detrimental, leading to undesirable renal, vascular, myocardial and other effects. This abnormal, sustained neurohumoral overactivity is believed to be a major cause of progression of CHF, and explains the steady haemodynamic and symptomatic decline that characterises the CHF syndrome. The focus of scientific attention has been on neurohumoral systems with potentially undesirable effects in CHF, but it is now recognised that other neurohumoral axes that could have beneficial effects are also activated in CHF, for example the natriuretic peptides system [6]. In addition to improving our understanding of the pathophysiology of CHF, this neurohumoral paradigm has provided a framework for understanding therapeutic interventions in CHF. Initially, the value of antagonising neurohumoral systems likely to have detrimental actions in CHF was recognised, while more recently it has come to be realised that the optimum strategy might be to achieve this while simultaneously augmenting potentially desirable neurohumoral mediators such as the natriuretic peptides. The 'neurohumoral model' of CHF has also now been broadened to include other mediators such as cytokines [7].

☐ DRUGS BLOCKING THE RENIN ANGIOTENSIN ALDOSTERONE SYSTEM

Angiotensin converting enzyme inhibitors

The prototype neurohumoral intervention in CHF was angiotensin-converting enzyme (ACE) inhibition. ACE inhibitors reduce the generation of angiotensin II from angiotensin I by ACE, thereby reducing the vasoconstrictor, mitogenic, renal and other undesirable actions of angiotensin II in CHF. Angiotensin II also stimulates aldosterone release from the adrenal cortex, and this hormone is also believed to have detrimental effects in CHF (see below). Lastly, as ACE is also kininase II, ACE inhibitors reduce the breakdown of bradykinin – although it is unknown whether or not this is beneficial. Bradykinin, however, augments nitric oxide production experimentally, which might be desirable in CHF.

The landmark CONSENSUS I trial [8] (see end of text for explanation of studies) showed that enalapril brought about symptomatic improvement (a reduction in New York Heart Association (NYHA) class) and reduction in mortality in patients with severe (NYHA class IV) CHF, treated with what was, at that time, full conventional therapy (proportion of patients taking other drugs: digoxin 93%, isosorbide dinitrate 46%, frusemide 98%, spironolactone 53%). It is also interesting to note that the mean doses of frusemide and of spironolactone were 205 mg and 80 mg, respectively.

Subsequently, the treatment arm of SOLVD (SOLVD-T) showed that enalapril also reduced mortality, decreased hospitalisation and improved NYHA class in a broader spectrum of patients (mainly NYHA classes II and III) with CHF and an LV ejection fraction (LVEF) of 35% or less (Table 1) [9]. These findings were supported by a meta-analysis of many other trials with ACE inhibitors in CHF [10].

It has been undisputed for a number of years that all patients with low LVEF CHF, no matter how mild or severe their symptoms, should be treated with an ACE inhibitor. There has, however, been debate about what dose should be used. The

Table 1 Summary of the benefits of angiotensin-converting enzyme inhibitors in heart failure.*

	Events prevented per 1,000 patient years of treatment	NNT for 3 years to prevent 1 event
Hospital admissions for worsening CHF	65	5
Hospital admissions – any cause	99	3
Deaths	13	26

* from treatment arm of SOLVD (67% of patients receiving digoxin).
CHF = chronic heart failure; NNT = number of patients needed to treat to prevent 1 event.

target dose of enalapril in CONSENSUS I was 20 mg twice daily, and the achieved dose was 18.4 mg; in SOLVD-T, the target dose was 10 mg twice daily, and the achieved dose was 16.6 mg. The landmark ACE inhibitor post-infarction studies and the recent HOPE trial had similarly high target and achieved doses [11–14]. Audits of clinical practice have, however, demonstrated the use of much lower doses by clinicians [15]. There has been concern that these unproven doses may have less benefit than those used in the key clinical trials. The recently reported ATLAS study set out to address this question by randomising patients with CHF to low (2.5–5.0 mg once daily) or high dose (32.5–35.0 mg) lisinopril [16]. There was no difference between the two treatment groups in terms of the primary end-point of all-cause mortality, but there was a significantly better outcome in the higher dose treatment group for the major secondary end-point of all-cause death or hospitalisation (a robust composite measure of mortality and morbidity). Close inspection of the ATLAS results suggests a real and valuable advantage to using higher dose ACE inhibition (Table 2).

Table 2 Summary of the benefits of higher versus lower dose angiotensin-converting enzyme inhibitor treatment in heart failure.*

	Events prevented per 1,000 patient years of treatment	NNT for 4 years to prevent 1 event
Hospital admissions for worsening CHF	59	4
Hospital admissions – any cause	84	3

* from ATLAS (median follow-up 3.8 years).
CHF = chronic heart failure; NNT = number of patients needed to treat to prevent 1 event.

Angiotensin II receptor antagonists

Angiotensin II receptor antagonists (AIIRAs) block the action of angiotensin II at its type I (AT_1) receptor which is believed to mediate all the conventionally understood actions of angiotensin II. The principal differences between AIIRAs and ACE inhibitors are:

1   AIIRAs do not block the breakdown of bradykinin by kininase II – although it is not clear whether this is good or bad. Bradykinin may directly or indirectly contribute to adverse effects of ACE inhibitors such as cough, yet be of benefit because of its nitric oxide stimulating action.

2   AIIRAs can block the action of angiotensin II generated from enzymes other than ACE. The physiological/pathophysiological significance of non-ACE angiotensin II generation is unclear.

3   AIIRAs leave AT_2 receptors (and other putative AT receptors) unblocked, and even hyperstimulated (by the reflex increase in angiotensin II that occurs during AT_1 receptor blockade). The function of the AT_2 receptor in humans is unknown.

The first head-to-head comparison between an ACE inhibitor (captopril) and an AT_1 receptor antagonist (losartan) showed survival to be no better with losartan [17]. The trial (ELITE II) had insufficient power to say whether or not losartan was as good as (equivalent to) or no worse than (non-inferior to) captopril. The place of AIIRAs in the treatment of CHF, therefore, remains far from clear. Two other trials may, however, shed some light on this issue:

1   Val HeFT is comparing placebo to valsartan added to full conventional therapy, including an ACE inhibitor [18].

2   CHARM is examining the effect of 'add on' or 'combination' therapy, and also whether candesartan is better than placebo:

☐   in ACE inhibitor intolerant patients with low LVEF CHF, and

☐   in patients with CHF and a preserved LVEF [19].

Spironolactone

Spironolactone is a synthetic steroid lactone that antagonises the effect of aldosterone by competitive inhibition. In addition to its recognised renal tubular actions (sodium and water retention/potassium and magnesium wastage), aldosterone seems to have growth effects (inducing fibrosis) and actions on autonomic and baroreceptor function [20]. Patients with CHF may exhibit 'aldosterone escape' despite treatment with an ACE inhibitor. Recently, the RALES study has shown that the addition of low dose spironolactone (mean dose 26 mg daily) to full conventional therapy (including an ACE inhibitor) improves NYHA class, reduces hospitalisations and increases survival in patients with severe (NYHA class III and IV), low LVEF CHF [21]. These benefits were substantial (Table 3).

☐ DRUGS BLOCKING THE SYMPATHETIC NERVOUS SYSTEM

In the same way as the RAAS is recognised to have actions that are potentially detrimental in CHF, the sympathetic nervous system (SNS) is seen as likely to be harmful if chronically activated [22]. Catecholamines may be directly cytotoxic to

Table 3 Summary of the benefits of spironolactone in severe heart failure.*

	Events prevented per 1,000 patient years of treatment	NNT for 2 years to prevent 1 event
Hospital admissions for worsening CHF	143	3
Hospital admissions – any cause	138	4
Deaths	57	9

* from RALES (mean follow-up 2 years).
CHF = chronic heart failure; NNT = number needed to treat to prevent 1 event.

myocytes, and the positive chronotropic and inotropic actions of the SNS may ultimately exhaust the failing heart. The SNS also has electrophysiological, renal (sodium and water retaining), hormonal (renin stimulating) and growth promoting actions that are probably disadvantageous in CHF. The risks of sudden and intense blockade of the SNS have also been recognised, however, perhaps even more so than with the RAAS. Although the tools to block the SNS (beta-blockers) have been available for many years, how to use them properly was not worked out, and only the risks of their misuse received attention. In the past few years, however, beta-blockers have been shown to be of clear benefit in CHF, and the trials demonstrating this have led to the greatest breakthrough in CHF therapeutics in the past decade [23].

Beta-adrenoceptor antagonists (beta-blockers)

In 1999, two major prospective randomised trials (CIBIS-2 and MERIT-HF), with all-cause mortality as the pre-specified end-point, clearly demonstrated that beta-blockers improve survival in patients with mild to moderately symptomatically severe (NYHA class II and III) low LVEF CHF (Table 4) [24,25]. NYHA class and quality of life are also improved and hospitalisation reduced [26]. All these benefits were obtained when beta-blockers were added to full conventional therapy,

Table 4 Summary of the benefits of beta-blocker therapy in mild to moderately symptomatically severe heart failure.*

	Events prevented per 1,000 patient years of treatment	NNT for 1 year** to prevent 1 event
Hospital admissions for worsening CHF	68	15
Hospital admissions – any cause	67	15
Deaths	37	27

* from MERIT-HF (mean follow-up 1 year).
** Shorter follow-up may exaggerate benefits of treatment: eg in SOLVD-T, the relative risk reduction in mortality at 3, 6 and 12 months was 33%, 29% and 23%, respectively, compared with 16% overall during the full 41.4 months of follow-up.
CHF = chronic heart failure; NNT = number of patients to treat to prevent 1 event.

including an ACE inhibitor. Figure 2 shows that dual neurohumoral blockade, antagonising both the RAAS and the SNS, has resulted in reducing by half the one-year mortality in patients with CHF. More recently, the COPERNICUS trial has reported that carvedilol reduces mortality in patients with severe CHF (NYHA class IIIb and IV). It is now clear that beta-blockers should be standard 'first-line' therapy, together with ACE inhibitors, in patients with NYHA class II and III low LVEF CHF [23]. Their place in patients with severe CHF is still not completely clear pending the publication of the final results of the COPERNICUS and BEST trials.

As with ACE inhibitors, it is important to use beta-blockers carefully in CHF. Sudden, intense neurohumoral inhibition is potentially dangerous. Gentle, gradual neurohumoral blockade is the correct strategy, which means cautious introduction of therapy in stable patients (ie not in patients with an acute exacerbation or who have been recently discharged) [23]. The three beta-blockers used in the landmark CHF trials should be preferred as they are available in the low dose strengths necessary for treatment initiation:

- ☐ bisoprolol 1.25 mg once daily

- ☐ carvedilol 3.125 mg twice daily, and

- ☐ metoprolol CR/XL 12.5–25 mg once daily.

☐ DIGOXIN

How digitalis glycosides work in CHF is unclear and difficult to resolve with the neurohumoral paradigm of CHF. Digoxin seems to inhibit the RAAS and SNS and

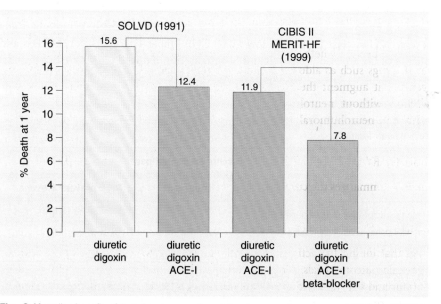

Fig. 2 Mortality benefit of beta-blockers and angiotensin-converting enzyme inhibitors (ACE-I) in chronic heart failure trials.

to augment parasympathetic activity. These effects are more likely to be of benefit than any modest inotropic action of digoxin in CHF. Digoxin is, however, of limited value in CHF. It is generally agreed that digoxin improves symptoms in patients with low LVEF CHF and sinus rhythm when added to a diuretic and an ACE inhibitor [1–3]. It also has a worthwhile effect on hospitalisation (Table 5) but no effect on mortality [27]. The benefit of digoxin seems to be greatest in patients with a very low LVEF, a high cardiothoracic ratio and more severe symptoms. Most authorities would now agree that the main place of digoxin is in the treatment of this subgroup of patients [1–3].

Table 5 Summary of the benefits of digoxin in heart failure.*

	Events prevented per 1,000 patient years of treatment	NNT for 3 years to prevent 1 event
Hospital admissions for worsening CHF	60	6
Hospital admissions – any cause	40	8
Deaths	0	N/A

* from DIG (94% of patients receiving an angiotensin-converting enzyme inhibitor).
CHF = chronic heart failure; N/A = not applicable; NNT = number of patients needed to treat to prevent 1 event.

☐ DIURETICS

Like digoxin, diuretics do not fit comfortably into the neurohumoral model of CHF, especially as they may actually cause neuroendocrine activation. Nevertheless, it is clear that patients who retain sodium and water gain symptomatic relief from diuretics and are at risk of deterioration if diuretics are withdrawn [28,29]. It remains to be seen whether there is a better alternative to conventional diuretics – that is, drugs such as aldosterone antagonists or neutral endopeptidase inhibitors (agents that augment the natriuretic peptides), which cause sodium and water excretion without neurohumoral activation (or even simultaneously suppress undesirable neurohumoral systems).

☐ SUMMARY OF CURRENT TREATMENT FOR CHRONIC HEART FAILURE

Figure 3 summarises the currently recommended management of CHF.

☐ FUTURE PHARMACOLOGICAL THERAPY

Drugs that inhibit the actions of endothelin-1 and cytokines are being studied in large-scale outcome trials. Similarly, omapatrilat, a molecule that is both an ACE inhibitor and a neutral endopeptidase inhibitor, is being compared to enalapril in a major mortality trial. With this agent, the neurohumoral paradigm of therapy has evolved from one of simply antagonising undesirable systems to that of trying to

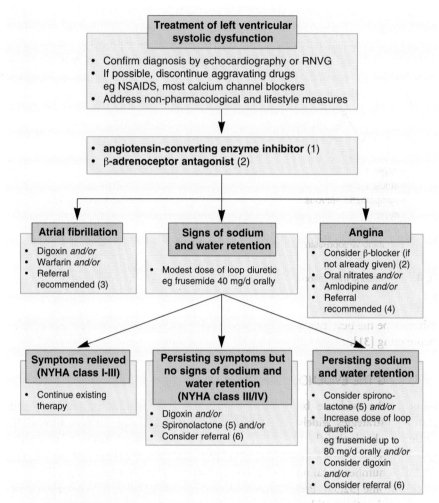

Fig. 3 Treatment algorithm (ACE = angiotensin-converting enzyme; NYHA = New York Heart Association; NSAID = non-steroidal anti-inflammatory drug; RNVG = radionuclide ventriculogram) (from [1], reproduced in [30]).

restore a more favourable neurohumoral balance (Fig. 4). In this approach, undesirable systems (eg the RAAS) are suppressed (ie blocked) at the same time as potentially favourable axes (eg natriuretic peptides) are stimulated (ie augmented).

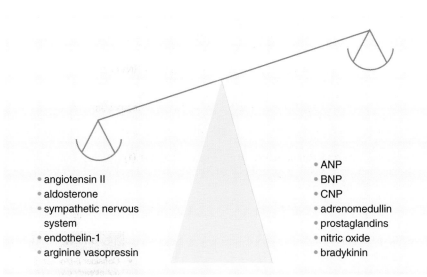

Fig 4. Neurohumoral modulation in heart failure (ANP, BNP, CNP = A-, B-, C-type natriuretic peptides).

This may be the best 'neurohumoral approach' to heart failure. Early experience is encouraging [31].

☐ PUTTING THE EVIDENCE INTO PRACTICE

Although the evidence base for CHF therapy is substantial and robust, and treatment strategies widely agreed upon and simple, many patients with CHF continue to be denied the benefit of modern pharmacological therapy. As a result, there has been a strong move towards better organised, rigorous systems of care [32,33]. A number of randomised trials have shown that such approaches lead to a better outcome [32,33]. Preliminary evidence suggests that titrating therapy against plasma natriuretic peptide concentrations may also improve outcome [34].

☐ TRIAL ACRONYMS

ATLAS	Assessment of Treatment with Lisinopril And Survival
BEST	Beta-blocker Evaluation Survival Trial
CHARM	Candesartan in Heart Failure: Assessment of Reduction in Mortality and Morbidity
CIBIS-II	The Cardiac Insufficiency Bisoprolol Study II
CONSENSUS-1	Cooperative North Scandinavian Enalapril Survival Study
COPERNICUS	Carvedilol Prospective Randomised Cumulative Survival Trial
DIG	Digitalis Investigation Group
ELITE II	Evaluation of Losartan In The Elderly
HOPE	Heart Outcomes Prevention Evaluation Study
MERIT-HF	Metoprolol CR/XL Randomised Intervention Trial in Congestive Heart Failure

RALES	Randomised Aldactone Evaluation Study
SOLVD-T	Treatment arm of the Studies Of Left Ventricular Dysfunction
Val HeFT	Valsartan Heart Failure Trial

REFERENCES

1   Scottish Intercollegiate Guidelines Network. *Diagnosis and treatment of heart failure due to left ventricular systolic dysfunction.* Edinburgh: SIGN, 1999. (www.show.scot.nhs.uk/sign/home.htm)

2   Consensus recommendations for the management of chronic heart failure. On behalf of the membership of the advisory council to improve outcomes nationwide in heart failure. *Am J Cardiol* 1999; **83**: 1A–38A.

3   Heart Failure Society of America (HFSA) practice guidelines. HFSA guidelines for management of patients with heart failure caused by left ventricular systolic dysfunction – pharmacological approaches. *J Card Fail* 1999; **5**: 357–82.

4   Cohn JN, Levine TB, Francis GS, Goldsmith S. Neurohumoral control mechanisms in congestive heart failure. *Am Heart J* 1981; **102**: 509–14.

5   Francis GS. Neurohumoral activation and progression of heart failure: hypothetical and clinical considerations. *J Cardiovasc Pharmacol* 1998; **32**(Suppl 1): S16–21.

6   Chen HH, Burnett JC Jr. The natriuretic peptides in heart failure: diagnostic and therapeutic potentials. *Proc Assoc Am Physicians* 1999; **111**: 406–16.

7   Seta Y, Shan K, Bozkurt B, *et al.* Basic mechanisms in heart failure: the cytokine hypothesis. *J Card Fail* 1996; **2**: 243–9.

8   Effects of enalapril on mortality in severe congestive heart failure. Results of the Cooperative North Scandinavian Enalapril Survival Study (CONSENSUS). The CONSENSUS Trial Study Group. *N Engl J Med* 1987; **316**: 1429–35.

9   Effect of enalapril on survival in patients with reduced left ventricular ejection fractions and congestive heart failure. The SOLVD Investigators. *N Engl J Med* 1991; **325**: 293–302.

10 Garg R, Yusuf S. Overview of randomized trials of angiotensin-converting enzyme inhibitors on mortality and morbidity in patients with heart failure. Collaborative Group on ACE Inhibitor Trials. *JAMA* 1995; **273**: 1450–6.

11 Pfeffer MA, Braunwald E, Moye LA, *et al.* Effect of captopril on mortality and morbidity in patients with left ventricular dysfunction after myocardial infarction. Results of the survival and ventricular enlargement trial. The SAVE Investigators. *N Engl J Med* 1992; **327**: 669–77.

12 Effect of ramipril on mortality and morbidity of survivors of acute myocardial infarction with clinical evidence of heart failure. The Acute Infarction Ramipril Efficacy (AIRE) Study Investigators. *Lancet* 1993; **342**: 821–8.

13 Kober L, Torp-Pedersen C, Carlsen JE, *et al.* A clinical trial of the angiotensin-converting-enzyme inhibitor trandolapril in patients with left ventricular dysfunction after myocardial infarction. Trandolapril Cardiac Evaluation (TRACE) Study Group. *N Engl J Med* 1995; **333**: 1670–6.

14 Yusuf S, Sleight P, Pogue J, *et al.* Effects of an angiotensin-converting-enzyme inhibitor, ramipril, on cardiovascular events in high-risk patients. The Heart Outcomes Prevention Evaluation Study Investigators. *N Engl J Med* 2000; **342**: 145–53.

15 McMurray JJ. Failure to practice evidence-based medicine: why do physicians not treat patients with heart failure with angiotensin-converting enzyme inhibitors? *Eur Heart J* 1998; **19**(Suppl L):L15–21.

16 Packer M, Poole-Wilson PA, Armstrong PW, *et al.* Comparative effects of low and high doses of the angiotensin-converting enzyme inhibitor, lisinopril, on morbidity and mortality in chronic heart failure. ATLAS Study Group. *Circulation* 1999; **100**: 2312–8.

17 Pitt B, Poole-Wilson PA, Segal R, *et al.* Effect of losartan compared with captopril on mortality in patients with symptomatic heart failure: randomised trial – the Losartan Heart Failure Survival Study ELITE II. *Lancet* 2000; **355**: 1582–7.

18 Cohn JN, Tognoni G, Glazer RD, *et al.* Rationale and design of the Valsartan Heart Failure Trial: a large multinational trial to assess the effects of valsartan, an angiotensin-receptor blocker, on morbidity and mortality in chronic congestive heart failure. *J Card Fail* 1999; **5**: 155–60.

19 Swedberg K, Pfeffer M, Granger C, *et al.* Candesartan in heart failure – assessment of reduction in mortality and morbidity (CHARM): rationale and design. Charm-Programme Investigators. *J Card Fail* 1999; **5**: 276–82.

20 Struthers AD. Why does spironolactone improve mortality over and above an ACE inhibitor in chronic heart failure? *Br J Clin Pharmacol* 1999; **47**: 479–82.

21 Pitt B, Zannad F, Remme WJ, *et al.* The effect of spironolactone on morbidity and mortality in patients with severe heart failure. Randomized Aldactone Evaluation Study Investigators. *N Engl J Med* 1999; **341**: 709–17.

22 Joseph J, Gilbert EM. The sympathetic nervous system in chronic heart failure. *Prog Cardiovasc Dis* 1998; **41**: 9–16.

23 McMurray JJ. Major beta blocker mortality trials in chronic heart failure: a critical review. *Heart* 1999; **82**(Suppl 4): IV14–22.

24 The Cardiac Insufficiency Bisoprolol Study II (CIBIS-II): a randomised trial. *Lancet* 1999; **353**: 9–13.

25 Effect of metoprolol CR/XL in chronic heart failure: Metoprolol CR/XL Randomised Intervention Trial in Congestive Heart Failure (MERIT-HF). *Lancet* 1999; **353**: 2001–7.

26 Hjalmarson A, Goldstein S, Fagerberg B, *et al.* Effects of controlled-release metoprolol on total mortality, hospitalizations, and well-being in patients with heart failure: the Metoprolol CR/XL Randomized Intervention Trial in congestive heart failure (MERIT-HF). MERIT-HF Study Group. *JAMA* 2000; **283**: 1295–302.

27 The effect of digoxin on mortality and morbidity in patients with heart failure. The Digitalis Investigation Group. *N Engl J Med* 1997; **336**: 525–33.

28 Anand IS, Kalra GS, Ferrari R, *et al.* Enalapril as initial and sole treatment in severe chronic heart failure with sodium retention. *Int J Cardiol* 1990; **28**: 341–6.

29 Richardson A, Bayliss J, Scriven AJ, *et al.* Double-blind comparison of captopril alone against frusemide plus amiloride in mild heart failure. *Lancet* 1987; **ii**: 709–11.

30 National Service Framework for Coronary Heart Disease. *Modern standards and service models.* London: Department of Health, 2000.

31 Rouleau JL, Pfeffer MA, Stewart DJ, *et al.* Comparison of vasopeptidase inhibitor, omapatrilat and lisinopril on exercise tolerance and morbidity in patients with heart failure. IMPRESS randomised trial. *Lancet* 2000; **356**: 615–20.

32 McMurray JJ, Stewart S. Nurse led, multidisciplinary intervention in chronic heart failure. *Heart* 1998; **80**: 430–1.

33 Stewart S, Marley JE, Horowitz JD. Effects of a multidisciplinary, home-based intervention on unplanned readmissions and survival among patients with chronic congestive heart failure: a randomised controlled study. *Lancet* 1999; **354**: 1077–83.

34 Troughton RW, Frampton CM, Yandle TG, *et al.* Treatment of heart failure guided by plasma aminoterminal brain natriuretic peptide (N-BNP) concentrations. *Lancet* 2000; **355**: 1126–30.

☐ SELF ASSESSMENT QUESTIONS

1 Activation of the following neurohumoral systems is detrimental in the syndrome of heart failure:
(a) Renin-angiotensin
(b) Natriuretic peptides
(c) Aldosterone
(d) Endothelin
(e) Catecholamines

2   Angiotensin-converting enzyme inhibitors:
    (a) Are associated with improved mortality in chronic heart failure (CHF)
    (b) Are associated with reduction of symptoms in CHF
    (c) Should be given to *all* patients with heart failure of any cause
    (d) Should be introduced rapidly at high dose
    (e) Are as effective at low dose as at high dose

3   Beta-blockers:
    (a) Are associated with reduced mortality and morbidity in CHF patients
    (b) Should be prescribed in all patients with any degree of heart failure
    (c) Are indicated only in patients with heart failure secondary to ischaemic heart disease
    (d) Introduction requires hospital admission
    (e) Should be introduced cautiously and only in patients with stable heart failure

4   Spironolactone, an aldosterone antagonist:
    (a) Is an outdated treatment in CHF
    (b) Has proven mortality benefit in patients with CHF
    (c) Does not reduce hospital admission rates in patients with heart failure
    (d) Can cause dangerously high serum potassium levels
    (e) Gynaecomastia and breast tenderness are the most common adverse effects of spironolactone in patients with heart failure

5   Digoxin:
    (a) Is indicated only in patients in atrial fibrillation
    (b) Is of benefit in patients with ongoing symptoms despite other medication
    (c) Does not reduce hospital admission rates in patients with heart failure
    (d) Has been shown to reduce mortality in CHF
    (e) Causes neurohumoural suppression in heart failure

ANSWERS

1a True	2a True	3a True	4a False	5a False
b False	b True	b False	b True	b True
c True	c False	c False	c False	c False
d True	d False	d False	d True	d False
e True	e False	e True	e True	e True

Cardiac arrhythmias – when to intervene

Edward Rowland and Aditya Kapoor

In the last 15 years interventional electrophysiology has transformed the practice of clinical electrophysiology from what was a predominantly diagnostic routine, occasionally leading to complex open heart surgery or anti-tachycardia pacemaker implantation, to a frequently curative procedure. Most electrophysiology procedures are now undertaken with a view to intervene by catheter ablation. This chapter reviews the results and indications for most catheter ablation procedures.

☐ SUPRAVENTRICULAR TACHYCARDIA

Patients with supraventricular tachycardia (SVT) still represent the predominant indication for catheter ablation [1] (Table 1). SVTs include all tachycardias that incorporate tissues proximal to the bifurcation of the bundle of His in the mechanism of the arrhythmia, but the term paroxysmal SVT is best restricted to those with junctional reentry. The commonest mechanism of paroxysmal SVT is atrioventricular nodal reentrant tachycardia (AVNRT), which accounts for about 65–70% of these cases. This is the commonest type of sustained supraventricular arrhythmia in adults, excluding atrial fibrillation. Junctional reentry mediated by an accessory pathway (AP) is the second most common cause of paroxysmal SVT, accounting for 25–30% of the cases. Other forms of SVT are rare, comprising unusual APs and mechanisms in the atria (atrial tachycardia (AT)) or around the sinus node (sinus node reentry).

Table 1 Indications for catheter ablation.

- Wolff-Parkinson-White syndrome
- Paroxysmal supraventricular tachycardia
    - concealed accessory pathways
    - atrioventricular nodal reentry tachycardia
- Atrial tachycardia
- Atrial flutter
- Atrial fibrillation
    - atrioventricular ablation and pacemaker implant
    - linear and focal ablation
- Ventricular tachycardia

☐ ATRIOVENTRICULAR NODAL REENTRANT TACHYCARDIA

Although the precise mechanism of atrioventricular (AV) nodal reentry continues to be debated, these patients can be considered to have two functionally distinct conduction pathways in the region of the AV node: one behaves like the normal AV node, and the other is referred to as the 'slow pathway'. In the typical form of AVNRT, the slow pathway, located more posteriorly, provides the antero-grade limb of the circuit, while the faster, anterior AV nodal pathway forms the retrograde limb of the circuit (Fig. 1). The recognition that these pathways are spatially separate has formed the basis for interventional solutions to AV nodal reentry [2].

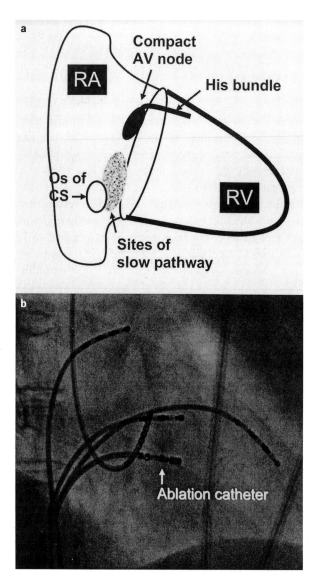

Fig. 1 (a) Diagram of the cardiac structures seen as if in the right anterior oblique (RAO) projection. This shows the area in which slow pathway potentials can be recorded relative to the right atrium (RA), right ventricle (RV), os of the coronary sinus (CS), the compact atrio-ventricular (AV) node and the bundle of His; **(b)** radiograph of the heart in the RAO projection showing catheters in the RA, RV, CS and adjacent to the bundle of His. The ablation catheter overlies the region of the slow pathway in a patient with AV nodal reentrant tachycardia.

Radiofrequency ablation in atrioventricular nodal reentrant tachycardia

Radiofrequency (RF) ablation of the slow pathway has become the preferred technique. Fast pathway ablation has fallen into disrepute because of the lower success rate and higher complication rate [3]. The reported success rate of slow pathway ablation is 98–100%, with a recurrence rate of 0–2%. The incidence of high-degree AV block is lower than in fast pathway ablation (0–1.3%). The Multicentre European Radiofrequency Survey [4] reported an incidence of inadvertent complete AV block in 5.3% of patients undergoing fast pathway ablation compared with only 2% in those undergoing slow pathway ablation. Since the efficacy of slow pathway ablation is nearly 100%, with a significantly lower chance of producing AV block, the Task Force of the American College of Cardiology/American Heart Association has recommended that slow pathway ablation should be the preferred approach in cases of AVNRT [5]. The cost-efficacy of this form of treatment compares favourably with competing therapies: over a projected 30-year follow-up, only successful prevention of attacks with digoxin or beta-blockers is cheaper [6].

Although highly effective for the long-term abolition of this form of SVT, the small risk of heart block requiring pacemaker implantation leads us to offer catheter ablation in young patients with AVNRT only when conventional anti-arrhythmic drugs (excluding amiodarone) have failed or when the patient does not wish to take drugs.

☐ SUPRAVENTRICULAR TACHYCARDIA MEDIATED BY ACCESSORY PATHWAYS

The abolition of pre-excitation by RF catheter ablation is one of the most potent images in clinical electrophysiology [7–9] (Fig. 2). With an operation performed under local anaesthetic, often taking little more than an hour, the patient can be

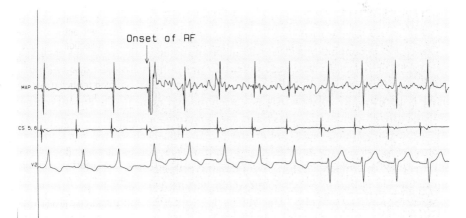

Fig. 2 Catheter ablation in a patient with the Wolff-Parkinson-White syndrome. Intracardiac electrograms (MAP D and CS 5,6), together with ECG lead V2 at the onset of radiofrequency (RF) energy. Three seconds after the delivery starts the delta wave disappears and the ECG shows normal conduction.

cured of a troublesome and occasionally life-threatening condition. Not all patients who have junctional reentry using an AP have pre-excitation in sinus rhythm. A significant number (at least 25%) have pathways that conduct only in the retrograde direction. Thus, the pathway supports tachycardia but does not conduct anterogradely and, therefore, when in sinus rhythm, the ECG is normal.

Irrespective of whether the AP is overt or concealed, the results of RF catheter ablation have been excellent. Some people would therefore advocate this as the treatment of first choice for those with symptoms.

Radiofrequency ablation of accessory pathways

In experienced hands, the procedural success rate is 90–100% – it is unusual to fail to ablate the pathway, irrespective of the location [9,10]. There is a small recurrence rate (ca 5%), a consequence of producing transient trauma to the pathway rather than functional destruction. The overall complication rate varies from 1–3%. Inadvertent AV block in patients undergoing ablation of septal APs remains the predominant concern (the risk of AV block in other pathway locations should be non-existent). Other complications should be rare, but they include cardiac tamponade (0.5%), transient cardiac ischaemia (0.8%), coronary artery spasm or thrombosis (0.2%), pulmonary or systemic embolism (0.2%), and access site complications (0.5%). The mortality rate as a direct result of the procedure is reported as 0.08%.

The Atakr Ablation System clinical trial [10] in 1,050 patients is the first prospective multicentre report on the efficacy and safety of RF ablation of supraventricular arrhythmias. The overall success rate was highest for patients undergoing ablation of AV junction (100%) and least for APs (93%). The acute success rate for AVNRT was 97%. In those with APs, the success rate was lower for right free wall and posteroseptal pathways (90% and 88%, respectively) than for left free wall pathways (95%). The recurrence rate was 7.8% among patients with APs (commoner with right free wall, septal and posteroseptal pathways) and 4.6% in AVNRT.

Based on contemporary evidence, RF ablation should be the treatment of choice for patients with symptomatic atrioventricular reentrant tachycardia due to Wolff-Parkinson-White syndrome. Since the risk of inadvertent AV block after ablation of an AP is quite low, RF ablation may also be considered as the first treatment option for patients with concealed bypass tracts and symptomatic tachycardia. Completely asymptomatic patients with pre-excitation do not need either a diagnostic electrophysiological study or an ablation procedure. Electrophysiological study may, however, be recommended for asymptomatic patients who are in a specific profession (eg airline pilots) and for young persons who wish to participate in competitive athletic activities. The aim is to determine both the number and location of APs and the risk of the development of threatening arrhythmias. If such a risk is substantial and the AP is in an easily accessible location with a low risk of causing AV block (eg left free wall AP), ablation would be a reasonable undertaking in this selected group of patients.

□ ATRIAL TACHYCARDIA

ATs may be unifocal or multifocal. Unifocal tachycardias are usually due to enhanced automaticity or triggered activity within a localised atrial focus [11]. These forms of tachycardia may be incessant and lead to development of ventricular dysfunction and a tachycardia-induced cardiomyopathy. Reentrant ATs are more common in patients with underlying structural heart disease and are usually paroxysmal. Multifocal AT is commonly due to enhanced automaticity and seen in the setting of underlying pulmonary disease.

Radiofrequency ablation of atrial tachycardia

RF ablation is usually more successful for unifocal tachycardias than for tachycardias arising from more than two foci [11]. In the latter situation, drug therapy rather than RF ablation is a better treatment option. However, if the ventricular rate is not controlled despite drugs, AV node ablation followed by pacemaker implantation may be performed. The overall short-term success rates are 85–95%, with a late recurrence rate of 5–10%.

Patients with unifocal AT may initially be treated with AV nodal blocking drugs, though it is unlikely that this will abolish the arrhythmia. RF ablation is a reasonable alternative to Class I or Class III drugs in patients who cannot tolerate, or are resistant to, these drugs.

□ ATRIAL FLUTTER

A precise definition of atrial flutter is important because the commonest type of flutter can be successfully treated by catheter ablation. The term 'typical atrial flutter' is best restricted to describe an atrial arrhythmia with a regular atrial rate, usually 200–340 beats per minute, and which produces a classical ECG pattern – that is, negative sawtooth flutter waves in leads II, III and aVF. There are other types of atrial flutter, but this type is usually due to a macroreentrant right atrial circuit, in which part of the circuit comprises the atrial myocardium between the tricuspid annulus (TA) and inferior vena cava (IVC). Proof of this cavotricuspid isthmus-dependent mechanism has allowed a technique for ablation of atrial flutter to be developed which prevents the arrhythmia by creating a line of block across the atrial wall between the TA and the IVC [12,13].

Atrial flutter can exist alone or concomitantly with other arrhythmias, notably atrial fibrillation. Treatment is often required on symptomatic grounds, and the options lie between anti-arrhythmic drugs, cardioversion and catheter ablation. The pharmacological strategy is essentially the same as for the treatment of atrial fibrillation: stabilise the atrium and/or control the ventricular response. The latter is often more difficult to achieve in atrial flutter than in atrial fibrillation, and the efficacy of atrial stabilising drugs is modest at best. The conventional approach has been to use Class IA drugs, often in combination with AV node blocking drugs such as digoxin. However, recent studies have shown that Class IC drugs may be more efficacious and have fewer adverse effects. Class III drugs offer a therapeutic alternative in cases resistant to other drugs. All these drugs may slow the atrial rate sufficiently to allow 1:1 AV conduction during atrial flutter, and paradoxically increase the ventricular rate. These factors have provided the impetus to the increased use of non-pharmacological methods for managing atrial flutter.

Radiofrequency ablation of atrial flutter

As with the other arrhythmias, transcatheter intervention in atrial flutter was preceded by successful cryosurgical ablation of the area of slow conduction in the low right atrium, and followed by encouraging results with DC ablation. RF catheter ablation has become the treatment of choice because of the high success and low complication rates. A successful procedure depends on identifying isthmus-dependent atrial flutter, creating a series of contiguous lesions between the TA and the IVC, and then demonstrating that there is conduction block in each direction across the ablation line (Fig. 3). Success rates in excess of 90% have been reported, with recurrence rates of less than 10% using the criteria of bidirectional conduction block in the isthmus rather than only non-inducibility of atrial flutter as the end-point [13].

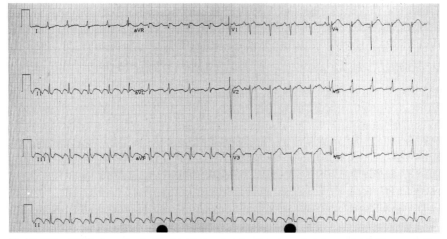

Fig. 3 12-lead ECG of a patient with atrial flutter showing the characteristic sawtooth P waves in the inferior leads. This pattern is generally associated with a counterclockwise reentrant wavefront in the right atrium which can be interrupted and prevented by isthmus ablation.

Because of the high success rates and low rates of complications, RF ablation of atrial flutter is suitable not only for patients refractory to drugs but also for those who do not wish to take drugs or undergo repeated cardioversion. The role of catheter ablation in those with both atrial fibrillation and atrial flutter is controversial. In our experience, patients continue to notice symptomatic palpitation during follow-up after flutter ablation due to continued paroxysms of atrial fibrillation, even though the attacks may be symptomatically less troublesome.

Others have found that flutter ablation in those with both flutter and fibrillation will improve control of paroxysmal atrial fibrillation [14]. We await the results of much longer follow-up to demonstrate whether atrial arrhythmias are abolished by these procedures or whether the natural history is simply delayed.

☐ ATRIAL FIBRILLATION

The decision whether to try to maintain or restore sinus rhythm, or to accept the inevitability or permanence of the fibrillating atria is complex and beyond the scope of this chapter [15]. The enthusiasm for non-pharmacological interventions has, in part, been driven by the limitations of drug treatment [16]. All anti-arrhythmic drugs have some limitations, whether attempting to maintain sinus rhythm or to control the ventricular rate. Their adverse effects are often given prominence, particularly because of a definite pro-arrhythmic risk with the Class I and Class III anti-arrhythmic drugs. Both the meta-analysis of the trials using quinidine [17] and the Stroke Prevention in Atrial Fibrillation (SPAF) trial [18] have shown an increased mortality with anti-arrhythmic drugs, particularly in patients with atrial fibrillation who also have heart failure [19]. Even the use of amiodarone in the recent Canadian Trial of Atrial Fibrillation (CTAF) showed that at 16 months 35% of patients had experienced a recurrence of atrial fibrillation [20].

Radiofrequency ablation for atrial fibrillation

Historically, ablation of AV conduction was the first technique to find a place in interventional electrophysiology using catheters [1]. It remains an effective method of achieving control of the ventricular rate, improving symptoms and reducing the need for anti-arrhythmic medication. It should, however, be reserved as a 'tactic of last resort' for those patients with permanent atrial fibrillation in whom the ventricular rate remains controlled despite drug therapy, and those with uncontrolled paroxysmal atrial fibrillation. After ablation of AV conduction and pacemaker implantation most patients will need to be anticoagulated, and they are dependent on the pacemaker for normal heart rate control. There remains a small incidence of sudden death after this technique. This has never been adequately explained, but may be related to bradycardia-dependent ventricular arrhythmias (VAs) in the weeks following the procedure. It may be prevented by pacing rates of 75 beats per minute or greater, at least for a month or two after the procedure.

The success of open heart surgery for the treatment of atrial fibrillation (MAZE surgery [21]) has encouraged the possibility that the same results can be achieved by catheter techniques. Initial attempts were undertaken to recreate multiple lines of block within the right and/or left atria. Success rates have, at best, been modest, and the procedure has been associated with a significant risk of thromboembolic events when ablation lines have been created in the left atrium.

The observation that has given such an impetus to the possibility of catheter ablation for atrial fibrillation was made by Haissaguerre [22]. Catheter mapping inside the left atrium in a patient who appeared to have repetitive paroxysmal atrial fibrillation, demonstrated early activity in one of the pulmonary veins. Ablation of the focal source raised the possibility that many episodes of atrial fibrillation are triggered by irritable foci within the pulmonary veins. Closer examination of the ECG in similar patients suggests that they have a rapid irregular AT, as well as possibly having atrial fibrillation (Fig. 4). However, more detailed observation of the ECG at the onset of the atrial arrhythmia in those with more typical features of atrial fibrillation may often reveal that the rhythm at the onset of attacks shows well formed atrial depolarisations before degenerating into the more classical appearances of atrial fibrillation.

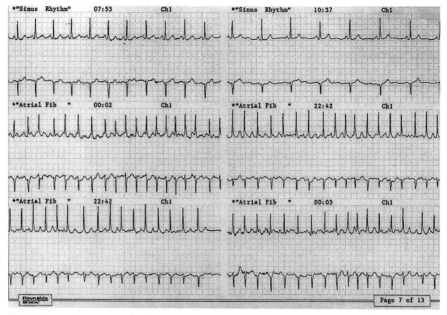

Fig. 4 Extract from an ambulatory ECG recording in a patient diagnosed as having paroxysmal atrial fibrillation. Close inspection of the ECG recordings shows the presence of a repetitive, rapid, irregular atrial tachycardia.

The results of the preliminary studies undertaken so far do not provide an accurate indication of what percentage of patients with typical atrial fibrillation have single focal sources amenable to ablation. Catheter mapping in these patients is not without its difficulties. Reliable ways of initiating atrial fibrillation that reproduce the precise electrophysiological features of spontaneous onsets have not yet been developed. The major complication that has occurred with RF catheter ablation in the pulmonary veins is pulmonary vein stenosis. The mechanisms by which this occurs, and specifically the techniques that must be employed to avoid it, are not clear.

Thus, focal ablation of atrial fibrillation remains a technique that should be restricted to those centres with high levels of expertise and experience in catheter mapping and interventional electrophysiological procedures, and where these new ablation techniques are being undertaken under the umbrella of new investigation techniques.

☐ VENTRICULAR ARRHYTHMIAS

Catheter ablation may provide a cure for selected patients with VA [23]. In most patients with idiopathic sustained ventricular tachycardia (VT), the heart is structurally normal and the substrate for the arrhythmia small and discrete. Mapping techniques are sufficiently accurate to identify the origin of the arrhythmia and to achieve success rates of over 90% with one or more RF deliveries. None of the patterns of idiopathic VT is common, but the morphologies of the ECG during the arrhythmia are archetypal. That arising from the outflow tract of the right ventricle has a left bundle branch block configuration and the frontal QRS axis is directed inferiorly (Fig. 5). The pattern of fascicular VT (so-called because it arises from the region of the left posterior fascicle of the left bundle) has a right bundle branch block pattern with a superior QRS axis (Fig. 6). Catheter ablation in such cases has increasingly been used as an early treatment option.

It has not so far been possible to achieve similar success rates for RF ablation in unselected patients with sustained monomorphic VT in the setting of coronary artery disease. Success in these patients must be measured in terms of prevention of further recurrences of arrhythmia but also of a benefit on prognosis. Increasing experience with both electrophysiological mapping and new technologies of mapping has achieved high success rates in selected small series [24,25]. However, in these patients, many of whom are at significant risk of sudden death because of

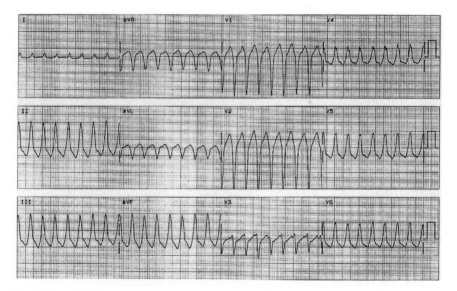

Fig. 5 12-lead ECG recorded during tachycardia in a patient with ventricular tachycardia arising from the outflow tract of the right ventricle.

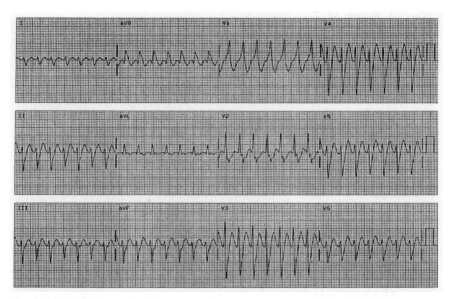

Fig. 6 12-lead ECG recorded during tachycardia in a patient with ventricular tachycardia arising from the left posterior fascicle.

impaired ventricular function and widespread electrical instability, catheter ablation is used as an adjunct to the implantable cardioverter-defibrillator and not as a substitute.

REFERENCES

1   Morady F. Radiofrequency ablation as treatment for cardiac arrhythmias. *N Engl J Med* 1999; **340**: 534–44.

2   Jackman WM, Beckman KJ, McClelland JH, *et al.* Treatment of supraventricular tachycardia due to atrioventricular nodal reentry by radiofrequency catheter ablation of slow pathway conduction. *N Engl J Med* 1992; **327**: 313–8.

3   Jazayeri MR, Hemper SL, Sra JS, *et al.* Selective transcatheter ablation of fast and slow pathways using radiofrequency energy in patients with atrioventricular nodal reentrant tachycardia. *Circulation* 1992; **85**: 1318–28.

4   Hindricks G. The multicentre European radiofrequency survey. Complications of radiofrequency catheter ablation of arrhythmias. *Eur Heart J* 1993; **14**: 256–61.

5   American College of Cardiology/American Heart Association Task Force Report: guidelines for clinical intracardiac electrophysiological and catheter ablation procedures. *J Am Coll Cardiol* 1995; **26**: 555–73.

6   Kalbfleisch SJ, Calkins H, Langberg JJ, *et al.* Comparison of the cost of radiofrequency catheter modification of the atrioventricular node and medical therapy for drug refractory atrioventricular node reentrant tachycardia. *J Am Coll Cardiol* 1992; **9**: 1583–7.

7   Jackman WM, Wang XZ, Friday KJ, *et al.* Catheter ablation of accessory atrioventricular pathways (Wolff-Parkinson-White syndrome) by radiofrequency current. *N Engl J Med* 1991; **324**: 1605–11.

8   Kuck KH, Schuter M, Geiger M, *et al.* Radiofrequency current catheter ablation of accessory atrioventricular pathways. *Lancet* 1991; **337**: 1557–61.

9   Kay GN, Epstein AE, Dailey SM, Plumb VJ. Role of radiofrequency ablation in the management of supraventricular arrhythmias: experience in 760 consecutive patients. *J Cardiovasc Electrophysiol* 1994; **5**: 219–31.

10 Calkins H, Yong P, Miller JM, *et al.* Catheter ablation of accessory pathways, atrioventricular nodal reentrant tachycardia, and the atrioventricular junction: final results of a prospective, multicenter clinical trial. The Atakr Multicenter Investigators Group. *Circulation* 1999; **99**: 262–70.

11 Chen SA, Chiang CE, Yang CJ, *et al.* Sustained atrial tachycardia in adult patients: electrophysiological characteristics, pharmacological response, possible mechanisms and effects of radiofrequency ablation. *Circulation* 1994; **90**: 1262–78.

12 Cosio FG, Lopez-Gil M, Goicolea A, *et al.* Radiofrequency ablation of the inferior vena cava-tricuspid valve isthmus in common atrial flutter. *Am J Cardiol* 1993; **71**: 705–9.

13 Poty H, Saoudi N, Nair M, *et al.* Radiofrequency catheter ablation of atrial flutter: further insights into various types of isthmus block: application to ablation during sinus rhythm. *Circulation* 1996; **94**: 3204–13.

14 Nabar A, Rodriguez LM, Timmermans C, *et al.* Effect of right atrial isthmus ablation on the occurrence of atrial fibrillation: observations in four patient groups having type 1 atrial flutter with or without associated atrial fibrillation. *Circulation* 1999; **99**: 1441–5.

15 Sopher SM, Camm AJ. Atrial fibrillation: maintenance of sinus rhythm versus rate control. Review. *Am J Cardiol* 1996; **77**: 24A–37A.

16 Coumel P, Thomas O, Leenhardt A. Drug therapy for prevention of atrial fibrillation. *Am J Cardiol* 1996; **77**: 3A–9A.

17 Coplen SE, Antman EM, Berlin JA, *et al.* Efficacy and safety of quinidine therapy for maintenance of sinus rhythm after cardioversion: a meta-analysis of randomised clinical trials. *Circulation* 1990; **82**: 1106–11.

18 Flaker GC, Blackshear JL, McBride R, *et al.* Antiarrhythmic drug therapy and cardiac mortality in atrial fibrillation. The Stroke Prevention in Atrial Fibrillation Investigators. *J Am Coll Cardiol* 1992; **20**: 527–32.

19 Effect of prophylactic amiodarone on mortality after acute myocardial infarction and in congestive heart failure: meta-analysis of individual data from 6500 patients in randomised trials. The Amiodarone Trials Meta-Analysis Investigators. *Lancet* 1997; **350**: 1417–24.

20 Roy D, Talajic M, Dorian P, *et al.* Amiodarone to prevent recurrence of atrial fibrillation. *N Engl J Med* 2000; **342**: 913–20.

21 Cox JL, Schuessler RB, Lappas DG, Boineau JP. An 8½ year clinical experience with surgery for atrial fibrillation. *Ann Surg* 1996; **224**: 267–75.

22 Haissaguerre M, Jais P, Shah DC, *et al.* Spontaneous initiation of atrial fibrillation by ectopic beats originating in the pulmonary veins. *N Engl J Med* 1998; **339**: 659–65.

23 Klein LS, Miles WM, Mirani RD, *et al.* Ablation of ventricular tachycardia in patients with structurally normal hearts. In: Zipes DP, Jalife J (eds). *Cardiac electrophysiology. From cell to bedside.* Philadelphia: WB Saunders, 1995: 1518–23.

24 Bogun F, Bahu M, Knight BP, *et al.* Comparison of effective and ineffective target sites that demonstrate concealed entrainment in patients with coronary artery disease undergoing radiofrequency ablation of ventricular tachycardia. *Circulation* 1997; **95**: 183–90.

25 Callans DJ, Zado E, Sarter BH, *et al.* Efficacy of radiofrequency catheter ablation for ventricular tachycardia in healed myocardial infarction. *Am J Cardiol* 1998; **82**: 429–32.

☐ SELF ASSESSMENT QUESTIONS

1   Slow pathway radiofrequency (RF) catheter ablation for atrioventricular (AV) nodal reentrant tachycardia:
    (a) Is successful in almost 100% of cases
    (b) Is complicated by heart block and the need for pacemaker implantation in more than 5% of cases

    (c) Is more expensive than most comparative drug therapies

    (d) Is associated with a recurrence rate of up to 5%

2   Concerning accessory AV pathways:

    (a) Pre-excitation is present in all patients with accessory pathways (APs)

    (b) At least a quarter of those with paroxysmal supraventricular ventricular tachycardia (VT) due to an AP will have a normal ECG in sinus rhythm

    (c) RF catheter ablation carries a mortality in excess of 1%

    (d) Ablation of free wall APs is associated with a negligible risk of heart block

3   Typical atrial flutter:

    (a) Is due to a right atrial focal mechanism

    (b) Can be ablated with a 90% success rate

    (c) Is ablated by creating a linear lesion between the inferior vena cava and the mitral annulus

    (d) Responds better to atrial stabilising drugs than atrial fibrillation

4   RF catheter ablation:

    (a) Of AV conduction removes the need for anticoagulation

    (b) Of AV conduction should be considered in those with atrial fibrillation in whom the ventricular rate remains uncontrolled

    (c) Achieves success rates of more than 90% in all forms of VT

    (d) When used for ablation of VT achieves the same improvement in prognosis as implantable cardioverter-defibrillator implantation

ANSWERS

1a True	2a False	3a False	4a False
b False	b True	b True	b True
c False	c False	c False	c False
d True	d True	d False	d False

Reducing risk of atherosclerotic vascular disease in the diabetic population

Christopher D Byrne

☐ ATHEROSCLEROTIC VASCULAR DISEASE AND DIABETES

Approximately 1.4 million people in the UK have diabetes, a number that is likely to double in the next decade because the prevalence of both type 1 and type 2 diabetes is increasing. The ratio of the number of people with type 2 diabetes to type 1 diabetes is approximately 10:1, with type 2 diabetes having a greater impact on health care resources. The epidemic of diabetes is rapidly becoming a global pandemic and it has been predicted that the number of people with type 2 diabetes will increase from 100 million in 1994 to 300 million in 2025.

Diabetes is associated with an increase in all-cause mortality of approximately three-fold and a three- to eight-fold increase in cardiovascular mortality. For reasons that are poorly understood the increase in cardiovascular mortality attributable to diabetes is greater in women than in men. Interestingly, in a group of people with diabetes, even after adjustment for other potential cardiovascular risk factors, those in the highest quartile of plasma glucose levels have a fourfold greater risk of all-cause mortality than those in the lowest quartile. Cardiovascular disease (CVD) accounts for almost 80% of all deaths in people with diabetes. Three-quarters of these deaths result from ischaemic heart disease (IHD). Not only is the case fatality rate higher after myocardial infarction (MI), but also the benefit derived from coronary revascularisation is reduced because peri-operative mortality is doubled and surgery is associated with reduced long-term survival.

There is increased risk of atherosclerotic vascular disease (AVD) causing MI and thrombotic stroke, regardless of whether individuals have type 1 or type 2 diabetes. Recently, the results of the BDACS (see end of chapter for explanation of studies) [1] provided important information on deaths and causes of deaths among people with type 1 diabetes (Table 1). The study retrospectively analysed the records of 23,752 people aged 1–84 years. Attributable risks, or the excess deaths in persons with diabetes compared with the general population, increased with age in both sexes. Most significantly, the study showed that CVD is the leading cause of death in people aged 30–50 years. In contrast to the general population, women in the 30–50 year age group lose the protective effect conferred by their gender and have the same risk of CVD as men of the same age [1].

People with type 2 diabetes also die mainly from the consequences of AVD manifest as CVD or cerebrovascular disease, causing MI or stroke. Often individuals

Table 1 Deaths in type 1 diabetes in the BDACS [1].

No. of patients at follow-up	Duration of diabetes (years)	No. of deaths		SMR	95% CI
22,803	4-25	Total:	949		
		M:	566	2.7	2.5–2.9
		W:	383	4.0	3.6–4.4

CI = confidence interval; M = men; SMR = standardised mortality rate; W = women.

with type 2 diabetes have relatively minor abnormalities of plasma glucose concentration. Indeed, risk of AVD increases not only with impaired glucose tolerance (IGT) but also with the minor increases in plasma glucose levels observed in some individuals in a 'normal' population. The explanation for this phenomenon is uncertain, but increasing evidence suggests that many of the features of the metabolic syndrome [2] (Table 2) independently predict development of AVD, and

Table 2 Features of the metabolic syndrome.

Factor	Cause

Insulin resistance (resistance to biological actions of insulin)	Insulin mediated:
	• glucose uptake into skeletal muscle
	• suppression of:
	  – adipocyte lipolysis
	  – protein catabolism
	  – VLDL production
	• vascular endothelial cell relaxation
	• enhancement of gene expression

Glucose intolerance	↑Plasma glucose concentration
Central adiposity	↑Waist measurement: • men >95 cm • women >80 cm
Atherogenic lipoprotein phenotype	↑VLDL ↑HDLc ↑Small dense LDLc
Hypertension	↑Blood pressure
Hyperuricaemia	↑Plasma urate
Abnormal fibrinolysis	↑PAI-1 ↑PAI activity
Abnormal haemostasis	↑Fibrinogen ↑Thrombin generation markers
Vascular inflammation	↑CRP ↑TNF-α ↑IL-6

CRP = C-reactive protein; HDLc = high-density lipoprotein c; IL = interleukin; LDLc = low-density lipoprotein c; PAI = plasminogen activator inhibitor; TNF = tumour necrosis factor; VLDL = very low-density lipoprotein.

features of the metabolic syndrome are frequently present in people with type 2 diabetes. The impact of many of these risk factors can be modified to attenuate risk of AVD. The purpose of this review is to discuss both non-pharmacological and pharmacological strategies for intervention.

☐ LIFESTYLE CHANGES TO REDUCE RISK OF ATHEROSCLEROTIC VASCULAR DISEASE

Diet, nutrition, smoking cessation and physical activity

Priority should be given to lifestyle changes, and these should be highlighted for everyone both with and without diabetes to emphasise the influence of behaviour on health.

It is uncertain whether dietary intervention strategies are helpful in the primary prevention of AVD in people with diabetes. Meta-analysis of cholesterol lowering by dietary modification has shown that cholesterol levels can be reduced by an average of 5% by diet alone. Furthermore, changes in diet result in a small but significant reduction in IHD mortality but seem to have minimal effect on all-cause mortality. Although there is limited evidence in individuals with diabetes and established AVD, increasing evidence supports the notion that adopting a Mediterranean-type diet is beneficial in reducing recurrent vascular events. The LDHS was a randomised secondary prevention trial to test whether a Mediterranean-type diet reduced the rate of recurrence after a first MI. After a mean follow-up of 46 months, cardiac death and non-fatal MI were markedly reduced (14 events versus 44 in the prudent Western-type diet group, $p = 0.0001$). Two other composite end-points were similarly reduced. Adjusted risk ratios ranged from 0.28–0.53, which were also highly significant relative risk reductions. Although these data were obtained from the general population, they highlight the need to consider dietary changes to improve nutrition as part of a strategy to decrease cardiovascular morbidity and mortality in people with diabetes.

Men and women who stop smoking experience a rapid decline in risk of AVD, by as much as 50% in one year, although 10 years' cessation may be required to reach the level of risk of someone who has never smoked. These data were obtained in individuals not known to have diabetes. However, it is reasonable to assume that the benefit of smoking cessation should be at least as marked in people with diabetes.

A well-recognised factor leading to increased risk of type 2 diabetes is a rapid transition from subsistence living to a more 'Westernised' high fat diet. This type of diet often causes marked obesity and an increase in the prevalence of type 2 diabetes, as has been observed in populations such as the Pima Indians and Nauruan Islanders. Obesity, specifically central obesity, is a major feature of the metabolic syndrome. The increase in prevalence of obesity in the last couple of decades is largely attributable to a decline in energy expenditure, a problem also evident in children. In preventing and controlling weight gain, it is important not only to regulate energy intake but also to increase energy expenditure. Given that energy expenditure improves insulin sensitivity both in subjects with normal glucose tolerance and in people with type 2 diabetes, patients should be encouraged to engage in activities that increase calorie consumption.

Measures that not only decrease insulin resistance but also lower plasma glucose levels should be useful in preventing retinopathy, nephropathy or neuropathy in type 2 diabetes. Thus, diet, weight reduction and exercise should be beneficial to patients with type 2 diabetes. Preventing or delaying excess mortality attributable to AVD in people with type 2 diabetes may be possible by utilising strategies that focus on dietary counselling and physical exercise. In Da Qing (China), 577 of 110,660 individuals (men and women) were classified (using World Health Organization criteria) as having IGT. Subjects were randomised either to a control group or to one of three active treatment groups: diet only, exercise only, or diet plus exercise. The relative decrease in rate of development of diabetes in the active treatment groups was similar regardless of whether subjects were initially stratified as being lean or overweight (body mass index ≥ 24 kg/m^2) [3]. Thus, diet and/or exercise interventions produce an important decrease in the incidence of diabetes amongst those with IGT, whether or not an individual is initially overweight.

☐ PHARMACOLOGICAL TREATMENT TO REDUCE RISK OF ATHEROSCLEROTIC VASCULAR DISEASE

The results from various randomised controlled trials (RCTs) show that six different classes of drugs (antiplatelet agents, anticoagulants, α-blockers, angiotensin-converting enzyme (ACE) inhibitors, lipid lowering agents and calcium antagonists) reduce the risk of recurrent vascular events in people with established IHD. Although there is evidence to support the use of thrombolytics, α-blockers, ACE inhibitors, lipid lowering agents and inhibitors of platelet aggregation in people with diabetes *and* established IHD, there is little evidence to date to support their use in the primary prevention of vascular disease in people with diabetes. Given the limited available data, it is often possible nevertheless to extrapolate from the available evidence and use clinical judgement to assess the likely impact of primary prevention strategies.

Treatment of obesity

Obesity predisposes to type 2 diabetes and is associated with a worsening in the features of the metabolic syndrome. Thus, measures directed at inducing weight loss might have an impact on AVD, although there is little evidence to support this suggestion at present. Orlistat, a lipase inhibitor, can achieve a small degree of weight loss in people with type 2 diabetes treated with a calorie-restricted diet. This drug inhibits lipases in the gastrointestinal tract, preventing the absorption of about 30% of dietary fat. Orlistat 120 mg three times daily for one year in conjunction with a hypocaloric diet, reduced weight by 7.9-10.2% in obese non-diabetic individuals, but was less effective (6.2%) in obese patients with type 2 diabetes. At present, it is uncertain whether this amount of weight loss will reduce risk of cardiovascular events.

Lipid lowering therapies

Various classes of drugs lower cholesterol levels. Classes of drugs in decreasing order of use in the UK include statins, fibrates, resins and niacin (Table 3).

A large body of evidence substantiates the notion that increased plasma cholesterol levels cause AVD. However, cholesterol is only one of many plasma lipids transported within lipoprotein particles produced by the liver and small intestine. Cholesterol exists in various forms in the circulation (Fig.1). The disturbance of

Table 3 Actions of drugs that predominantly lower plasma cholesterol concentration.

Drug	Action
Statins	Inhibit HMG CoA reductase in the liver Inhibit cholesterol synthesis Lower total plasma cholesterol by an average of 23%
Fibrates	Activate the nuclear receptor PPARα that influences enzymes involved in triglyceride metabolism, resulting in both enhanced catabolism of TGRPs and reduced production of VLDL Lower total cholesterol by an average of 16% Lower triglyceride by ca 35% (more marked effect than statins)
Resins	Bile acid sequestrants that interfere with the entero-hepatic circulation of cholesterol in the gut Lower total cholesterol by an average of 9%, but may be associated with increased triglyceride levels and gastrointestinal side effects
Niacin	Reduces lipolysis in adipocytes, and so reduces the plasma non-esterified fatty acid levels (a powerful substrate and stimulus for hepatic VLDL production); therefore, lowers both plasma triglyceride and cholesterol levels

HMG CoA = hydroxymethylglutaryl coenzyme A; PPAR = peroxisomal proliferator-activated receptor; TGRP = triglyceride-rich particle; VLDL = very low-density lipoprotein.

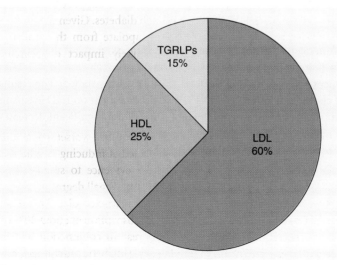

Fig. 1 Percentage of plasma cholesterol located in the major lipoprotein classes (HDL = high-density lipoprotein; LDL = low-density lipoprotein; TGRLP = triglyceride-rich lipoprotein particle.

lipid metabolism associated with the metabolic syndrome and type 2 diabetes is principally an abnormality of triglyceride metabolism, leading to the atherogenic lipoprotein phenotype (ALP) with relatively normal plasma cholesterol levels (Table 2). The precise mechanism by which abnormalities of triglyceride metabolism contribute to development of AVD is uncertain. However, increasing evidence suggests that the ALP is associated with vascular inflammation and disturbances of haemostasis [4].

Statin therapy

The results of large RCTs using 3-hydroxymethylglutaryl coenzyme A reductase inhibitors (statins) that reduce total cholesterol concentration by about 30% show a similar reduction in risk of first vascular event (primary prevention) and recurrent vascular events (secondary prevention), and an improvement in survival by 20–30%. In individuals with type 1 diabetes with albuminuria and/or renal impairment and in many people with type 2 diabetes, risk of a first vascular event often exceeds 3% per year. Thus, there is an acceptable case for treating these individuals with lipid lowering agents based upon their absolute risk of AVD. In order to achieve this aim, many guidelines have been established. Guidelines such as the Joint British Guidelines [5] illustrate the need to measure many risk factors associated with diabetes before assigning a level of overall risk for a first vascular event. These guidelines take into account risk factors such as gender, blood pressure, age and the cholesterol to high-density lipoprotein (HDL) c ratio.

The evidence supporting the use of lipid lowering therapy in people with diabetes is limited to results of subgroup analysis from the large trials. The numbers of diabetic subjects recruited to the statin trials were relatively small: 202 to the 4S, 586 to the CARE study, and 782 to the LIPID study. These data suggest that treatment with either 20 mg or 40 mg of simvastatin (in 4S) or 40 mg of pravastatin (in CARE and LIPID) is as effective in people with diabetes as in individuals with normal glucose tolerance.

Using the 1997 American Diabetes Association criteria for diagnosis of diabetes, the effect of simvastatin therapy in 4S patients with normal fasting glucose (n = 3,237), impaired fasting glucose (n = 678), and diabetes (n = 483) was studied. The results suggest a benefit of cholesterol lowering with simvastatin treatment on IHD events in subjects with varying degrees of glucose intolerance. In addition, significant decreases in total mortality, major coronary events and revascularisations were observed in simvastatin-treated patients with impaired fasting glucose levels [6] (Table 4).

Fibrate therapy

At present, the available data suggest that, despite little effect on low-density lipoprotein (LDL) c concentration, treatment with fibrates may also be effective in preventing AVD, particularly in subgroups of patients with high triglyceride and low HDLc levels. The fibrate group of lipid lowering agents have many beneficial effects on triglyceride metabolism but should not be used in subjects with renal

Table 4 Effect of simvastatin on risk reduction, reduction in cost and length of hospital stay in normal fasting glucose, impaired fasting glucose and diabetes mellitus participants in the 4S [6].

Subgroup	Reduction in average cost of CV disease-related hospitalisations	No.	Relative risk (MCE) reduction		Reduction in cost of CV hospitalisations		Reduction in length of stay (CV disease)	
			%	*p* value	%	*p* value	%	*p* value
Normal fasting glucose	Reduced costs and offset 60% of the cost of simvastatin therapy	3,237	40	<0.001	23	0.001	28	<0.001
Impaired fasting glucose	Reduced costs and offset 74% of the cost of simvastatin therapy	678	38	0.003	30	0.015	38	0.005
Diabetes mellitus	Net cost saving of ca £1,000 per subject in the trial	483	42	0.001	40	0.007	55	<0.001

CV = cardiovascular; MCE = major cardiovascular event.

impairment. These compounds, peroxisomal proliferator-activated receptor α agonists, lower plasma triglyceride levels by about 30% and increase HDLc by about 10%. There is limited evidence so far to support their use, although both the primary prevention HHS and the secondary prevention VA-HIT showed a reduction in risk of coronary events of 35% ($p = 0.02$) and 22% ($p = 0.006$), respectively. In both studies, individuals were randomised to gemfibrozil 1,200 mg/day and there was minimal change in LDLc levels [7] (Table 5). Several angiographic studies also support the use of fibrates in individuals at high risk of a vascular event. It should be noted, however, that one secondary prevention RCT with bezafibrate versus placebo, the BIP trial, showed a 9% (non-significant) reduction in vascular events in individuals randomised to 400 mg bezafibrate retard versus placebo. A total of 3,122 men and women recruited to BIP were randomised *a priori* because they had evidence of IHD and because of their cholesterol levels. Despite little effect on the pre-specified end-points, a *post hoc* subgroup analysis of hypertriglyceridaemic patients showed that bezafibrate treatment reduced fatal and non-fatal MI by 40% ($p = 0.03$).

Combination therapy with statins and fibrates

At present, it is uncertain whether combination therapy with a fibrate and a statin confers additional benefit to reduce risk of AVD. These drugs are not currently licensed for use together, but increasing evidence suggests that combined use of the newer statins and newer fibrates is safe. To address the issues of effectiveness and safety, the effect of combination therapy to reduce incident vascular events in subjects with type 2 diabetes is being examined in the LDS.

□ CONTROL OF HYPERGLYCAEMIA

The DCCT was the first large RCT designed to study the link between metabolic control and complications in type 1 diabetes. A total of 1,441 patients with type 1 diabetes, ranging in age from 13–39 years, were assigned randomly to either intensive or conventional diabetes therapy. Intensive therapy, which aimed at achieving a glucose level as close as possible to the normal range, included three or more daily insulin injections or a continuous subcutaneous insulin infusion, guided by four or more glucose tests daily. Conventional therapy included one or two daily insulin injections. Intensive insulin therapy, compared with conventional therapy, significantly reduced the risk of developing microvascular and neuropathic complications. In both the primary prevention and secondary intervention arms of the trial, intensified control reduced retinopathy risk by about 50%, and also reduced nephropathy and neuropathy risks. By contrast, there were no differences in quality of life, neurocognitive or emotional assessments between the two groups. However, the risk of hypoglycaemia increased threefold in the intensive treatment group, and in some patients this outweighed the relative benefit of intensive insulin therapy. The results of the DCCT have raised many questions that remain unanswered about intensive treatment indications, risk to benefit ratios and cost to

Table 5 Results of the secondary prevention VA-HIT randomised controlled trial with gemfibrozil 1,200 mg/day in 2,531 men, 25% of whom had diabetes [7].

Lipid values at recruitment	Median follow-up	Lipid values at 1 year		Primary events		Relative risk reduction		
		Lipid	%	No.	%	%	95% CI	p value
HDLc <1.0 mmol/l	5.1 years	HDLc	↑6	Placebo: 275/1,267	21.7	22	7–35	0.006
LDLc <3.6 mmol/l		Cholesterol	↓4	Gemfibrozil: 219/1,264	17.3			
		Triglyceride	↓31					
		LDL	no change					

CI = confidence interval; HDLc = high-density lipoprotein c; LDLc = low-density lipoprotein c.

benefit ratios. To date, results of various analyses suggest that DCCT-type intensive therapy is more expensive than conventional therapy, but that intensive therapy offers the hope of cost savings as a result of averted complications [8].

Achieving optimal metabolic control in the peri-infarct period by using an insulin infusion has been recommended for several years for patients with acute MI. The results of the DIGAMI study suggested that better metabolic control using intravenous infusion of insulin and glucose followed by long-term intensive therapy with insulin improves prognosis following MI [9] (Tables 6(a) and (b)). Better metabolic control may be of importance during the acute cardiac event because it is assumed that fatty acid metabolism is increased and glycolysis inhibited both in ischaemic tissue as well as in the non-ischaemic areas.

The effects of intensive blood glucose control with either sulphonylurea or insulin and of conventional treatment on the risk of microvascular and macrovascular complications in patients with type 2 diabetes were compared in the UKPDS [10]. Despite the favourable outcome for reduction in microvascular disease, it should be noted that subjects in the intensive group had more hypoglycaemic episodes ($p <0.0001$) and significantly higher weight gain (mean 2.9 kg) than the conventional treatment group ($p <0.001$) (Table 7). Disappointingly, there was little evidence that improved blood glucose control in type 2 diabetes in UKPDS reduced morbidity and mortality from IHD.

Table 6(a) DIGAMI study after 3.4 years' follow-up (n = 620) [9].

	Intensive insulin (n = 306)		Control group (n = 314)				
	No.	%	No.	%	*p* value	Relative risk reduction	NNT (3.4 years)
Deaths	102	33	138	44	0.01	Total mortality: 11%	9

The effect was most pronounced among the pre-defined group that included 272 patients without previous insulin treatment and at low cardiovascular risk: 0.49 (confidence interval 0.30-0.80, *p* = 0.004).
NNT = numbers needed to treat.

Table 6(b) Independent predictors of total mortality in the DIGAMI study after 3.4 years' follow-up (n = 620) [9].

Independent factors	Non-independent factors
Old age	Previous myocardial infarction
Previous heart failure	Hypertension
Diabetes duration	Smoking
Admission blood glucose	Female sex
Admission HbA1c	

HbAlc = glycated haemoglobin.

Table 7 Effect of intensive glycaemic control in the UKPDS at 10-year follow-up (glucose) and 8.4-year follow-up (blood pressure) (n = 3,867) [10,11].

	Intensive glycaemic treatment (FBG <6 mmol/l)		Intensive BP treatment (BP <150/85 mmHg)	
	Level	CI	Level	CI
HbA1c (%)	7.0 (Control 7.9)	6.2–8.2 (Control 6.9–8.8)		
Blood pressure (mmHg)			144/82 (Control 154/87) p <0.001	
Diabetes-related end-points	0.88	0.78–0.99	0.76	0.62–0.92
All-cause mortality	0.94	0.80–1.10	0.82	0.63–1.08
Diabetes-related deaths	0.90	0.73–1.11	0.68	0.49–0.94
Microvascular end-points	0.75	0.60–0.93	0.63	0.44–0.89
Weight gain (kg)	2.9 (overall p <0.001) 4.0 (insulin) 1.7 (glibenclamide) 2.6 (chlorpropamide)			
Stroke	1.1	0.89–1.51	0.56	0.35–0.89
Myocardial infarction	0.84	0.71–1.0	0.79	0.56–1.07

Relative risk (95% CI) experimental group vs control group

BP = blood pressure; CI = confidence interval; FBG = fasting blood glucose; HbA1c = glycated haemoglobin.

□ CONTROL OF BLOOD PRESSURE

Increasing evidence suggests that tight blood pressure control reduces vascular complications in people with diabetes [11]. Whether tight control of blood pressure can specifically prevent both macrovascular and microvascular complications in people with type 2 diabetes was recently investigated. Long-term follow-up of the cohort of individuals with newly diagnosed type 2 diabetes recruited to the UKPDS showed a 24% relative risk reduction in diabetes-related end-points in the group assigned to tight control [11] (Table 7). The data from UKPDS provide evidence that tight blood pressure control in patients with hypertension and type 2 diabetes achieves a clinically important reduction in the risk of death related to diabetes, complications related to diabetes, progression of diabetic retinopathy, and deterioration in visual acuity.

Recent trials have linked calcium antagonists with adverse cardiovascular events in hypertensive patients with diabetes. A closer examination of these trials, in particular the ABCD trial and the FACET, reveals a lack of data from which to draw conclusions of harm. In fact, based on the results of these trials and the recent HOT trial [12], it may be concluded that the combination of a calcium antagonist with an ACE inhibitor is a rational therapeutic choice for patients with coexisting hypertension and diabetes. There were 1,501 people with diabetes in the HOT trial. Treatment, primarily with the calcium channel blocker felodipine, in which target diastolic blood pressure was 90 mmHg or lower, reduced risk of major vascular events over four years by 51%. In subjects achieving a target diastolic blood pressure of less than 80 mmHg, the incidence of stroke was reduced by 30% (Table 8).

Results from the HOPE RCT in patients at high risk of AVD, which used 10 mg of the ACE inhibitor ramipril, showed an impressive reduction in stroke, MI and all-cause mortality [13] (Table 9). The study was stopped prematurely because of the

Table 8 Effect of aspirin therapy in the HOT study (n = 18,790, mean age 61.5 years, diastolic blood pressure (BP) 100-115 mmHg) [12].

At baseline	Diastolic BP (mmHg)		
Target diastolic BP (mmHg) with felodipine ± other agents	<90 (n = 6,264)	<85 (n = 6,264)	<80 (n = 6,262)
	Randomisation to aspirin or placebo		
		Placebo (n = 9,391)	Aspirin (75 mg) (n = 9,399)
Reduction in all major CV events (%) p = 0.03		–	15
Reduction in MI (%) p = 0.002		–	36
No. of non-fatal major bleeds p <0.001		70	129

1,501 participants had diabetes. Reduction in all major cardiovascular (CV) events and in myocardial infarction (MI) is presented as a percentage reduction for aspirin treatment versus placebo.

Table 9 Effect of ramipril on death from cardiovascular (CV) disease, HOPE study (n = 9,297, aged 55 years) [13].

HOPE study design:
- 2 x 2 factorial evaluating ramipril and vitamin E
- randomisation to ramipril 10 mg or placebo
- inclusion criteria:
  - evidence of vascular disease or diabetes *plus*
    - 1 CV risk factor (hypertension, ↑cholesterol, low HDLc, cigarette smoking, microalbuminuria) *plus*
    - no known low ejection fraction or heart failure

Outcome	Event	Ramipril (n = 4,645)		Placebo (n = 4,652)		RR	
		No.	%	No.	%	RR	95% CI
Primary	MI, stroke or CV death	653	14.1	824	17.7	0.78	0.70–0.86
	MI	460	9.9	567	12.2	0.80	0.71–0.91
	Stroke	157	3.4	226	4.9	0.69	0.56–0.84
Secondary	All-cause mortality*	486	10.4	568	12.2	0.84	0.75–0.95

* eg revascularisation, hospitalisation for unstable angina or heart failure, diabetic complications.
CI = confidence interval; HDL = high-density lipoprotein c; MI = myocardial infarction; RR = relative risk.

beneficial effect of ramipril. Relative risk reductions were approximately 20% for a range of vascular end-points and, interestingly, 38% of the 9,297 recruited patients had diabetes. The mechanism responsible for the improvement in outcomes with treatment is uncertain. It seems unlikely that the benefit was due to blood pressure reduction, which was only 2 mmHg systolic and 3 mmHg diastolic in the treatment group versus no reduction in systolic blood pressure and 2 mmHg diastolic in the placebo group at the end of the study.

The effect of low-dose, diuretic-based antihypertensive treatment on major CVD event rates in older patients with type 2 diabetes and isolated systolic hypertension and in non-diabetic patients was compared in the SHEP trial. This study randomised 583 people with type 2 diabetes and 4,149 non-diabetic patients. The active treatment group received a low dose of chlorthalidone (12.5-25.0 mg/day) with a step-up to atenolol (25.0-50.0 mg/day) or reserpine (0.05-0.10 mg/day) if needed. The five-year major CVD rate was reduced by 34% for active treatment compared with placebo, both for diabetic patients (95% confidence interval (CI) 6-54%) and for non-diabetic patients (95% CI 21-45%). Absolute risk reduction with active treatment compared with placebo was twice as great for diabetic as for non-diabetic patients (101/1,000 vs 51/1,000 randomised participants at the five-year follow-up), reflecting the higher risk of CVD in diabetic patients.

Thus, it seems reasonable to suggest a target blood pressure of 130/85 mmHg for people with diabetes at increased absolute risk of a first or recurrent vascular event. Unfortunately, achieving this goal is unrealistic for many individuals. Treatment involves using several different classes of antihypertensive agents at high doses, with consequences for cost-effectiveness and patient compliance.

☐ INHIBITION OF PLATELET FUNCTION

At present, it is uncertain whether subjects with diabetes will specifically benefit from treatment with antiplatelet agents in the primary prevention of vascular disease. However, given that subjects with diabetes are at higher absolute risk of vascular events than people with normal glucose tolerance, it is reasonable to extrapolate from evidence obtained in other high risk subgroups randomised to aspirin versus placebo. In the HOT study, treatment with aspirin significantly reduced major cardiovascular events (Table 8), and the benefit was similar in people with diabetes compared to those not known to have diabetes.

☐ COST-EFFECTIVENESS

Numbers needed to treat to prevent one vascular event by lowering plasma glucose, reducing blood pressure or treating plasma lipids

Although the UKPDS study was primarily designed to determine the effect of tight glucose control, the effect of lowering blood pressure was the more effective intervention for reducing vascular complications. A recent analysis shows that the effect of tight versus less exact glucose control produced a 'numbers needed to treat' (NNT) of 200 to reduce a diabetes-related end-point. This compares with an NNT of 61 for the intensive control of blood pressure. Tight glucose control was more effective than less exact glucose control in reducing microvascular complications, but the NNT was 357 and the NNT for intensive blood pressure regulation was 138. Tight glucose control was no more effective than less exact glucose control in reducing incident strokes, whereas the NNT to prevent stroke for intensive blood pressure reduction was 196.

Limited NNT data are available for specific treatment with lipid lowering agents in subjects with diabetes. The costs of simvastatin treatment and of CVD-related hospitalisations in three subgroups of glucose tolerance have recently been analysed in the 4S [14] (Table 4). Relative risk reductions for vascular events with statin treatment are consistent in both men and women at different absolute risks of a vascular event. In 4S, the NNT was 13, and the absolute risk of a vascular event was approximately 5% in the placebo group. Since the absolute risk of a recurrent vascular event is about 8% for people who have established IHD and diabetes, the NNT may be lower than 13, and thus cost-effectiveness of statin treatment may be even better.

☐ CONCLUSIONS

AVD is the major cause of morbidity and mortality in people with diabetes. Effective treatment of diabetes must address the increased absolute risk of AVD by aggressive treatment of each individual risk factor with both lifestyle and pharmacological measures.

Acknowledgements

I acknowledge and thank the Medical Research Council and the British Diabetic Association for their support, my mentor Professor C N Hales for his encouragement and support over many years, members of my laboratory for their hard work and loyalty, and Christine Kyme for help in compiling this review.

□ TRIAL ACRONYMS

4S	Scandinavian Simvastatin Survival Study
ABCD	Appropriate Blood Pressure Control in Diabetes
BDACS	British Diabetic Association Cohort Study
BIP	Bezafibrate Infarction Prevention
CARE	Cholesterol and Recurrent Events
DCCT	Diabetes Control and Complications Trial
DIGAMI	Diabetes Mellitus Insulin Glucose Infusion in Acute Myocardial Infarction
FACET	Fosinopril versus Amlodipine Cardiovascular Events Trial
HHS	Helsinki Heart Study
HOPE	Heart Outcomes Prevention Evaluation
HOT	Hypertension Optimal Treatment
LDHS	Lyon Diet Heart Study
LDS	Lipid and Diabetes Study
LIPID	Long Term Intervention with Pravastatin in Ischaemic Disease
SHEP	Systolic Hypertension in the Elderly Program
UKPDS	UK Prospective Diabetes Study
VA-HIT	Veterans Administration High density lipoprotein Intervention Trial

REFERENCES

1   Laing SP, Swerdlow AJ, Slater SD, *et al.* The British Diabetic Association Cohort Study, I: all-cause mortality in patients with insulin-treated diabetes mellitus. *Diabetic Med* 1999; **16**: 459–65.

2   Reaven GM. Role of insulin resistance in human disease. *Diabetes* 1988; **37**: 1595–607.

3   Pan XR, Li GW, Hu YH, *et al.* Effects of diet and exercise in preventing NIDDM in people with impaired glucose tolerance. The Da Qing IGT and Diabetes Study. *Diabetes Care* 1997; **20**: 537–44.

4   Byrne CD. Triglyceride-rich lipoproteins: are links with atherosclerosis mediated by a procoagulant and proinflammatory phenotype? *Atherosclerosis* 1999; **145**: 1–15.

5   Joint British recommendations on prevention of coronary heart disease in clinical practice. *Heart* 1998; **80**: S1–26.

6   Haffner SM, Alexander CM, Cook TJ, *et al.* Reduced coronary events in simvastatin-treated patients with coronary heart disease and diabetes or impaired fasting glucose levels: subgroup analyses in the Scandinavian Simvastatin Survival Study. *Arch Intern Med* 1999; **159**: 2661–7.

7   Rubins HB, Robins SJ, Collins D, *et al.* Gemfibrozil for the secondary prevention of coronary heart disease in men with low levels of high-density lipoprotein cholesterol. Veterans Affairs High-Density Lipoprotein Cholesterol Intervention Trial Study Group. *N Engl J Med* 1999; **341**: 410–8.

8   The Diabetes Control and Complications Trial Research Group. The effect of intensive treatment of diabetes on the development and progression of long-term complications in insulin-dependent diabetes mellitus. *N Engl J Med* 1993; **329**: 977–86.

9   Malmberg K. Prospective randomised study of intensive insulin treatment on long term survival after acute myocardial infarction in patients with diabetes mellitus. DIGAMI (Diabetes Mellitus Insulin Glucose Infusion in Acute Myocardial Infarction) Study Group. *Br Med J* 1997; **314**: 1512–5.

10   UK Prospective Diabetes Study (UKPDS) Group. Intensive blood-glucose control with sulphonylureas or insulin compared with conventional treatment and risk of complications in patients with type 2 diabetes (UKPDS 33). *Lancet* 1998; **352**: 837–53.

11   UK Prospective Diabetes Study (UKPDS) Group. Tight blood pressure control and risk of macrovascular and microvascular complications in type 2 diabetes: UKPDS 38. *Br Med J* 1998; **317**: 703–13.

12   Hansson L, Zanchetti A, Carruthers SG, *et al*. Effects of intensive blood-pressure lowering and low-dose aspirin in patients with hypertension: principal results of the Hypertension Optimal Treatment (HOT) randomised trial. HOT Study Group. *Lancet* 1998; **351**: 1755–62.

13   The Heart Outcomes Prevention Evaluation (HOPE) Study Investigators. Effects of an angiotensin-converting-enzyme inhibitor, ramipril, on death from cardiovascular causes, MI, and stroke in high-risk patients. *N Engl J Med* 2000; **342**: 145–53.

14   Herman WH, Alexander CM, Cook JR, *et al*. Effect of simvastatin treatment on cardiovascular resource utilization in impaired fasting glucose and diabetes. Findings from the Scandinavian Simvastatin Survival Study. *Diabetes Care* 1999; **22**: 1771–8.

□ SELF ASSESSMENT QUESTIONS

1   What level of risk per annum should be considered appropriate for implementing pharmacological strategies to reduce risk of a first vascular event with lipid lowering therapy in people with diabetes?
 (a) 0%
 (b) 0.1%
 (c) 3%
 (d) 10%
 (e) 100%

2   What blood pressure target is desirable for individuals with diabetes at increased risk of a vascular event?
 (a) No target
 (b) <100/<60 mmHg
 (c) <120/<80 mmHg
 (d) <140/<80 mmHg
 (e) <160/<90 mmHg

3   What are the minimum lipid measurements required to assess risk of a vascular event in people with diabetes?
 (b) Total plasma cholesterol
 (c) Total plasma cholesterol and HDLc levels
 (d) Non-fasting plasma triglyceride concentrations
 (e) Total plasma cholesterol, HDLc levels and fasting plasma triglyceride concentrations
 (f) LDLc concentrations

4   What is the level of absolute risk per year for a first vascular event per annum in a 57 year old man with type 2 diabetes, HbA1c 7.5%, blood pressure 165/90 mmHg, in whom fasting lipids are total cholesterol 6.0 mmol/l, HDLc 0.8 mmol/l, LDLc 4.5 mmol/l, triglyceride 4.0 mmol/l?

(a) 0.1%
(b) 3%
(c) 10%
(d) 50%
(e) 100%

5   Will a 70 year old woman with type 2 diabetes, creatinine 200 mmol/l, blood
pressure 210/110 mmHg, fasting plasma triglyceride 4 mmol/l and LDLc
2.8 mmol/l benefit from treatment of her blood pressure and treatment with a
statin if she continues to smoke 30 cigarettes per day?
(a) No
(b) No, she should be treated with a fibrate
(c) Yes, but she should also be treated with a fibrate
(d) No, her blood pressure should be treated
(e) Yes

ANSWERS

1a False	2a False	3a False	4a False	5a False
b False	b False	b True	b True	b False
c True	c False	c False	c False	c False
d False	d True	d False	d False	d False
e False	e False	e False	e False	e True

Strategies for reducing cardiovascular risk in the NHS

Jane Flint and David A Wood

Coronary heart disease (CHD) is a national priority. The government White Paper, *Saving lives: our healthier nation* [1], has set the national target of reducing the death rate from heart disease by two-fifths by 2010. The blueprint to achieve this is the *National Service Framework for Coronary Heart Disease* (NSF) [2] which establishes clear standards for prevention:

☐ public health: reducing the overall population burden of disease

☐ identification and management of high risk individuals

☐ appropriate cardiological assessment and intervention for those who develop symptomatic disease and, finally,

☐ the provision of cardiac prevention and rehabilitation.

CHD is important to the overall public health strategy because it is common, frequently fatal and largely preventable. It is a leading cause of death, killing over 110,000 people in England in 1998, including more than 41,000 under the age of 75. Although death rates for CHD have been falling since the late 1970s, the UK's position is still high in international terms and rates have fallen less than in comparable countries such as the USA and Australia. There are inequalities in the disease burden across social class, ethnic groups and regions. Professional men have experienced much greater declines in death rates compared with unskilled men, with the result that the social class gradient for CHD mortality has become dramatically steeper. The 1998 Health Survey for England [3] emphasised the inverse relationship between CHD or its major risk factors and household income, albeit somewhat less marked for women. South Asians living in England have a much higher rate of premature mortality from CHD than the general population, and the fall in their death rates has been much slower.

The lifestyle risk factors for CHD are well described in the NSF, and the public health strategy aims to:

☐ reduce smoking

☐ promote healthy eating (and reduce overweight and obesity), and

☐ promote physical activity.

In the context of this public health strategy, general practitioners (GPs) and primary care teams are to identify and treat those individuals at greatest risk from CHD:

- [ ] *Step one*: identifying, advising and treating those with clinical evidence of CHD (eg past history of heart attack, angina or coronary revascularisation) or who have other clinical manifestations of occlusive arterial disease (eg peripheral vascular disease, transient cerebral ischaemic attack or ischaemic stroke). For patients admitted to hospital with coronary disease (angina, myocardial infarction (MI) or for coronary revascularisation), a multidisciplinary programme of secondary prevention and cardiac rehabilitation is to be offered. The aim is to reduce the risk of subsequent cardiac problems and to promote a return to a full and normal life.

- [ ] *Step two*: identifying, advising and treating people without clinical evidence of CHD or other occlusive arterial disease, but whose risk of a cardiac event is greater than 30% over 10 years.

The NSF has set standards, priorities, milestones and goals for coronary prevention in the population, both for high risk individuals and for those with overt disease.

☐ JOINT BRITISH SOCIETIES RECOMMENDATIONS ON CORONARY PREVENTION

Early during the evolution of this national strategy, the British Cardiac Society co-operated with the British Hyperlipidaemia Association, the British Hypertension Society and the British Diabetic Association in preparing national guidance on coronary prevention [4–6]. The principal recommendations were embraced by the NSF. In putting forward joint recommendations it was hoped that this professional collaboration would result in a more unified, and hence effective, approach to prevention of CHD in clinical practice. To achieve a common approach, the recommendations stated that:

- [ ] All cardiovascular risk factors must be addressed, rather than focusing on a single risk factor (eg blood pressure (BP)) and treating it in isolation.

- [ ] Hospital specialists and GPs need to co-ordinate their efforts and, with the support of other health professionals, create an integrated hospital and community based clinical strategy for prevention of CHD and other atherosclerotic diseases.

- [ ] Specialists and GPs should recognise their responsibilities for preventive medicine in routine clinical practice.

The objectives for physicians are different, but complementary, to those of public health medicine. Clinicians regularly see patients who have presented with either CHD or other atherosclerotic disease, or are found to be at high risk of developing atherosclerotic disease because of hypertension, dyslipidaemia, diabetes or a combination of these risk factors. In defining the objectives for CHD prevention in clinical practice, it is implicit that priority is given to those patients at highest risk of developing CHD rather than attempting to reach every adult in the population.

The order of priorities proposed for CHD prevention in clinical practice is given in Table 1. The aim of the joint British societies' recommendations is to encourage a unified approach to the management of patients in these categories. The specific objectives of prevention both of CHD and of other major atherosclerotic disease are:

1   *In patients with established CHD and/or other atherosclerotic disease*: to reduce the risk of a further major cardiac event – that is, unstable angina, MI or reinfarction, the need for coronary revascularisation procedures – and to reduce overall mortality.

2   *In high-risk individuals in the general population*: to reduce substantially the risk of such individuals developing coronary disease or other major atherosclerotic disease.

Table 1. Order of priorities for coronary heart disease (CHD) prevention in clinical practice (adapted from [5]).

1	(a)	Patients with established CHD
	(b)	Patients with other major atherosclerotic disease
2		Patients at high risk of developing CHD or other atherosclerotic disease because of:
	(a)	hypertension, dyslipidaemia, diabetes mellitus,* family history of premature CHD, or a combination of these risk factors

* patients with diabetes mellitus are at particularly high risk of CHD.

☐ CONCEPT OF RISK

Patients with angina or a history of MI or other major atherosclerotic disease are at high risk of death from CHD. They have the highest priority for coronary prevention because the quality of evidence that their lives can be extended and their morbidity decreased is among the best available for any aspect of medical practice. Such patients identify themselves to medical services, and it is not necessary to measure absolute coronary risk before deciding on intervention. Although patients with CHD are at high absolute risk of a further (or new) event compared with the healthy population, some individuals without any clinical manifestation of CHD, such as those with diabetes mellitus, may be at greater risk because of the coexistence of multiple predisposing factors [7].

The division of prevention into primary and secondary is therefore somewhat arbitrary in terms of the biology of atherosclerotic disease and its complications. In medicine, this distinction reflects the reality of clinical practice because patients with symptomatic disease present to medical services, and thus are already receiving care which should include secondary prevention and rehabilitation. High risk individuals in the general population have to be sought through screening, whether opportunistic or systematic, in order to deliver primary prevention. For those individuals without symptomatic disease, it is important to assess their absolute risk of developing CHD – that is, the probability of developing non-fatal MI or fatal

CHD over a defined time period, given a particular combination of risk factors – and to intervene appropriately depending on the degree to which they are at risk.

Taking account of all major cardiovascular risk factors avoids undue emphasis being placed on an individual risk factor at the expense of overall or absolute risk. Risk factors often exert a cumulative effect on absolute CHD risk. An individual with a number of mildly abnormal risk factors may have a level of absolute CHD risk greater than that of someone with only one high risk factor. An estimate of absolute risk of developing CHD or other atherosclerotic disease should always be made *before* the decision to introduce medication, for example, to decrease BP or serum cholesterol.

☐ PATIENTS WITH CORONARY HEART DISEASE OR OTHER MAJOR ATHEROSCLEROTIC DISEASE

For all patients with CHD (angina, MI) or other major atherosclerotic disease, every effort should be made to achieve the lifestyle, risk factor and therapeutic targets listed in Table 2. The care of coronary patients should embrace all aspects of cardiac prevention and rehabilitation [8]. Interventions that should be offered in rehabilitation are summarised in Table 3 (from the NSF). This process should begin as soon as possible after someone is admitted to hospital with CHD (Phase 1), continue through the early discharge period (Phase 2) and the formal prevention and rehabilitation programme (Phase 3), and extend into long-term maintenance of best possible health (Phase 4). The provision of skilled help, support and supervision tailored to individual patients can:

- ☐ help people understand their illness and its treatment

- ☐ improve success in making beneficial lifestyle changes (eg smoking cessation, physical activity)

- ☐ modify risk factors (eg hypertension, hyperlipidaemia and hyperglycaemia)

- ☐ improve compliance with prophylactic drug therapies and other interventions

- ☐ provide psychological and emotional support, and

- ☐ help people make the transition back to as full and normal a life as possible.

Multidisciplinary cardiac rehabilitation is therefore seen as an integral component both of the acute stages of care and of secondary prevention, and should be integrated closely with other services provided in primary and secondary care over the long term. The NSF calls for a systematic approach in identifying CHD patients who will benefit from this service, with an individualised risk assessment and documentation of advice, treatment, compliance and outcomes. Local implementation teams should ensure that there is commitment to this service in the local delivery plan, reflected in the health improvement plan and long-term service agreement.

Table 2. Lifestyle, risk factor and therapeutic targets for prevention of coronary heart disease (CHD) in patients with established CHD or other atherosclerotic disease and in healthy people at high risk of developing CHD (adapted from [5]).

Patients with CHD or other atherosclerotic disease	People without overt CHD or atherosclerotic disease at high risk (absolute CHD risk ≥15% over 10 years)
	Lifestyle targets for all patients
	Stop smoking, make healthier food choices, increase aerobic exercise, moderate alcohol consumption BMI <25 kg/m^2 is desirable, with no central obesity
	Targets for other risk factors
	Systolic BP <140 mmHg, diastolic BP <85 mmHg
• *All patients to have BP reduced to consistently <140/85 mmHg*	• *Systolic BP ≥160 mmHg or diastolic BP ≥100 mmHg:* lifestyle advice and drug treatment if BP is sustained at these levels on repeat measurements, regardless of absolute CHD risk
	• *Systolic BP 140–159 mmHg or diastolic BP 90–99 mmHg:*
	CHD risk ≥15% or target organ damage: lifestyle advice and drug treatment if BP is sustained at these levels on repeat measurements
	CHD risk <15% and no target organ damage: lifestyle advice, reassess annually
	• *Systolic BP <140 mmHg, diastolic BP <90 mmHg:* lifestyle advice, reassess in 5 years
	Total cholesterol <5.0 mmol/l (LDL cholesterol <3.0 mmol/l)
• *All patients to have total cholesterol reduced to consistently <5.0 mmol/l (LDL cholesterol <3.0 mmol/l)*	• *Familial hypercholesterolaemia or other inherited dyslipidaemia:* lifestyle advice and drug treatment
	• *Total cholesterol >5.0 mmol/l:*
	CHD risk ≥15%: lifestyle advice and drug treatment* if cholesterol sustained on repeat measurements
	CHD risk <15%: lifestyle advice, reassess annually if risk is close to 15% *continued over*

Table 2 *continued*

Patients with diabetes mellitus

Total cholesterol <5.0 mmol/l (LDL cholesterol <3.0 mmol/l)

Systolic BP <130 mmHg, diastolic BP <80 mmHg (systolic BP <125 mm, diastolic BP <75 mmHg when there is proteinuria)

Optimal glycaemic control: HbA₁c <7%

Cardioprotective drug treatment

- Aspirin (75 mg daily) in individuals aged >50 years whose hypertension, if present, is controlled

- Aspirin for all patients
- β-blockers at doses prescribed in clinical trials after MI, particularly in high risk coronary patients and for at least 3 years
- Cholesterol lowering agents (statins) at doses prescribed in clinical trials
- ACE inhibitors at doses prescribed in clinical trials for patients with symptoms or signs of heart failure at time of MI, or in those with persistent LV systolic dysfunction (ejection fraction <40%)
- Anticoagulants for patients at risk of systemic embolisation with large anterior infarctions, severe heart failure, LV aneurysm or paroxysmal tachyarrhythmias

Screening of first-degree blood relatives

- Screen close relatives if familial hypercholesterolaemia or other inherited dyslipidaemia is suspected

- Screening of first-degree blood relatives (principally siblings and offspring aged ≥18 years) of patients with premature CHD (men <55 years, women <65 years) or other atherosclerotic disease is encouraged, and essential in the context of familial dyslipidaemias

* If resources do not permit drug treatment at 15%, then 30% is the minimum acceptable standard of care.

ACE = angiotensin-converting enzyme; BMI = body mass index; BP = blood pressure; HbA₁c = glycated haemoglobin; LDL = low-density lipoprotein; LV = left ventricular; MI = myocardial infarction.

Table 3. The investigations and interventions that candidates for cardiac rehabilitation should be offered, unless contraindicated (adapted from [2]).

Phase 1: before discharge from hospital
to be offered as soon as is practical as an integral part of the acute care of someone admitted (or planned to be admitted) to

- assessment of physical, psychological and social needs for cardiac rehabilitation
- negotiation of a written individual plan for meeting these identified needs (copies should be given to the patient and the general practitioner)
- initial advice on lifestyle (eg smoking cessation, physical activity (including sexual activity), diet, alcohol consumption and employment)
- prescription of effective medication, and education about its use, benefits and harms
- involvement of relevant informal carer(s)
- provision of information about cardiac support groups
- provision of locally relevant written information about cardiac rehabilitation

Phase 2: early post-discharge period
- comprehensive assessment of cardiac risk, including physical, psychological and social needs for cardiac rehabilitation, and review of the initial plan for meeting these needs
- provision of lifestyle advice and psychological interventions according to the agreed plan, from relevant trained therapists who have access to support from a cardiologist
- maintain involvement of relevant informal carer(s)
- review involvement with cardiac support groups
- offer resuscitation training for family members

Phase 3: four weeks after an acute cardiac event, as Phase 2 plus
- structured exercise sessions to meet the assessed needs of individual patients
- maintain access to relevant advice and support from people trained to offer advice about exercise, relaxation, psychological interventions, health promotion and vocational advice

Phase 4: long-term maintenance of changed behaviour
- long-term follow-up in primary care
- offer involvement with local cardiac support groups
- referral to specialist cardiac, behavioural (eg exercise, smoking cessation) or psychological services as clinically indicated

☐ PEOPLE AT HIGH RISK WITHOUT CLINICALLY OVERT CORONARY HEART DISEASE OR OTHER MAJOR ATHEROSCLEROTIC DISEASE

For people without clinical atherosclerotic disease, the absolute risk of developing CHD (non-fatal MI or coronary death) or other atherosclerotic disease during the next 10 years strongly influences the intensity of lifestyle and therapeutic interventions. As absolute CHD risk increases, the intensity of intervention also increases, thus maximising potential benefit from risk factor reduction, while the threshold for drug treatment of BP and dyslipidaemia is lowered. A decision not to introduce a particular therapy for a given individual needs to be reviewed regularly. With advancing age and over time, the absolute risk associated with any one risk factor or combination of risk factors may become sufficiently great to justify intervention.

The joint British societies' coronary risk prediction charts (Fig. 1) are the preferred method [2,5] for estimating the 10-year risk of CHD (non-fatal MI or coronary death) in individuals with or without diabetes and, when formally evaluated, were found to be popular with the primary care team [9]. (See Appendix 1 for instructions on how to use these charts.) These charts enable the identification of those presently healthy individuals at highest CHD risk (red band: ≥30%), those at the next level of CHD risk (orange band: ≥15%) and, finally, those whose CHD risk is less than 15% (green band). A 'cardiac risk assessor' computer program was also developed for these recommendations. Using a personal computer, absolute 10-year CHD risk can be calculated for an individual, based on the Framingham function [7], and also cardiovascular risk (including stroke) over the same period.

Exceptions to treatment based on absolute risk, where drug treatment is required to reduce CHD and cardiovascular risk, are the presence of:

☐ hypertension (systolic BP ≥160 mmHg or diastolic BP ≥100 mmHg) or hypertension with associated target organ damage

☐ familial hypercholesterolaemia or other inherited dyslipidaemia, and

☐ diabetes mellitus with associated target organ damage.

An absolute risk of CHD ≥15% (equivalent to a cardiovascular risk of 20%) over 10 years is considered sufficiently high in the joint British recommendations to justify drug treatment for both BP (Fig. 2) and blood lipids (Fig. 3). In these high risk individuals, every effort should be made to achieve the lifestyle, risk factor and therapeutic targets given in Table 1.

Identification, investigation and management of everyone at this level of risk, particularly with some drug therapies, would be hugely demanding on NHS resources, so a staged approach to coronary and other atherosclerotic disease prevention is advised. After managing patients with established CHD or other atherosclerotic disease, those individuals with a 30% or higher CHD risk over 10 years should all be identified and treated appropriately and effectively *now*. This is the minimum target for the healthy population, and consistent with the recommendation of the NSF and with other advice, including that from the Standing Medical Advisory Committee on the use of statins [10] and the Scottish

Intercollegiate Guidelines Network (SIGN) guidelines on lipids and primary CHD prevention [11].

However, the scientific evidence clearly justifies risk factor intervention in healthy individuals with a CHD risk below 30%. As the next step, therefore, it is entirely appropriate for physicians progressively to expand opportunistic screening and risk factor intervention down to individuals with a 15% CHD risk over 10 years – provided that those with higher levels of risk have already received effective preventive care. Taking a progressive, staged approach to coronary prevention in this way ensures that those at highest risk are targeted first, and that the delivery of care is commensurate with the ability of medical services to identify, investigate and manage patients properly over the long term.

The NSF recommends that such high risk people should be sought initially among those with established diagnoses of diabetes and hypertension, not by unselected screening of the whole population. The NSF has also set standards, priorities, milestones and goals for preventing CHD in high risk individuals. Primary care groups are asked to set up not only CHD but 'at risk' registers and audit.

☐ DEVELOPMENT AND IMPLEMENTATION OF PREVENTION STRATEGIES IN CLINICAL PRACTICE

Although the evidence base for coronary prevention in those with established atherosclerotic disease and for those at high risk of developing this disease is amongst the best of any aspect of clinical medicine, the delivery of care often falls short of professional standards. The NSF has set minimum standards, priorities, milestones and goals over the next five years. Cardiac prevention and rehabilitation are currently not available for many patients who would benefit from such a service [12,13]. The extent and nature of provision vary dramatically around the country, and there are marked inequalities in the way patients access the services that are available. Patients with more severe CHD, the elderly, women and minority ethnic groups are underrepresented among users of rehabilitation services. In many parts of the country those who do attend may have to wait several weeks after being ready to benefit from cardiac prevention and rehabilitation, thereby delaying their return to normal life. Risk factor management is inadequate, as is the use of prophylactic drug therapies which have been shown to reduce morbidity and mortality [14]. There is thus considerable scope for improving cardiac prevention and rehabilitation services. A British Association for Cardiac Rehabilitation survey in 1998 [15] found that under half of UK rehabilitation programmes have any linked secondary prevention network, although these are developing rapidly.

The joint British societies' recommendation is that care of coronary patients and other patients with atherosclerotic disease should embrace all aspects of cardiac prevention and rehabilitation, and that such an integrated service should be available to all patients following MI, treated unstable angina, exertional angina, and revascularisation by angioplasty or coronary surgery. Integrating the care of patients

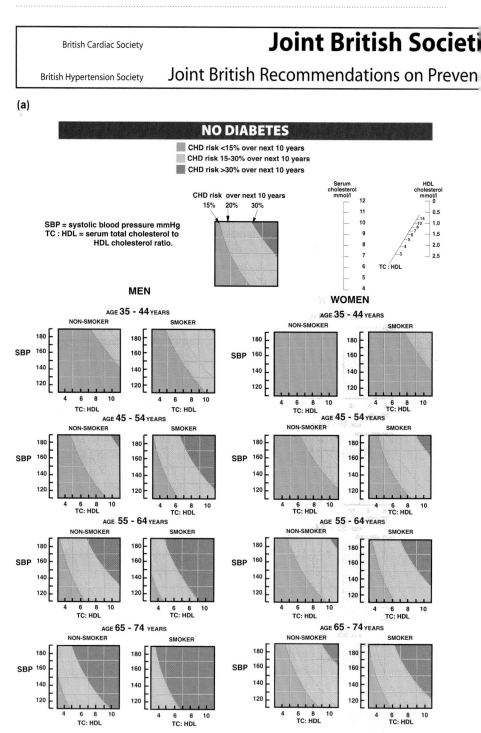

Fig. 1 Coronary risk prediction charts for men and women, aged 35–74 years (a) without and (b) with diabetes (BP = blood pressure; CHD = coronary heart disease).

onary Risk Prediction Chart
British Hyperlipidaemia Association

oronary Heart Disease in Clinical Practice
British Diabetic Association

(b)

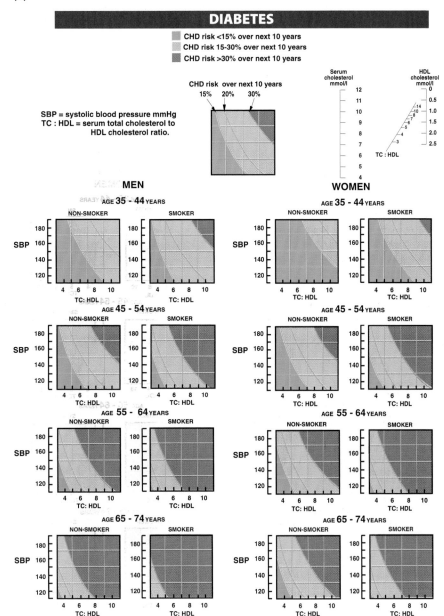

DIABETES

- CHD risk <15% over next 10 years
- CHD risk 15-30% over next 10 years
- CHD risk >30% over next 10 years

SBP = systolic blood pressure mmHg
TC : HDL = serum total cholesterol to HDL cholesterol ratio.

CHD risk over next 10 years
15%   20%   30%

Serum cholesterol mmol/l

HDL cholesterol mmol/l

TC : HDL

MEN
AGE 35 - 44 YEARS
NON-SMOKER   SMOKER

AGE 45 - 54 YEARS
NON-SMOKER   SMOKER

AGE 55 - 64 YEARS
NON-SMOKER   SMOKER

AGE 65 - 74 YEARS
NON-SMOKER   SMOKER

WOMEN
AGE 35 - 44 YEARS
NON-SMOKER   SMOKER

AGE 45 - 54 YEARS
NON-SMOKER   SMOKER

AGE 55 - 64 YEARS
NON-SMOKER   SMOKER

AGE 65 - 74 YEARS
NON-SMOKER   SMOKER

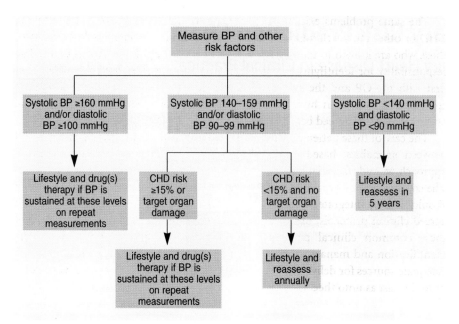

Fig. 2 Absolute coronary heart disease (CHD) risk and management of blood pressure (BP) in primary prevention of CHD and other atherosclerotic disease. CHD risk: non-fatal myocardial infarction and coronary death over 10 years (from [5]).

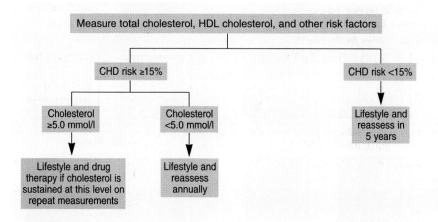

Fig. 3 Absolute coronary heart (CHD) risk and management of blood lipids in primary prevention of CHD. CHD risk: non-fatal myocardial infarction and coronary death over 10 years (from [5]) (HDL = high-density lipoprotein).

with atherosclerotic disease between hospital and general practice is essential, and can be achieved by using common protocols to ensure optimal long-term lifestyle, risk factor and therapeutic management. Auditing the impact of these common clinical protocols on the management of patients with CHD and other atherosclerotic disease between hospital and general practice is strongly recommended.

The same problems exist for those people who are at high risk of developing CHD or other atherosclerotic disease, in that many are not identified and many of those who are known to the medical services are not optimally managed [16]. The responsibility for identifying, investigating and treating these high risk people lies first with the GP and the primary health care team. Some of them will require specialist assessment in hypertension, lipid and diabetic clinics, and the referral criteria need to be agreed between primary and secondary care.

The care of these patients at high multifactorial risk should also be co-ordinated between specialists, based on agreed protocols, to ensure a common clinical approach to multifactorial risk assessment, lifestyle and therapeutic interventions. The continuing care of such high risk patients assessed in specialised hospital clinics should then be integrated with general practice to ensure, also through the use of agreed clinical protocols, optimal long-term management. Auditing the impact of these common clinical protocols for hospital and general practice for the identification and management of high risk individuals is strongly recommended. Adequate sources for delivery of NSF must be realised: 'There is no wealth but life ... unto this last as unto thee' (John Ruskin, *Ad Valorem*, 1860).

REFERENCES

1   Department of Health. *Saving lives: our healthier nation.* White Paper on public health. London: The Stationery Office, 1999.

2   National Service Framework for Coronary Heart Disease. *Modern standards and service models.* London: Department of Health, 2000.

3   *Health Survey for England, 1998.* London: Department of Health, 1998.

4   Wood DA, Durrington P, McInnes G, *et al.* Joint British recommendations on prevention of coronary heart disease in clinical practice. *Heart* 1998; **80**(Suppl): S1–29.

5   Joint British recommendations on prevention of coronary heart disease in clinical practice: summary. British Cardiac Society, British Hyperlipidaemia Association, British Hypertension Society, British Diabetic Association. *Br Med J* 2000; **320**: 705–8.

6   Ramsay LE, Williams B, Johnston GD, *et al.* British Hypertension Society guidelines for hypertension management 1999: summary. *Br Med J* 1999; **319**: 630–5.

7   Anderson KV, Odell PM, Wilson PWF, Kannel WB. Cardiovascular disease risk profiles. *Am Heart J* 1991; **121**: 293–8.

8   Thompson DR, Bowman GS, Kitson AL, *et al.* Cardiac rehabilitation in the United Kingdom: guidelines and audit standards. National Institute for Nursing, British Cardiac Society, Royal College of Physicians of London. *Heart* 1996; **75**: 89–93.

9   Isles CG, Ritchie LD, Murchie P, Norrie J. Risk assessment in primary prevention of coronary heart disease: randomised comparison of three scoring methods. *Br Med J* 2000; **320**: 690–1.

10 NHS Executive. *Standing Medical Advisory Committee statement on the use of statins.* EL (97) 41. London: Department of Health, 1997.

11 Scottish Intercollegiate Guidelines Network (SIGN). *Lipids and the primary prevention of coronary heart disease: a national clinical guideline.* SIGN publication No. 40. Edinburgh: Royal College of Physicians of Edinburgh, 1999.

12 Thompson DR, Bowman GS, Kitson AL, *et al.* Cardiac rehabilitation services in England and Wales: a national survey. *Int J Cardiol* 1997; **59**: 299–304.

13 Lewin RJ, Ingleton R, Newtrias AS, *et al.* Adherence to cardiac rehabilitation guidelines: a survey of cardiac rehabilitation guidelines in the United Kingdom. *Br Med J* 1999; **316**: 1254–5.

14   Action on Secondary Prevention by Intervention to Reduce Events (ASPIRE) Steering Group. A British Cardiac Society survey of the potential for the secondary prevention of coronary disease: principal results. *Heart* 1996; 75: 334–42.

15   Bethell H, Turner S, Flint EJ, Rose L. The BACR database of cardiac rehabilitation units in the UK. *Coronary Health Care* 2000; 4: 92–5.

16   Colhoun HM, Dong W, Poulter NR. Blood pressure screening, management and control in England: result from the health survey for England 1994. *J Hypertens* 1998; 16: 747–53.

☐ APPENDIX 1
(reproduced, with permission, from [5]).

Using the coronary risk prediction charts for primary prevention

These charts are for estimating the risk of coronary heart disease (non-fatal myocardial infarction and death from coronary heart disease) for individuals who have not developed symptoms of coronary heart disease or other major atherosclerotic disease. These charts are not appropriate for patients who have existing disease which already puts them at high risk. Such diseases are:

☐   Coronary heart disease or other major atherosclerotic disease

☐   Familial hypercholesterolaemia or other inherited dyslipidaemia

☐   Established hypertension (systolic BP >160 mmHg or diastolic BP >100 mmHg) or associated target organ damage

☐   Diabetes mellitus with associated target organ damage

☐   Renal dysfunction

Drug treatment is required for all these patients to reduce risk of coronary heart disease.

Estimating risk

To estimate an individual's absolute 10 year risk of developing coronary heart disease, find the table for their sex, diabetes (yes/no), smoking (smoker/non-smoker), and age. Within this square define the level of risk according to systolic blood pressure and the ratio of total cholesterol to high density lipoprotein (HDL) cholesterol. If there is no HDL cholesterol result, assume this is 1.0 mmol/l; then the lipid scale can be used for total cholesterol alone.

High risk individuals are defined as those whose 10 year risk of coronary heart disease exceeds 15% (equivalent to a cardiovascular risk of 20% over the same period). As a minimum, those at highest risk (≥30%; red) should be targeted and treated now; and as resources allow others with a risk of >15% (orange) should be progressively targeted.

Smoking status should reflect lifetime exposure to tobacco and not simply tobacco use at the same time as risk assessment.

The initial blood pressure and the first random (non-fasting) total cholesterol and HDL cholesterol measurement can be used to estimate an individual's risk. However, the decision on using drug treatment should be based on repeat measurements of risk factors over a period of time. The chart should not be used to estimate risk if treatment of hyperlipidaemia or blood pressure has already been started.

Risk of coronary heart disease is higher than indicated in the charts for:

☐   Patients with a family history of premature coronary heart disease (<55 years in men and <65 years in women), which increases the risk by a factor of approximately 1.5

☐   Those with raised triglyceride concentrations

☐   Those who are not diabetic but have impaired glucose tolerance

☐   Women with premature menopause

☐   Ages approaching the next age category: as risk increases exponentially with age, the risk will be closer to the higher decennium for the last four years of each decade.

In ethnic minorities the risk chart should be used with caution as it has not been validated in these populations.

The estimates of risk from the chart are based on groups of people, and in managing an individual patient the doctor has also to use clinical judgement in deciding how intensively to intervene on lifestyle and whether or not to use drug treatment.

A patient can be shown on the chart the direction in which the risk of coronary heart disease can be reduced by changing smoking status, blood pressure, or cholesterol.

☐ SELF ASSESSMENT QUESTIONS

1   The priorities for prevention of cardiovascular disease include:
   (a) Patients following myocardial infarction
   (b) Patients with exertional angina
   (c) Patients with peripheral arterial disease
   (d) Patients with hypertension and end-organ damage
   (e) Patients with familial dyslipidaemias

2   Absolute risk of developing coronary heart disease (CHD) is:
   (a) a rate
   (b) a probability of a cardiac event over a defined period of time
   (c) expressed as a ratio
   (d) a mathematical function of several risk factors and their relation to a disease end-point
   (e) used for patients with established CHD or other atherosclerotic disease

3   The use of drug therapies to manage blood pressure (BP) and blood cholesterol in primary prevention of CHD is justified in the following patients:
   (a) 58 year old patient with a sustained BP 154/96 mmHg, no target organ damage and an absolute risk of CHD of 12%
   (b) 64 year old patient with diabetes mellitus, no target organ damage, total cholesterol 5.9 mmol/l (high-density lipoprotein (HDL) cholesterol 0.9 mmol/l), triglycerides 1.8 mmol/l and an absolute risk of CHD of 19%
   (c) 43 year old patient with a sustained total cholesterol 6.8 mmol/l (HDL cholesterol 1.0 mmol/l), no family history of CHD and an absolute CHD risk of 14%
   (d) 39 year old patient with a sustained total cholesterol 5.8 mmol/l (HDL cholesterol 0.9 mmol/l), no family history of CHD and an absolute CHD risk of 20%
   (e) 52 year old patient with a sustained BP 146/92 mmHg, no target organ damage and an absolute CHD risk of 16%

4   The risk factor targets in the Joint British Recommendations on coronary prevention for CHD patients are:
   (a) BP <140/90 mmHg

(b) Total cholesterol <5.0 mmol/l
(c) Total cholesterol <5.2 mmol/l
(d) BP <140/85 mmHg
(e) BP <130/85 mmHg in patients with diabetes mellitus

5   The risk factor targets in the Joint British Recommendations on coronary prevention for high risk individuals (absolute CHD risk >15% over 10 years) are:
(a) BP <140/90 mmHg
(b) Total cholesterol <6.5 mmol/l
(c) BP <140/85 mmHg
(d) Total cholesterol <5.0 mmol/l
(e) Total cholesterol <5.0 mmol/l in diabetes mellitus

ANSWERS

1a True	2a True	3a False	4a False	5a False
b True	b True	b True	b True	b False
c True	c False	c False	c False	c True
d True	d True	d True	d True	d True
e True	e False	e True	e True	e True

The treatment of asthma in adults

Philip W Ind

☐ INTRODUCTION

Asthma prevalence continues to increase worldwide. In the UK asthma is now estimated to affect 3.4 million (6.8%) of the population with a prevalence of 10–12% in children aged 5–15 years [1].

☐ PROBLEMS OF ASTHMA MANAGEMENT

It is clearly essential to establish the diagnosis of asthma accurately and unequivocally since there are lifelong implications, including those for treatment. Asthma is a chronic, heterogeneous condition with a variable nature and no prospect of pharmacological cure. The absence of an integrated long-term measure of control (eg the equivalent of the HbA1c in diabetes) makes continued monitoring essential. Many patients require multiple inhalers and complex drug regimens which reduce compliance (adherence). Steroid phobia is widespread and unfortunately extends to low doses of inhaled steroids, and to some doctors as well as patients. Severe asthma affects perhaps 10% of patients. Asthma treatment consumes significant amounts of healthcare budgets of all industrialised countries. It is estimated that the total cost of asthma [1] to the UK is now in excess of £2 billion per year (Table 1).

Table 1 Estimated average annual costs of asthma (1995–1996).

	£ million
GP consultations	57
GP prescriptions	557
Total primary care costs	614
Cost of hospital admissions	52
Outpatient costs	5.5
Social security costs	161
Lost productivity nationally	1.2 billion
(18.3 million work days lost)	
*Total annual costs	2.03 billion

*Cost of asthma treatment per patient £192.
GP = general practitioner.

□ ASTHMA MORBIDITY AND MORTALITY

A number of morbidity surveys have documented the extent of the problem. The situation has not improved a great deal over 25 years, despite major advances in understanding of asthma pathogenesis and treatment. Asthma has a marked effect on quality of life [1], limiting daily activities in approximately 50% of adult patients. Symptoms are experienced daily by 42% of asthmatics, with 71% having symptoms at least once weekly. Up to 31% of patients suffer sleep disturbance at least once weekly. Perhaps 20% of all asthmatics have severe or very severe symptoms with frequent time off work, poor quality of life and repeated hospital visits. In 1995 there were 85,585 hospital admissions relating to asthma, each averaging 3.2 days. Each year, 2.5 million asthmatics consult their general practitioner an average of 2.4 times [1], and the number of prescriptions for asthma has approximately doubled over the last 10 years.

The death rate from asthma in England and Wales has fallen from a high of nearly 2,000 per year in the 1980s to 1,347 in 1998, but 33–42% of UK deaths occur in asthmatics under the age of 65 years [1]. This all emphasises that in many patients asthma remains a severe, potentially disabling condition.

□ ASTHMA MANAGEMENT

Asthma therapy

Discussion of asthma therapy is confined here to the consideration of newer aspects of the treatment of chronic asthma in adults, excluding the treatment of acute severe asthma, difficult asthma and asthma in childhood.

Aims of treatment

The aims of therapy and asthma control are summarised in Table 2. Arbitrary measures of success can be included but may not be attainable in a substantial minority of patients despite the many different classes of drugs and large number of different asthma preparations available (Table 3).

Table 2 Aims of asthma therapy.

- □ Minimal asthma symptoms (day and night)
- □ Normal level of activity
- □ Normal quality of life
- □ Normal/maximal lung function
- □ Normal/minimal peak flow variability
- □ Minimal use of 'rescue' β2-agonist
- □ Minimal/no exacerbations
- □ Normal life expectancy
- □ No/minimal side effects

Table 3 Asthma treatment: numbers of drugs and preparations available [2].

Therapeutic class	Agents	Preparations
Inhaled β2-agonists	4	16
Inhaled anticholinergics	2	9
Inhaled long-acting β2-agonists	2	9
Oral β2-agonists	4	12
Theophyllines	3	18
Leukotriene receptor antagonists	2	3
Inhaled corticosteroids	3	51
Inhaled cromones	2	8
Miscellaneous: antihistamines, nasal/ocular steroids, antitussives		

Classification of severity

A robust classification of asthma severity remains elusive. The best single indicator is the individual level of asthma treatment required for control.

Asthma guidelines

There are now multiple sets of approved management guidelines, both national and international. All are based on incomplete/poor evidence [3]. Most stress the importance of patient education and the role of the asthma nurse as a partner in healthcare, the use of a peak expiratory flow (PEF) meter and the benefits of self-management plans [4]. Guideline steps in asthma therapy are shown in Table 4.

Non-pharmacological management

Non-pharmacological aspects of management include removing offending allergens, and avoiding other precipitants (particularly if patients are aspirin intolerant or have occupational asthma). Smoking cessation, recognising concurrent anxiety/depression, counselling and appropriate management of coincidental conditions, including chronic obstructive pulmonary disease (COPD), remain important.

Complementary therapy

Alternative or complementary therapies, particularly breathing exercises, are popular with, and widely used by, asthma patients. To date, controlled clinical trials are few, but not promising [5].

Inhaler devices

Most asthma medication is given by the inhaled route. Many devices are available including conventional metered dose inhalers (MDIs), separate or integral spacers, a

Table 4 Steps in asthma therapy.

Step	Recommended	(Alternative)	Comment
Step 1	Inh β2-agonists	Individualise device	Use as required
Step 2	Inh β2-agonists + inh steroids (low dose)	(inh cromone) (?LTRA)	Threshold >1 puff β2-agonist daily Advice to start with high doses Not supported by clinical trials Step dose down after 2–3 months
Step 3	Inh β2-agonists + inh steroids (low dose) + long-acting β2-agonist	(High dose inh steroid) + theophylline +LTRA	Clinical trials support use of inh long-acting β2-agonist Step down as possible
Step 4	Inh β2-agonists + inh steroids (high dose) + trial of long-acting β2-agonist, +/theophylline, +/anticholinergic, +/LTRA		Sequential trial of different agents in combination unless side effects
Step 5	All of the above + oral prednisolone		Step down as possible
Step 6	All of the above + oral prednisolone + non-steroid immunosuppressive		3–6 month trial with close monitoring

inh = inhaled; LTRA = leukotriene receptor antagonist.

variety of breath-activated devices (autohalers, clickhaler) and dry powder inhalers (DPIs). The latter include rotacaps, turbohalers, diskhalers, accuhalers and the Easybreathe. Others are under development, including hand-held nebulisers. The need to replace chlorofluorocarbon propellants (CFCs) and the advent of new oral treatment (leukotriene modifiers) has focused attention on devices. CFC-free MDIs are available for salbutamol (two brands) and one each for beclomethasone and fluticasone. DPIs are available for all drug classes. It seems sensible, practical and pragmatic to match patient and inhaler device, bearing in mind cost, patient ability, ease of use and patient preference, aiming to enhance compliance. Cost alone should not be the determining factor, as the most expensive inhaler is one that is unused.

☐ BETA 2-AGONISTS

Inhaled conventional short-acting β2-agonists remain the bronchodilators of choice because of their efficacy, rapidity of action, convenience, safety (acutely, even in high doses) and low cost. The current emphasis is on 'as required' rather than 'regular' use with the aim of decreasing demand to a few puffs per week. Consumption is then a useful clinical measure of asthma control.

Inhaled long-acting beta 2-agonists

Salmeterol and formoterol are the two available inhaled long-acting β2-agonists (Table 5). This drug class has recently acquired new importance in asthma therapy. An increasing number of clinical trials have demonstrated better control, with improved lung function, particularly morning PEF, reduced diurnal variation of PEF, fewer symptoms, less usage of rescue salbutamol and reduced frequency of severe exacerbations. This last effect strongly supports a non-bronchodilator action of the drugs and emphasises their long-term safety. They are additive to inhaled steroids and superior to increasing steroid dose over a range of starting doses (200–1,000 µg/day) in different degrees of asthma severity (Table 6). Their addition at Step 3 of the guidelines (Table 4) is the most evidence-based step.

Table 5 Comparison of inhaled long-acting β2-agonists.

	Salmeterol	Formoterol
Onset of action	Slow	Rapid
Duration of action	Long (intrinsic)	Long (by inhalation)
Agonist activity	Partial	Full
Receptor affinity	High	High
Receptor selectivity	High	High
Lipid solubility	Very high	High
Available device	Metered dose Diskhaler Accuhaler	Dry powder Turbohaler
Dose range	25–50 µg bd	6–24 µg bd
Children	>4 years	Not recommended

Table 6 Addition of a long-acting β2 agonist compared with increasing the dose of inhaled steroids.

Reference	No. of patients	Drugs	Reference	No. of patients	Drugs
		LAβ2/ICS (initial dose)	12	274	Salm/FP200/500
6	429	Salm/BDP400	13	437	Salm/FP200
7	738	Salm/BDP1000	14	514	Salm/BDP400
8	852	Form/Bud200/800	15	680	Salm/FP176
9	514	Salm/BDP400	16	483	Salm/BDP336
10	496	Salm/FP500	17	132	Form/BDP500
11	177*	Salm/BDP400			

BDP = beclomethasone dipropionate; Bud = budesonide; Form = formoterol; FP = fluticasone propionate; ICS = inhaled corticosteroid (initial dose = baseline dose during run-in period); LAβ2 = inhaled long-acting β2-agonist; Salm = salmeterol.

The oral prodrug bambuterol is effective in nocturnal asthma and compares well with inhaled salmeterol [18].

□ INHALED CORTICOSTEROIDS

Inhaled steroids have long been recognised as the cornerstone of the modern treatment of asthma [19]. The current hypothesis is that their effects on symptoms, airway function (calibre and bronchial hyperresponsiveness), short-acting bronchodilator use and asthma control (including exacerbations) reflect their anti-inflammatory activity. In fact, the relationship between airway inflammation and anti-asthma effects is complex and incompletely understood. The hope is that good control and suppression of bronchial inflammation can prevent the development of airway remodelling and irreversible airflow obstruction.

Three compounds are currently available for treating asthma by the inhaled route in the UK; beclomethasone, budesonide and fluticasone, with a fourth, mometasone, shortly to be launched. In the USA, older steroids including triamcinolone and flunisolide are quite widely used. There is a large literature on dose comparisons, but it is difficult to draw firm quantitative conclusions.

Dose response

There is considerable confusion regarding dose-response to inhaled steroids. A dose response undoubtedly exists across the population. The difficulty in demonstrating this in many clinical studies relates to the study design, patient selection, end-point(s), duration of treatment, previous steroid therapy, the numbers required and the problems of measurement of steroid effects. Hence it is relatively easy to demonstrate dose-response effects (Fig. 1) on bronchial responsiveness, but more difficult in patients with mild asthma.

Starting inhaled steroids

There are few controlled data on the threshold of lung function or asthma symptoms for initiating steroid therapy. Available studies show that patients over a range of severities taking inhaled steroids for up to three years do better than patients taking inhaled β2-agonists alone. Several studies now also suggest that delay in instituting steroid therapy may adversely affect the subsequent maximal response. This is potentially of major importance. Large ongoing prospective studies may shed further light on this. In clinical practice, the usual threshold adopted is the requirement for more than one daily dose of an inhaled β2-agonist. This is a simple practical guide for most patients, in contrast to lower thresholds that have been proposed [3].

Initial dose, duration of treatment and stepping down

The current British Thoracic Society guidelines advocate starting inhaled steroids at high doses and tailing down rather than starting low and stepping up. This is based on no more than clinical practice and common sense aiming to achieve rapid control

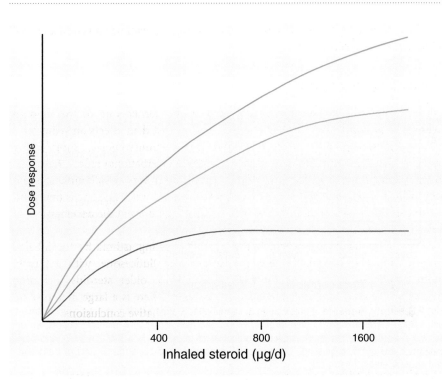

Fig. 1 Schematic illustration of inhaled steroid dose-response curves. The different lines indicate different patients and/or different steroid effects eg response is steeper and over a greater range in severe asthma or when bronchial responsiveness is measured as opposed to lung function (green = severe asthma inflammation and exacerbations; blue = bronchial responsiveness; red = symptoms, lung function and exhaled nitric oxide).

to enhance compliance before stepping down the dose. In fact, two recent studies which have addressed this issue have reported negative results. In the first study [20] in 84 very mild, steroid naïve, general practice patients (mean baseline FEV_1 84% predicted), budesonide 200 µg/day was no different from 800 µg/day. In the second study [21], with 24 more severe patients (mean baseline FEV_1 67% predicted), fluticasone 1,000 µg/day produced greater improvement in symptoms, β2-agonist use and induced sputum eosinophil suppression, but not in peak flow, FEV_1 or bronchial responsiveness compared to 100 µg/day. Low and high doses did not differ in rapidity of onset in these trials (Fig. 2).

There is remarkably little information to guide protocols for adjusting doses of inhaled steroids. In general, alterations are made on the basis of symptoms, β2-agonist use and lung function. Recently, the adoption of a strategy of using bronchial responsiveness determinations to guide treatment has resulted in higher doses of inhaled steroids yielding greater benefit in terms of improved FEV_1, reduced (mild) exacerbations, mast cell numbers and basement membrane thickness of the reticular layer on bronchial biopsy [22]. In clinical practice, patients are usually advised to step steroid doses down at 2–3 month intervals, though clinical trials usually adopt more rapid protocols. Once-daily regimens for budesonide and

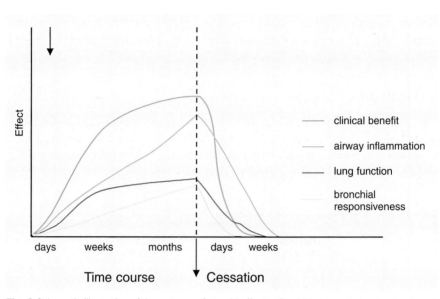

Fig. 2 Schematic illustration of time course of steroid effects after initiating and stopping treatment with inhaled steroids (x-axis = time in days, weeks and months; y-axis = different effects, eg on asthma exacerbations, asthma symptoms, bronchial inflammation, lung function (FEV_1 and peak expiratory flow not distinguished), and bronchial responsiveness; 1st arrow = start of treatment; 2nd arrow = end of treatment).

fluticasone are effective in mild patients and can be used to step down. When inhaled steroids are stopped the effects wear off rapidly (Fig. 2).

Safety of high doses of inhaled steroids

The dangers of high doses of oral steroids are well known. Justifiable concern persists about the safety of high-dose inhaled steroids taken over long periods. Fears regarding weight gain, chest infections, hypertension, diabetes, etc appear groundless. Concerns regarding osteoporosis, skin thinning, posterior subcapsular cataracts and glaucoma are shared by doctors as well as patients. The exact risks are not known and a long-term, prospective controlled study is probably impossible. However, there is no doubt that inhaled steroids are much safer than oral steroids, even in repeated short courses. Local side effects, which include hoarseness, sore throat, induced cough and oropharyngeal thrush, are well known but are usually a minor inconvenience to be circumvented by a change of inhaler device and gargling.

☐ THEOPHYLLINES

In addition to their traditional actions as bronchodilators, it is now clear that theophyllines have other clinical benefits which may relate to their anti-inflammatory or immunomodulatory effects. It is as yet unclear whether recently developed phosphodiesterase inhibitors will be more effective in asthma treatment.

Modern strategies include adding low-dose theophyllines to low-dose inhaled steroids [23]. There are no controlled trials as yet of adding theophylline to inhaled steroids as well as long-acting β2-agonists.

☐ LEUKOTRIENE MODIFIERS

Anti-leukotriene drugs include leukotriene receptor antagonists (LTRAs) which block Cys-LT1 receptors, and biosynthesis inhibitors (eg zileuton) which are not yet licensed in Europe. Zafirlukast and montelukast are potent, highly selective antagonists available worldwide (Table 7); pranlukast is licensed only in Japan [24].

Table 7 Comparison of leukotriene modifier drugs.

	Montelukast (*Singulair*)	Zafirlukast (*Accolate*)
Dose	Oral 10 mg od	Oral 20 mg bd
Patients	Adults	Adults
Children	>6 years (5 mg)	>12 years
Indication	Add in mild-moderate asthma Exercise-induced asthma	Asthma treatment
Interactions	CYP3A (inducers)	CYP2C9 (warfarin)
Daily cost	£0.92	£0.92

bd = twice daily; od = once daily.

Leukotriene receptor antagonists

Clinically important actions of LTRAs are compared with inhaled steroids in Table 8. The place of LTRAs in asthma guidelines is unclear. Oral medication removes difficulties with inhaler technique and may be preferred by some patients. Rapid onset of action and once-daily treatment may also improve compliance. In the USA, zafirlukast and montelukast are both approved as first-line monotherapy for persistent asthma. In general, LTRAs achieve similar efficacy to low-dose inhaled steroids (<400 µg/day beclomethasone dipropionate equivalent). However, it is not yet clear whether LTRAs can substantially alter the natural history of asthma. Two studies have examined the role of LTRAs at Step 3. In a 16-week study of 642 mild to moderate asthmatics the combination of montelukast 10 mg od and beclomethasone 200 µg bd was more effective than beclomethasone alone, which was more effective than montelukast monotherapy, which was superior to placebo [25]. There is early evidence to suggest that LTRAs offer additional benefit to high-dose inhaled steroids at Step 4.

Side effects of LTRAs

LTRAs are well tolerated and safe, but there is no information about long-term use. Higher than licensed doses of zafirlukast may have adverse effects on the liver. The

Table 8 Comparison of important clinical effects of inhaled steroids and leukotriene receptor antagonists (LTRAs).

	Inhaled steroids	LTRAs
Onset of action	Days to weeks	Days
Daily dosing	bd (od)	od/bd
Symptoms	Reduce	Reduce
Nocturnal symptoms	Reduce	Reduce
Lung function	Gradual increase	Modest bronchodilatation
Reliever use	Reduce	Reduce
Asthma exacerbations	Reduce	Reduce
Laboratory bronchial challenge:		
Acute protection exercise (+cold air)	−	+
aspirin	+	+
antigen early phase	+	+
late phase	+	+
Bronchial responsiveness	Reduce	Reduce
Oral steroid sparing	+	+
Airways inflammation	Reduce	Reduce
Quality of life	Improve	Improve
Emergency health contacts	Reduce	?
Hospital admissions	Reduce	?

bd = twice daily; od = once daily; + = protection; − = no protection; ? = not tested.

development of a Churg-Strauss-like syndrome seems more likely to be related to unmasking the occult condition, as it has usually been associated with oral corticosteroid withdrawal or pre-existing features. Drug interactions are a potential problem with LTRAs. Zafirlukast inhibits the CYP2C9 isoenzyme of hepatic cytochrome P450 and may interfere with drugs such as warfarin, phenytoin, carbamazepine, terfenadine, cyclosporin and cisapride. The plasma concentration of montelukast is reduced by CYP3A inducers (eg phenytoin, rifampicin etc).

☐ COMBINED THERAPY

The trend is to combine therapy with lower doses of inhaled steroids together with other drugs including long-acting β2-agonists or theophyllines or LTRAs. This reflects treatment Step 3 onwards (Table 4).

Combination inhaler therapy applied to a long-acting β2-agonist and an inhaled steroid (Seretide; salmeterol/fluticasone) is an attractive concept: two complementary therapies both taken on a twice daily basis. A single inhaler is simpler, more convenient, cheaper, prevents differential non-compliance and may improve compliance with the steroid component. Symbicort (a turbohaler combination of formoterol and budesonide) should be available in the future.

☐ CHRONIC SEVERE ASTHMA

Treatment of chronic severe asthma in oral steroid-dependent patients (Table 4) should probably be undertaken in a specialist hospital clinic. Various immunosuppressive steroid-sparing strategies (Table 9) may be employed.

Table 9 Non-steroid immunosuppressive agents for chronic asthma.

- ☐ Methotrexate
- ☐ Oral gold
- ☐ Cyclosporin
- ☐ Azathioprine
- ☐ Cyclophosphamide
- ☐ Immunoglobulin
- ☐ Plasma exchange

☐ FUTURE THERAPEUTIC DEVELOPMENTS

New drugs

A range of new agents aimed at a variety of therapeutic targets are under development including phosphodiesterase inhibitors, nitrosodilators, new steroids, various enzyme inhibitors, agents directed at particular cytokines, chemokines, and their receptors, adhesion molecules, immunoglobulin E etc. However, in addition to advances in different classes of new drugs, developments can be expected in how we presently assess and utilise current treatment.

Responders versus non-responders

More attention should be paid to 'responders' and 'non-responders' to particular drugs; for example, approximately 40% patients respond to LTRAs. We need to know what the important determinants are and whether patients can change from one category to another with time. Advances in pharmacogenetics, β2-receptor and leukotriene synthase polymorphisms are likely to be important.

Trials of effectiveness of medication

Conventional controlled clinical trials are widely accepted as the gold standard for evaluation of therapy. Whilst these are unparalleled for studying efficacy, they suffer from some limitations. They produce few data about rarer side effects, and little information regarding the place of the drug in comparison with other established treatments, rates of response, costs and relative costs. They tell us little about clinical effectiveness because individual patients often differ radically from patients included in clinical trials. 'Real world' studies in 'real world' patients are required.

REFERENCES

1 *National asthma audit 1999/2000.* London: National Asthma Campaign.

2 *Monthly Index of Medical Specialities.* London: Haymarket Publishing Services Ltd, July 2000.

3 British Thoracic Society. The British guidelines on asthma management: 1995 review and position statement. *Thorax* 1997; **52**: S1–21.

4 Gibson PG, Coughlan J, Wilson AJ, *et al.* Self-management education and regular practitioner review for adults with asthma. In: *Cochrane Collaboration. Cochrane Library.* Issue 2. Oxford: Update Software, 2000.

5 Balon J, Aker PD, Crouther ER, *et al.* A comparison of active and simulated chiropractic manipulation as adjunctive treatment for childhood asthma. *New Engl J Med* 1998; **339**: 1013–20.

6 Greening AP, Ind PW, Northfield M, Shaw G. Added salmeterol versus higher-dose corticosteroids in asthma patients. *Lancet* 1994; **344**: 219–24.

7 Woolcock A, Lundback B, Ringdal N, Jacques LA. Comparison of addition of salmeterol to inhaled steroids with doubling of the dose of the inhaled steroids. *Am J Respir Crit Care Med* 1996; **153**: 1481–8.

8 Pauwels RA, Lofdahl C-G, Postma DS, *et al.* Effect of inhaled formoterol and budesonide on exacerbations of asthma. *N Engl J Med* 1997; **337**: 1405–11.

9 Weinstein SF, Murray JJ, Kerwin E, *et al.* The effect of adding Serevent to Beclovent versus doubling the dose of Beclovent on pulmonary function in symptomatic asthmatic patients ≥18 years of age. *Am J Resp Crit Care Med* 1997; **155**: A347.

10 Ind PW, Dal Negro R, Colman N, *et al.* Inhaled fluticasone propionate and salmeterol in moderate adult asthma I. Lung function and symptoms. *Am J Resp Crit Care Med* 1998; **157**: A416.

11 Verberne AAPH, Frost C, Duiverman EJ, *et al.* Addition of salmeterol versus doubling the dose of beclomethasone in children with asthma. Dutch Paediatric Asthma Study Group. *Am J Resp Crit Care* 1998; **158**: 213–9.

12 Van Noord JA, Schreurs AJM, Mol SJM, Mulder PGH. Addition of salmeterol versus doubling the dose of fluticasone propionate in patients with mid to moderate asthma. *Thorax* 1999; **54**: 207–12.

13 Condemi JJ, Goldstein S, Kalberg C, *et al.* The addition of salmeterol to fluticasone propionate versus increasing the dose of fluticasone propionate in patients with persistent asthma. Salmeterol Study Groups. *Ann Allergy Asthma Immunol* 1999; **82**: 383–9.

14 Murray JJ, Church NL, Anderson WH, *et al.* Concurrent use of salmeterol with inhaled corticosteroids is more effective than inhaled corticosteroid dose increases. *Allergy Asthma Proc* 1999; **20**: 173–80.

15 Baraniuk J, Murray JJ, Nathan RA, *et al.* Fluticasone alone or in combination with salmeterol vs triamcinolone in asthma. *Chest* 1999; **116**: 625–32.

16 Kelsen SG, Church NL, Gilman SA, *et al.* Salmeterol added to inhaled corticosteroid therapy is superior to doubling the dose of inhaled corticosteroids: a randomised clinical trial. *J Asthma* 1999; **36**: 703–15.

17 Bouros D, Bachlitzanakis N, Kottakis J, *et al.* Formoterol and beclomethasone versus higher dose beclomethasone as maintenance therapy in adult asthma. *Eur Respir J* 1999; **14**: 627–32.

18 Crompton GK, Ayres JG, Basran G, *et al.* Comparison of oral bambuterol and inhaled salmeterol in patients with symptomatic asthma and using inhaled corticosteroids. *Am J Respir Crit Care Med* 1999; **159**: 824–8.

19 Barnes PJ, Pedersen S, Busse WW. Efficacy and safety of inhaled corticosteroids. *Am J Respir Crit Care Med* 1998; **157**: S1–53.

20 Van der Molen, Kerstjens HAM. Starting inhaled corticosteroids in asthma: when, how high, and how long. *Eur Respir J* 2000; **15**: 3–4.

21 Gershman NH, Wong HH, Liu JT, Fahy JV. Low- and high-dose fluticasone propionate in asthma; effects during and after treatment. *Eur Respir J* 2000; **15**: 11–18.

22 Sont JK, Willems LNA, Bel EH, *et al.* Clinical control and histopathologic outcome of asthma when using airway hyperresponsiveness as an additional guide to long term treatment. *Am J Respir Crit Care Med* 1999; **159**: 1043–51.

23 Evans DJ, Taylor DA, Zetterstrom O, *et al.* A comparison of low-dose inhaled budesonide plus theophylline and high-dose inhaled budesonide for moderate asthma. *N Engl J Med* 1997; **337**: 1412–8.

24 Lipworth BJ. Leukotriene-receptor antagonists. *Lancet* 1999; **353**: 57–62.

25 Laviolette M, Malmstrom K, Lu S, *et al.* Montelukast added to inhaled beclomethasone in treatment of asthma. *Am J Respir Crit Care Med* 1999; **160**: 1862–8.

☐ SELF ASSESSMENT QUESTIONS

1 Asthma:
(a) Has increasing prevalence, severity and mortality in the UK
(b) Prescribing has doubled in 10 years
(c) Is associated with increased FEV_1 decline over time
(d) Management is improved by measuring bronchial responsiveness
(e) Control is usually not easy in routine clinical practice

2 Inhaled corticosteroids:
(a) Can normalise bronchial hyperresponsiveness in mild asthma
(b) Reduce hospital admissions due to asthma
(c) Are associated with pulmonary infection
(d) Can cause adverse systemic effects even at <1,000 μg/day beclomethasone (or equivalent)
(e) With inhaled β2-agonists produce maximal achievable benefit in asthma, providing a sufficient dose is given for an adequate time

3 Long-acting inhaled β2-agonists:
(a) Are potent physiological antagonists
(b) Are steroid sparing
(c) Reduce bronchial hyperresponsiveness
(d) Exhibit tachyphylaxis in laboratory challenge studies
(e) Increase mild and severe exacerbations of asthma

4 Current leukotriene receptor antagonists (LTRAs):
(a) Inhibit LT cys 1 and cys 2 receptors
(b) Inhibit exercise-induced asthma
(c) Are potent bronchodilators
(d) Provide additional benefit to high-dose inhaled steroids
(e) Provide additional benefit to low-dose inhaled steroids

5 LTRAs:
(a) May be particularly useful in aspirin-induced asthma
(b) Are not associated with vasculitis
(c) Usually reduce counts of circulating eosinophils

(d) May interact with other drugs
(e) Are steroid sparing

ANSWERS

1a False	2a True	3a True	4a False	5a True
b True	b True	b True	b True	b False
c False	c False	c True	c False	c True
d True	d True	d True	d True	d True
e True	e False	e False	e True	e True

The clinical management of pulmonary hypertension

J Simon R Gibbs

☐ INTRODUCTION

Advances in the treatment of primary pulmonary hypertension have transformed the lives of patients in the last decade, although the disease is still perceived as untreatable by many doctors. Treatment is now being extended to other forms of pulmonary hypertension. The implication is that early recognition and diagnosis of pulmonary hypertension will enable patients to receive new specialised therapies which may improve symptoms and prolong life.

Pulmonary hypertension is defined as a mean pulmonary artery pressure greater than 25 mmHg at rest or 30 mmHg on exercise. The definition does not require elevated pulmonary vascular resistance, which is the underlying mechanism of most aetiologies apart from high output heart failure.

A new classification of pulmonary hypertension has been proposed by the World Health Organization (WHO) [1], to replace the previous pathologically based classification which lacked practical clinical relevance. The new WHO Evian system is founded on common pathophysiological mechanisms and clinical features (Table 1), and emphasises the similarities between primary pulmonary hypertension and pulmonary hypertension caused by some other known conditions. The commonest forms of pulmonary hypertension are caused by acquired chronic heart and lung diseases. These are not considered in this article since their treatment currently focuses on management of the underlying disease. The major advances in treatment of pulmonary vascular disease itself affect pulmonary arterial and thromboembolic pulmonary hypertension.

Primary pulmonary hypertension is rare, with an annual incidence of approximately 1–2 cases per million population. Secondary causes account for a similar number. A small number of cases of primary pulmonary hypertension are familial and the gene has been identified as a mutation of the *BMPR2* gene which encodes the type III morphogenetic protein receptor (BMPRII), and is located on chromosome 2q31–32. The pathophysiology involves pulmonary vasoconstriction, thrombosis and vascular remodelling. These are the main targets for treatments.

☐ CLINICAL FEATURES

It is disappointing that the average delay from onset of symptoms to diagnosis (three years) has not improved over the last 10 years. The symptoms of

Table 1 Classification of pulmonary hypertension according to the World Health Organization Evian system 1998 (for more details see [1]).

Pulmonary arterial hypertension:
- Primary pulmonary hypertension
- Sporadic
- Familial

Related to:
- Collagen vascular disease
- Congenital systemic to pulmonary shunts
- Portal hypertension
- HIV infection
- Drugs/Toxins
  - Anorexigens (aminorex, fenfluramine, dexfenfluramine)
  - Other
    - Definite: toxic rapeseed oil
    - Very likely: amphetamines, L-tryptophan
    - Possible: meta-amphetamines, cocaine, chemotherapeutic agents
- Persistent pulmonary hypertension of the newborn
- Other

Pulmonary venous hypertension:
- Left-sided atrial or ventricular heart disease
- Left-sided valvular heart disease
- Pulmonary veno-occlusive disease
- Pulmonary capillary haemangiomatosis
- Other

Pulmonary hypertension associated with disorders of the respiratory system and/or hypoxaemia:
- Chronic obstructive lung disease
- Interstitial lung disease
- Sleep disordered breathing
- Alveolar hypoventilation disorders
- Chronic exposure to high altitude
- Neonatal lung disease
- Alveolar capillary dysplasia
- Other

Pulmonary hypertension due to chronic thrombotic and/or embolic disease:
- Thromboembolic obstruction of proximal pulmonary arteries
- Obstruction of distal pulmonary arteries
  - Pulmonary embolism
    - Thrombus, tumour, ova/parasites, foreign material
  - *In situ* thrombosis
  - Sickle cell disease

Pulmonary hypertension associated with miscellaneous diseases:
- Inflammatory
  - Schistosomiasis
  - Sarcoidosis
  - Other
- Extrinsic compression of the central pulmonary veins
  - Fibrosing mediastinitis
  - Adenopathy/tumours

breathlessness, chest pain and syncope are non-specific and physical signs may be subtle, but an ECG and chest radiograph are likely to demonstrate an abnormality in most cases. Symptomatic limitation is measured using a modified New York Heart Association (NYHA) scale [1] (Table 2).

The symptoms correlate with the severity of the reduction in cardiac output. Cardiac output falls with compression of the left ventricle by the pressure overloaded right ventricle (Figs. 1 and 2). In addition, there is asynchrony between the ventricles: right ventricular systole is prolonged into early diastole in the left ventricle, which reduces forward flow through the mitral valve and impairs filling of the left ventricle.

Table 2 Functional classification of pulmonary hypertension modified after the New York Heart Association Functional Classification according to the World Health Organization Evian system 1998 (for more details see [1]).

A	**Class I**	Patients with pulmonary hypertension but without resulting limitation of physical activity. Ordinary physical activity does not cause undue dyspnoea or fatigue, chest pain or near syncope.
B	**Class II**	Patients with pulmonary hypertension resulting in slight limitation of physical activity. They are comfortable at rest. Ordinary physical activity causes undue dyspnoea or fatigue, chest pain or near syncope.
C	**Class III**	Patients with pulmonary hypertension resulting in marked limitation of physical activity. They are comfortable at rest. Less than ordinary activity causes undue dyspnoea or fatigue, chest pain or near syncope.
D	**Class IV**	Patients with pulmonary hypertension with inability to carry out any physical activity without symptoms. These patients manifest signs of right heart failure. Dyspnoea and/or fatigue may even be present at rest. Discomfort is increased by any physical activity.

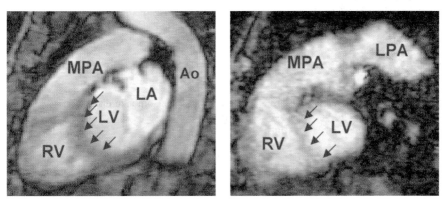

Normal   Hypertension

Fig. 1 Magnetic resonance (sagittal view) of the heart and main pulmonary artery (MPA) in a normal subject and a pulmonary hypertensive patient shown at the same stage in the cardiac cycle. Note the enlargement of the right ventricle (RV) and pulmonary arteries in the patient. The interventricular septum (highlighted by arrows) is flattened by the high pressure in the RV, and does not deviate towards the RV as in the normal subject (Ao = aorta; LA = left atrium; LPA = left pulmonary artery; LV = left ventricle). (Courtesy Dr Philip Kilner, Cardiac Magnetic Resonance Unit, Royal Brompton Hospital, London.)

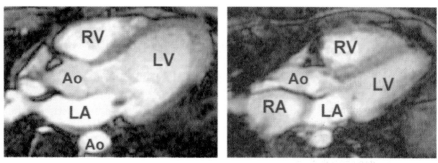

Normal   Hypertension

Fig. 2 Magnetic resonance (left ventricular (LV) outflow tract view) of the heart in a normal subject and a pulmonary hypertensive patient shown at the same stage in the cardiac cycle. The LV is seen to be compressed by the right ventricle (RV). This impairs LV filling during early diastole, and hence reduces cardiac output. Distortion of the heart by the enlarged right-sided chambers has brought the right atrium (RA) into view. (Courtesy Dr Philip Kilner, Cardiac Magnetic Resonance Unit, Royal Brompton Hospital, London.)

☐ INVESTIGATION

Where pulmonary hypertension is suspected, the patient should undergo echocardiography to estimate systolic pulmonary artery pressure from the tricuspid regurgitant jet and evidence sought of right ventricular pressure overload. Following the demonstration of echocardiographic abnormalities, further investigation (Table 3) is required to confirm the diagnosis and determine the classification according to the WHO criteria. Cardiac catheterisation confirms the diagnosis and provides important prognostic information, while the haemodynamic data guide treatment (Table 4). An acute pulmonary vasodilator study should be carried out during the same procedure to determine whether the pulmonary vascular resistance falls. This is done using an infusion of adenosine, inhaled nitric oxide or nebulised prostacyclin. The test is positive if there is a fall in pulmonary vascular resistance and/or a mean pulmonary artery pressure of at least 20% without a fall in cardiac output. This is found in up to 25% of patients, and identifies those who may respond to calcium antagonists (Fig. 3).

Lung biopsy, which has been used to aid diagnosis in many patients in the past, has been abandoned in all but a few cases because the pathological findings rarely alter treatment.

☐ PROGNOSIS

The prognosis of pulmonary hypertension in the National Institutes of Health registry used to be a median of 2.8 years from diagnosis [2]. With anticoagulants and supportive medical therapy, the median survival is now 4.3 years, while prostaglandin therapy (see below) has extended median survival to 12 years. Lung transplantation improves survival to six years, but prostaglandin therapy with the addition of transplantation when prostaglandin therapy fails has a median survival of 15.2 years.

Table 3 Investigation of pulmonary hypertension.

Screening:
- ECG
- Chest radiograph
- Echocardiography

Detailed investigation:

Respiratory   Ventilation perfusion scan
High-resolution CT lungs
Contrast helical CT pulmonary arteries with pulmonary angiography (to delineate thromboembolic disease)
Arterial blood gases in room air
Lung function
Nocturnal oxygen saturation monitoring

Cardiology   Submaximal exercise test (six-minute walk or incremental shuttle test)
Cardiac catheterisation (including measurement of mixed venous and systemic oxygen saturation, right heart pressures, cardiac output, pulmonary and systemic vascular resistance, and acute pulmonary vasodilator test)

Other   Routine biochemistry and haematology
Thrombophilia screen
Thyroid function
Autoimmune screen (including anti-centromere antibody, anti-SCL70 and RNP, phospholipid antibodies)
Hepatitis serology
Serum angiotensin-converting enzyme
HIV
Urine beta-HCG (women)
Abdominal ultrasound

Follow-up:
- Submaximal exercise test (3–6 monthly)
- Echocardiography
- Chest radiograph
- Arterial blood gases
- (Cardiac catheterisation may be required if there is clinical deterioration)

CT = computed tomography; HCG = human chorionic gonadotrophin; RNP = ribonucleoprotein; SCL = scleroderma.

Table 4 Prognostic indicators obtained at cardiac catheterisation.

Indicator	Value	Survival
Pulmonary arterial oxygen saturation	<63%	17% at 3 years
	>63%	55% at 3 years
Cardiac index	<2.1 l/min/m^2	median, 17 months
Right atrial pressure	<10 mmHg	mean, 4 years
	>20 mmHg	mean, 1 month

Lack of pulmonary vasodilator response to acute pulmonary vasodilator study indicates a worse prognosis

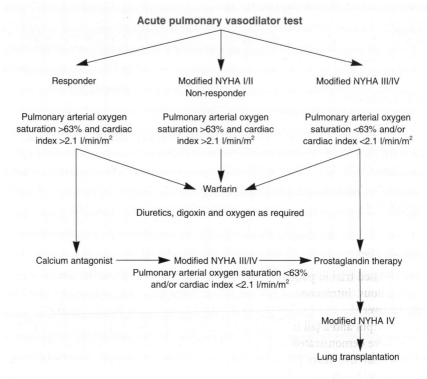

Fig. 3 Management of primary pulmonary arterial hypertension (NYHA = New York Heart Association).

☐ TREATMENT

Primary pulmonary hypertension

General measures

Warfarin is recommended for all patients because it has been shown to almost double three-year survival [3]. Diuretics are used to control fluid balance, and digoxin is used in patients in sinus rhythm whose symptoms persist despite optimal therapy. Oxygen is used to relieve symptoms since continuous oxygen does not improve outcome except in chronic lung disease. Oxygen may be given during the night in patients who desaturate below 90% at night to reduce any hypoxic vasoconstriction. Chest infections in these patients may have serious consequences, so all patients should receive a one-off pneumococcal immunisation and regular influenza immunisations. Women require contraceptive advice because pregnancy places the patient at high risk both during the pregnancy and in the postpartum period.

There is little public knowledge about this disease and many patients want more information. A patients' association was established in the UK in 2000 to help support patients and their families [4]. These patients frequently require psychological and social support. Those with more severe limitations may need help with mobility and financial benefits such as the disability living allowance. Advice from specialist palliative care should be considered if symptoms cannot be adequately controlled in end-stage disease.

Calcium antagonists

Calcium antagonists improve outcome in patients with a positive vasodilator response at cardiac catheterisation [5] (Fig. 3). The best evidence is for diltiazem and nifedipine. Calcium antagonists are contraindicated in patients with a negative vasodilator response, a low cardiac output or pulmonary venous disease. Not only do they not improve outcome in these conditions but they may even cause deterioration.

Prostaglandins

A randomised trial in patients in modified NYHA classes II and IV has shown that a continuous intravenous infusion of epoprostenol improved symptoms and survival over the three months of the trial [6], and was associated with a rise in cardiac output and a fall in pulmonary vascular resistance. Other registry and open studies have demonstrated a long-term beneficial effect, including almost doubling survival after five years [7]. Symptomatic benefit is dramatic in many cases, and patients may return to work on a continuous infusion.

Although epoprostenol may cause some improvement acutely by virtue of its vasodilating effect, its main action appears to be progressive reduction of pulmonary vascular resistance over years [8]. Patients with a negative acute vasodilator response derive the greatest benefit from this treatment. Improvement is probably achieved by modulation of the process of vascular remodelling; this would be consistent with the known antiproliferative and cytoprotective actions, and inhibition of platelet aggregation. Once started, prostaglandin therapy needs to be continued for life or until transplantation; no patients have yet been able to stop therapy and show continued improvement. Similar improvement is seen with iloprost.

The side effects of prostaglandin therapy vary in severity but are worst when dose uptitration is undertaken. A lancinating jaw pain is almost universal, and loose bowel motions, diarrhoea, abdominal pain, headache, flushing, arthralgia and muscle pain are also seen.

Serious complications may occur with the tunnelled central venous catheter and battery-driven pump for delivering the drug. Patients may develop catheter infection and septicaemia, catheter thrombosis and paradoxical embolism. Pump or catheter malfunction may occur up to an average of 2.5 times per year.

In view of the risks and complexity of managing continuous intravenous delivery systems, other methods of prostaglandin delivery to the pulmonary circulation have been sought. Uniprost (UT-15), an analogue of epoprostenol which can be delivered by subcutaneous infusion with frequent switching of the injection site to avoid infection, is currently undergoing clinical trials. Oral beraprost is also being investigated. Both nebulised epoprostenol and iloprost improve haemodynamics acutely. The results are awaited from a randomised trial in Germany in which iloprost has been administered chronically via the nebulised route.

Prostaglandins are also effective in several other types of pulmonary hypertension (Table 5).

The cost of prostaglandin therapy in Europe is high, although prices are already starting to fall below £20,000 per year. The cheaper pricing in the USA is a consequence of the orphan drug status of epoprostenol.

Table 5 Types of pulmonary hypertension which may respond to prostaglandin therapy

---

Primary sporadic and familial
Related to:
- Collagen vascular disease
- Congenital systemic to pulmonary shunts
- Portal hypertension
- HIV infection
- Drugs/Toxins
- Portal hypertension

Thromboembolic*
Sarcoidosis

---

* where surgical thromboendarterectomy is not feasible.

Lung transplantation

Heart-lung or lung transplantation has not proved to be a cure for pulmonary hypertension. Survival at five years is 54%, and is no better than long-term prostaglandin therapy. The main problems are related, first, to obliterative bronchiolitis in the grafted organ and, secondly, to the falling number of transplant donors so that the wait for a donor may be longer than the patient's prognosis.

Patients with pulmonary hypertension being considered for lung transplantation must meet the internationally agreed criteria [9]. The best results are obtained in patients treated with prostaglandin infusions [10]. Lung transplantation should be reserved for patients who deteriorate despite prostaglandins.

Atrial septostomy

The creation of a hole in the atrial septum using a catheter approach has been reported anecdotally and in one small series [11]. The rationale for this comes from the observation that pulmonary hypertensive patients with a patent foramen ovale and those with Eisenmenger's syndrome live longer than those with an intact atrial septum. Atrial septostomy reduces right ventricular end-diastolic pressure and increases cardiac output, but it is not clear which of these mechanisms improves survival. The formation of a shunt is at the expense of more severe hypoxaemia. There are no randomised trial data to support this form of treatment. It does not alter pulmonary vascular resistance, so its use may be as an adjunctive therapy to those already described above. It is unsafe in severely ill patients.

Connective tissue diseases

Although pulmonary hypertension may occur in association with a number of connective tissue diseases, including systemic lupus erythematosus, mixed connective tissue disease and the antiphospholipid syndrome, it is most commonly seen in scleroderma associated with the anti-centromere antibody. Pulmonary artery pressure tends to be lower than in primary pulmonary hypertension. Unlike primary pulmonary hypertension, a positive acute pulmonary vasodilator response is common but does not appear to improve survival. There is a paucity of data on the results of treatment. A randomised trial of epoprostenol over three months in scleroderma showed improved symptoms and exercise capacity, but was not powered to detect survival benefit [12]. Connective tissue diseases increase the risks of transplantation [9].

Thromboembolic disease

Pulmonary hypertension in thromboembolic disease is the result of recurrent thromboembolic events which have failed to resolve completely. Diagnosis is made by lung computed tomography imaging, pulmonary angiography and magnetic resonance angiography. Its recognition is important because selected cases may be suitable for surgical thromboendarterectomy at which pulmonary endothelium and thrombi are removed from the pulmonary circulation bilaterally, starting with the central pulmonary arteries and working peripherally [13]. This procedure restores pulmonary artery pressure to normal, with an increase in cardiac output. The operative mortality is 10%, and the long-term results show sustained improvement. Patients in whom the disease is not amenable to surgery may benefit from prostaglandin therapy.

New therapies

New agents are being developed and tested in pulmonary hypertension, and it is likely that the choice of therapies will increase in the next decade. These include the use of subcutaneous and oral prostaglandins, nitric oxide and endothelin antagonists, as well as novel agents. Ultimately, tissue engineering of the lung may help to provide a solution.

REFERENCES

1   Executive summary from the World Symposium on Primary Pulmonary Hypertension, 1998. http://www.who.int/ncd/cvd/pph.htm

2   D'Alonzo GE, Barst RJ, Ayres SM, *et al*. Survival in patients with primary pulmonary hypertension. Results from a national prospective registry. *Ann Intern Med* 1991; **115**: 343–9.

3   Fuster V, Steele PM, Edwards WD, *et al*. Primary pulmonary hypertension: natural history and the importance of thrombosis. *Circulation* 1984; **70**: 580–7.

4   http://www.pha-uk.com

5   Rich S, Kaufmann E, Levy PS. The effect of high doses of calcium-channel blockers on survival in primary pulmonary hypertension. *N Engl J Med* 1992; **327**: 76–81.

6   Barst RJ, Rubin LJ, Long WA, *et al.* A comparison of continuous intravenous epoprostenol (prostacyclin) with conventional therapy for primary pulmonary hypertension. The Primary Pulmonary Hypertension Study Group. *N Engl J Med* 1996; **334**: 296–302.

7   Higenbottam TW, Spiegelhalter D, Scott JP, *et al.* Prostacyclin (epoprostenol) and heart-lung transplantation as treatments for severe pulmonary hypertension. *Br Heart J* 1993; **70**: 366–70.

8   McLaughlin VV, Genthner DE, Panella MM, Rich S. Reduction in pulmonary vascular resistance with long-term epoprostenol (prostacyclin) therapy in primary pulmonary hypertension. *N Engl J Med* 1998; **338**: 273–7.

9   International guidelines for the selection of lung transplant candidates. The American Society for Transplant Physicians (ASTP)/American Thoracic Society(ATS)/European Respiratory Society(ERS)/International Society for Heart and Lung Transplantation (ISHLT). *Am J Respir Crit Care Med* 1998; **158**: 335–9.

10 Conte JV, Gaine SP, Orens JB, *et al.* The influence of continuous intravenous prostacyclin therapy for primary pulmonary hypertension on the timing and outcome of transplantation. *J Heart Lung Transplant* 1998; **17**: 679–85.

11 Sandoval J, Gaspar J, Pulido T, *et al.* Graded balloon dilation atrial septostomy in severe primary pulmonary hypertension. A therapeutic alternative for patients nonresponsive to vasodilator treatment. *J Am Coll Cardiol* 1998; **32**: 297–304.

12 Badesch DB, Tapson VF, McGoon MD, *et al.* Continuous intravenous epoprostenol for pulmonary hypertension due to the scleroderma spectrum of disease. A randomized, controlled trial. *Ann Intern Med* 2000; **132**: 425–34.

13 Jamieson SW. Pulmonary thromboendarterectomy. *Heart* 1998; **79**: 118–20.

FURTHER READING

Rubin LJ. Primary pulmonary hypertension. *N Engl J Med* 1997; **336**: 111–7.

Drug resistant tuberculosis

Peter Ormerod

□ INTRODUCTION

Drug resistance in tuberculosis (TB) has been around as long as TB drugs. With the introduction of streptomycin, isoniazid and *para*-aminosalicylic acid (PAS), it took several years to realise that spontaneous mutations allowed drug resistance to develop at an approximate rate of one in 10^7 organisms. Combination chemotherapy was needed to treat TB effectively, and to prevent the emergence of drug resistance. In 1960 [1] over 10% of patients with TB and a history of prior treatment had drug resistance.

The use of newer drugs, rifampicin, pyrazinamide and ethambutol has also been followed by drug resistance, through the same failure of doctors to give adequate and appropriate treatment and to monitor compliance, and the patients' failure to comply with or complete medication.

Developments in molecular biology and genetics have enabled the mechanisms of drug resistance to most of the first-line anti-TB drugs to be worked out (Table 1). However, definitions of both non-multidrug resistance TB (NMDR-TB) and multidrug resistance TB (MDR-TB) are needed.

□ INCIDENCE OF DRUG RESISTANCE

In the UK, mycobacterial drug resistance is monitored by Mycobnet, a small section of the Public Health Laboratory Service (PHLS) Communicable Diseases Surveillance Centre. All positive culture data for TB for the UK are collated and monitored on a continuing basis. Data from 1993 onwards show the current level of

Table 1 Genetic sites for drug resistance in tuberculosis.

Drug	Target	Gene
Isoniazid	catalase-peroxidase enzyme	*katG*
Isoniazid/Ethionamide	mycolic acid synthesis	*inhA*
Rifampicin	RNA polymerase	*rpoB*
Streptomycin	ribosomal S12 protein	*rpsL*
	16S rRNA	*rrs*
Quinolones	DNA gyrase	*gyrA*

drug resistance and also give information on risk factors [2]. Rates of isoniazid resistance are 5–6% overall. Separate risk factors for resistance from multivariate analysis are:

- ☐ a history of previous treatment (x3)
- ☐ HIV infection (x4)
- ☐ Indian subcontinent (ISC) ethnic origin (x3)
- ☐ Black African ethnic origin (x4)
- ☐ residence in London (x 2).

☐ CLINICAL EPIDEMIOLOGY

Before drug resistance can be diagnosed, two steps are required: first, an appreciation that the diagnosis is, or could be, TB and, secondly, the sending of appropriate samples for mycobacterial culture, drug resistance being diagnosable only in those with positive bacteriology.

In 1998, a national notification survey [3] showed approximately 6,000 total cases of TB in England and Wales, with wide variations in the rates in different ethnic groups. The overall population rate was 10.9/100,000, the rate in the white population was 4.4/100,000, that in the ISC ethnic group 120/100,000 and in the Black African ethnic group 210/100,000. Over 50% of people in non-white ethnic groups with TB had been born abroad, and their rates were highest within 2–3 years of first arrival in the UK. Overall, the white ethnic group contributed 37% of cases, the ISC ethnic group 40%, and the Black Africans 13%. Over half the white ethnic cases were aged over 55 years, and are thought to represent reactivation of disease acquired earlier in life.

Because the majority of cases are now in ethnic minority groups, the geographical breakdown of cases strongly reflects the distribution of those groups. In 1998, Greater London had a rate of 32/100,000, whereas in the rest of England and Wales it was 7.7/100,000 [3]. Such wide geographical variation has also been shown in previous surveys [4]. The much higher rates of TB in ethnic minority groups mean that certain clinical presentations should be regarded as TB until proved otherwise, and investigated appropriately with this as the working diagnosis (Table 2, Figs. 1 and 2).

Table 2 High probability clinical presentations in ethnic minority patients.

- mediastinal lymphadenopathy
- pleural effusion
- persistent cervical lymphadenopathy >4 weeks
- monoarthritis

Note: tuberculosis should also be very high on the differential diagnosis of pyrexia of unknown origin.

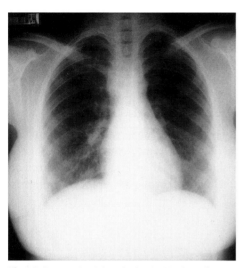

Fig. 1 Paratracheal lymphadenopathy in a female from the Indian subcontinent. Resolved with anti-tuberculosis therapy.

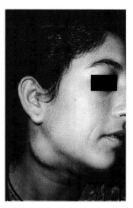

Fig. 2 Persistent cervical adenopathy in a female from the Indian sub-continent. Tuberculosis confirmed on biopsy and culture.

☐ BACTERIOLOGICAL CONFIRMATION

Because of the rates of drug resistance, every effort should be made to obtain bacteriological confirmation of the diagnosis. This also provides drug susceptibility data. Three sputum samples, obtained on separate mornings, should be sent for pulmonary cases. If a patient is unable to produce sputum, fibreoptic bronchoscopy and washings of the appropriate lung segment(s) should be undertaken. Samples from serous sites, pleura, peritoneum and pericardium, also pus obtained from neck glands and other sites, should be sent for TB culture. Surgeons biopsying lesions for suspected TB should be reminded to send half the sample for TB culture *without* preservative (eg formalin).

☐ TREATMENT OF TUBERCULOSIS

The current rates of isoniazid resistance are approximately 1% in previously untreated white ethnic patients, but 4–10% in other ethnic groups. The national treatment recommendations have been designed with this information in mind [5]. Standard treatment for all sites of disease except the central nervous system (CNS) comprises an initial phase of four drugs – rifampicin, isoniazid, pyrazinamide and ethambutol – for two months, followed by a continuation of rifampicin and isoniazid for a further four months [5]. CNS TB should be treated with the same initial phase, but the continuation phase should be prolonged to a further 10 months [5]. All patients should have the four-drug initial phase including ethambutol, except the following groups who have a low probability of drug resistance in whom ethambutol may be omitted:

☐   patients of white ethnic origin

☐   those previously untreated

☐   patients known, or thought likely, to be HIV-negative on risk assessment, and

☐   those who are not contacts of known drug resistance.

Treatment for all forms of TB should be given only under the supervision of a chest physician or other appropriately qualified and trained consultant with direct working access to TB nurses or health visitors [5]. National audit has shown that chest physicians are more likely to give treatment according to protocol than other types of doctor [6].

☐ TREATMENT OF DRUG RESISTANCE

Patients admitted to hospital should have an assessment of their infectivity and risk of drug resistance, and be placed in appropriate isolation taking into account the immune status of other patients on the ward [7]. Initial treatment should follow national guidance [5] unless there are concerns/risk factors for MDR-TB (see later). If cultures show full susceptibility, ethambutol and/or pyrazinamide can be stopped after two months. If susceptibility results are still outstanding at two months, the initial three or four drug phase of treatment should be continued until these results are available. If there is resistance to specific drugs, the drug regimen and duration require modification. Detailed guidance on NMDR-TB resistances is given in the national guidelines [5] (summarised in Table 3). Patients should be followed up for at least 12 months after completion of treatment [5].

☐ MULTIDRUG RESISTANT TUBERCULOSIS

Incidence

MDR-TB is found worldwide. Combined resistance to rifampicin and isoniazid, with or without additional resistance, is a particular concern. Certain countries, such as the Baltic Republics, Russia, the Dominican Republic and Côte D'Ivoire, are 'hot-spots' for MDR-TB [8]. MDR-TB occurred infrequently in England and Wales between 1982 and 1991, being reported in only 0.6% of isolates [9]. This rose to 1.3–1.9% of isolates between 1993 and 1997, and the current rate is 1.3% [9]. This represents approximately 50 cases per annum in the UK, two-thirds of them occurring in Greater London.

Risk factors

The risk factors for MDR-TB are those for drug resistance in all TB, but are even more marked [2]. The independent factors are:

☐   male sex (x2)

☐   birth in India (x4)

Table 3 Management of non-multidrug resistant tuberculosis (NMDR) resistance.

Resistance	Regimen	Comments
Streptomycin	2RHZ(E)/4RH	Does not alter standard treatment
Isoniazid	If known pre-treatment: 2RZSE/7RE If on treatment, ensure 2RZE/10RE	Fully supervised (ie DOT)
Pyrazinamide	Usually *Mycobacterium bovis* If had 2RHZE: stop ZE, then 7RH If had 2RHZ, then 2RHE/7RH	
Ethambutol	2RHZ/4RH	Uncommon Standard treatment unaffected
Rifampicin	Uncommon Under 10% of rifampicin resistance is *mono*-resistance Should be treated as MDR-TB until *full* sensitivity pattern available If *true* mono-resistance: 2HZE/16HE	
Streptomycin/ Isoniazid	As for H resistance during treatment	Fully supervised (ie DOT)
Other combination	Other NMDR-TB combinations are uncommon An individual regimen would need to be devised	Advice from PHLS Mycobacterium Reference Unit and experienced clinician

Note: The number in front of the letters is the number of months for that part of the regimen.
DOT = direct observation throughout; E = ethambutol; H = isoniazid; PHLS = Public Health Laboratory Service; R = rifampicin; S = streptomycin; Z = pyrazinamide.

- □ previous treatment (x12)
- □ HIV infection (x9), and
- □ residence in London (x2).

Clinical suspicion should also be raised by failure of clinical response on treatment and prolonged sputum smear or culture positivity whilst on treatment.

Detection

If a risk assessment using these factors raises concerns, rapid molecular tests for rifampicin resistance are available on either microscopy-positive or culture-positive samples via the PHLS mycobacteriology units. These tests can be performed within 1–2 working days and are 95% accurate. A report of rifampicin resistance in a patient with *Mycobacterium tuberculosis* confirmed on probe should be treated and isolated as for MDR-TB, for which separate isolation criteria are advised [7].

Management

The management of suspected or proven MDR-TB cases is complex. Treatment should be undertaken:

☐ only by a physician highly experienced in complex drug resistant cases

☐ for respiratory cases in a negative pressure ventilated room

☐ in close collaboration with the PHLS mycobacteriology units.

If the first two are not available in the same hospital, the patient must be transferred to a hospital where they are both available. The Health Service Management Executive includes services for such patients on the list of those which should be provided on a regional or supraregional basis.

The principles of management of such cases are:

1   A minimum of five drugs, including one injectable, to which the patient is known or thought likely to be susceptible, should be given until culture negative.

2   A minimum of three drugs should be continued for a minimum of nine further months.

Each patient's regimen has to be individually tailored, depending on previous drugs used and drug resistance pattern, and will have to include reserve drugs (Table 4). All treatment, both inpatient and outpatient, has to be under direct observation throughout.

Prognosis

Mortality is high in HIV-positive MDR-TB cases, with over 70% mortality reported in the USA before the diagnosis is made [10]. The prognosis is better in

Table 4 Reserve drugs for multidrug resistant tuberculosis [7].

Injectable	Tablet
Streptomycin	Ciprofloxacin
	Ofloxacin
Capreomycin	Clarithromycin
	Azithromycin
Kanamycin	Ethionamide
	Prothionamide
Amikacin	Cycloserine
	Rifabutin
	Thioacetazone
	PAS sodium

PAS = *para*-aminosalicylic acid.

HIV-negative individuals, but mortality and morbidity are still high. Patients who complete treatment should be on indefinite follow-up [5].

☐ PREDICTIONS FOR THE FUTURE

The proportion of cases of TB in the UK with drug resistance is likely to rise over the next 10 years, first because ethnic minority groups, who have higher rates of drug resistance, are providing an increasing proportion of cases. Secondly, drug resistance is increasing worldwide, with an increased chance of this being acquired by travel or imported with refugees. The global problem of MDR-TB will need a global response, and is a major potential problem for the future. Research is underway to try to develop new drugs, but to date none is near clinical trials.

REFERENCES

1   British Tuberculosis Association. Acquired drug resistance in patients with pulmonary tuberculosis in Great Britain – a national survey 1960–61. *Tubercle* 1963; **44**: 1–26.
2   Hayward AC, Bennett DE, Herbert J, Watson JM. Risk factors for drug resistance in patients with tuberculosis in England and Wales 1993–94. *Thorax* 1996; **51**(Suppl 3): A8.
3   Rose AM. 1998 National TB survey in England and Wales: final results. *Thorax* 1999; **54** (Suppl 3):S9.
4   Ormerod LP, Charlett A, Gilham C, *et al*. Geographical distribution of tuberculosis notifications in national surveys of England and Wales in 1988 and 1993: report of the Public Health Laboratory Service/British Thoracic Society/Department of Health Collaborative Group. *Thorax* 1998; **53**: 176–81.
5   Joint Tuberculosis Committee of the British Thoracic Society. Chemotherapy and management of tuberculosis in the United Kingdom: recommendations 1998. *Thorax* 1998; **53**: 536–48.
6   Ormerod LP, Bentley C. The management of pulmonary tuberculosis notified in England and Wales in 1993. *J R Coll Physicians Lond* 1997; **31**: 662–5.
7   The Interdepartmental Working Group on Tuberculosis. The prevention and control of tuberculosis in the United Kingdom: UK guidance on the prevention and control of transmission of 1. HIV-related tuberculosis, 2. Drug-resistant, including multiple drug-resistant, tuberculosis. London: Department of Health, The Scottish Office, The Welsh Office, September 1998.
8   Pablos-Mendez A, Raviglione MC, Laszlo A, *et al*. Global surveillance for antituberculosis-drug resistance 1994–97. World Health Organization-International Union against Tuberculosis and Lung Disease Working Group on Anti-Tuberculosis Drug Resistance Surveillance. *N Engl J Med* 1998; **338**: 1641–9.
9   Warburton AR, Jenkins PA, Waight PA, Watson JM. Drug resistance in initial isolates of Mycobacterium tuberculosis in England and Wales, 1982–1991. *Comm Dis Rev* 1993; **3**: R175–9.
10 Centers for Disease Control. Nosocomial transmission of multi-drug resistant tuberculosis among HIV-infected persons – Florida and New York, 1988–1991. *MMWR* 1991; **40**: 585–90.

☐ SELF ASSESSMENT QUESTIONS

1   Risk factors for drug resistance include:
    (a) A history of previous treatment
    (b) Being in an ethnic minority group

(c) Female sex
(d) HIV-infected
(e) Residence outside London

2   Tuberculosis should be strongly suspected in ethnic minority patients with:
(a) Pleural effusion
(b) Cervical glands persisting for longer than four weeks
(c) Polyarthropathy
(d) Mediastinal lymphadenopathy
(e) Pyrexia of unknown origin

3   Ethambutol can be omitted from the initial phase of treatment if:
(a) The patient is of non-white ethnic origin
(b) There is a history of previous treatment
(c) The patient is known or suspected to be HIV-infected
(d) The patient is a known contact of drug resistant disease
(e) None of the above apply

4   Isoniazid resistance:
(a) Occurs in 4–6% of white previously untreated cases
(b) Occurs in approximately 1% of ethnic minority groups
(c) Requires treatment modification
(d) Is found in *Mycobacterium bovis*
(e) If combined with streptomycin resistance, requires supervised treatment

5   Multidrug resistant tuberculosis:
(a) Is defined as combined resistance to rifampicin and isoniazid
(b) Is found in 4–6% of UK isolates
(c) Can be treated by standard isolation in respiratory cases
(d) Requires specialised management, including reserve drugs
(e) Has a very high mortality in HIV-infected patients

ANSWERS

1a True	2a True	3a False	4a False	5a True
b True	b True	b False	b False	b False
c False	c False	c False	c True	c False
d True	d True	d False	d False	d True
e False	e True	e True	e True	e True

Peanut and other food allergies

Pamela W Ewan

□ MECHANISM

The mechanism underlying acute allergic reactions to foods is the type I (immediate hypersensitivity) reaction. This requires production of specific immunoglobulin (Ig) E to the food in question, which binds via the high affinity Fcε receptor I to mast cells (Fig. 1). Mast cells are widely distributed in the skin, mucosal surfaces and around blood vessels. They are packed with granules containing stored mediators, particularly histamine. Cross-linking of adjacent IgE molecules by allergen (eg a food) activates the mast cell, leading to degranulation and mediator release. Degranulation occurs quickly and, within minutes, substantial quantities of histamine are released into the extracellular fluid. Other mediators (leukotriene (LTs), prostaglandins) are synthesised by the mast cell soon after activation and have similar effects to histamine.

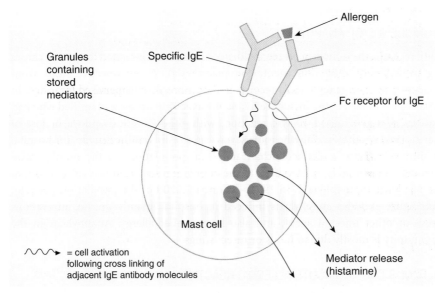

Fig. 1 The type I allergic reaction (Ig = immunoglobulin).

□ EFFECTS OF HISTAMINE

The effects of histamine account for the symptoms seen in allergic reactions. Histamine causes dilation of small veins and capillary leak, resulting in venous congestion and mucosal oedema, and also causes increased secretions. Mucosal oedema and secretions in the upper respiratory tract (particularly the larynx) contribute to airway obstruction, the main cause of acute dyspnoea in food-induced reactions. Histamine also induces smooth muscle contraction and bronchoconstriction. Other mediators, newly generated on mast cell activation, are released more slowly than histamine. Of these, the LTs (LTC4, LTD4 and LTE4) are potent bronchoconstrictors (1,000 times more potent than histamine). Histamine-induced systemic capillary leak will lead to hypotension and cardiovascular collapse.

☐ INCIDENCE

The incidence of food allergy is not well known, but the perception is that it is increasing. A study from the Isle of Wight in 1996 [1] found that 15 of 1,218 four year old children had specific IgE to peanut or tree nut, shown by positive skin-prick test (see later). Eight of these were clinically allergic to nuts, six of them to peanut (equivalent to one in 200, or 0.5% of this population, with confirmed peanut allergy). More recently, a telephone survey in the USA of over 12,000 subjects found an incidence of 1.14% for peanut or nut allergy. Even allowing for the fact that this study, based on self-diagnosis, is likely to be an overestimate, peanut and nut allergy is clearly a substantial problem.

☐ INCIDENCE OF ANAPHYLAXIS

Until recently, the only data on the incidence of anaphylaxis related to specific causes (eg penicillin or induction agents for anaesthesia). A retrospective study from accident and emergency (A&E) records in Addenbrooke's Hospital, Cambridge, in 1993–94 [2] looked at the incidence of anaphylaxis. Patients were identified who had features of a generalised allergic reaction, with either severe dyspnoea or loss of consciousness – that is, only the most severe cases. This was the only major hospital in the area serving a defined urban and rural population, so the number who attended A&E could be related back to the population served. It was calculated that the incidence of anaphylaxis in 1994 was one in 3,500 of the population per year. This figure excludes anaphylaxis induced in hospital, mainly due to intravenous drugs or other injected agent, and also latex rubber allergy. Anaphylaxis in the community is mostly due to foods or insect stings.

☐ FOODS CAUSING ACUTE ALLERGIC REACTIONS

Many foods may cause allergic reactions, the commonest of which are shown in Table 1. Fruits, especially apple, may cause reactions, commonly the milder oral allergy syndrome, but they may also cause anaphylaxis. Examples of foods which are rare causes of anaphylaxis are mustard seeds and green pepper.

Table 1 Foods most commonly causing allergic reactions.

• Peanut	• Milk	• Soya
• Tree nuts	• Fish	• Wheat
• Egg	• Shellfish	

□ AGE OF ONSET

Peanut and nut allergy begins at an early age (Table 2), mostly by the age of seven, and over half by the age of three. Egg and milk allergies develop mainly in infants and toddlers.

Table 2 Age of onset of peanut or tree nut allergy in 60 unselected consecutive referrals (adapted, with permission, from data in [3]).

Age (years)	Cumulative no.	%
<1	11	18
2	24	40
3	33	55
5	52	87
7	55	92

□ CLINICAL FEATURES

Foods may cause reactions ranging from mild to severe. Cutaneous features, especially of the mouth and face, are common: pruritus, erythema, urticaria or angio-oedema. The angio-oedema may be superficial, affecting the lips or face, but may also involve the oral mucosa. A more serious problem is oedema at the back of the throat and involving the larynx. This presents with a sensation of tightening of the throat, followed by closing up of the throat. This may lead to upper airway obstruction, with severe dyspnoea, stridor, voice change and cyanosis. Asthma may be associated, but laryngeal oedema and asthma occur independently. These respiratory features are the most important problem in acute severe food allergy. Patients may rapidly develop severe dyspnoea with cyanosis, which may go on to respiratory arrest.

Less commonly, patients may also develop hypotension, which causes weakness, collapse, faintness or loss of consciousness. Study of the progression of the allergic reaction shows that hypotension is almost always secondary to severe respiratory difficulty and anoxia. Patients do not develop hypotension as an early feature, as occurs in other situations in which a larger bolus of allergen is given systemically (eg intravenous drugs or bee or wasp stings).

Other possible symptoms are nausea and vomiting. These seem to be commoner in young children, and are rare in teenagers and adults. Children who vomit (eg in peanut, egg or milk allergy) often then improve quickly. Vomiting will limit absorption of allergen, and is beneficial. Young children sometimes become lethargic. Conjunctivitis and rhinitis, which are features of anaphylactic reactions, are rare in food-induced anaphylaxis.

The clinical features in an unselected series of 62 patients with peanut and/or tree nut allergy are shown in Table 3, listing the most severe reaction each patient has ever suffered [3]. In about one-third of patients the most severe reaction was cutaneous only. This varied in severity from trivial (a few patches of perioral

Table 3 Clinical features of peanut and tree nut allergy in 62 patients, listing the most severe reaction suffered by each patient (adapted, with permission, from data in [3]).

| Category | Cutaneous only | *Respiratory | |
		Respiratory	Respiratory and cardiovascular
Range of features	A few urticarial wheals Erythema (facial) Generalised urticaria Lip, oral mucosal or facial angio-oedema	Mild to severe laryngeal oedema Mild to severe asthma	Severe dyspnoea/ anoxia Respiratory arrest Hypotension Loss of consciousness (cardiovascular always followed severe respiratory symptoms)
No. (%) of patients	20 (32)	33 (53)	9 (15)

* Also included cutaneous features.

urticaria or facial erythema) to quite marked and alarming for the patient (eg angiooedema of the entire face or severe generalised urticaria). These reactions are, however, not life-threatening.

Importantly, two-thirds of the patients had respiratory involvement – the key potentially life-threatening feature. Again, this varied in severity from mild laryngeal oedema (felt as a slight closing up of the throat) to severe laryngeal oedema and/or asthma, with marked dyspnoea. Only 9% of patients had hypotension, always secondary to severe dyspnoea.

The same clinical features are seen in other food allergies, although the proportions may vary. Acute milk and egg allergy presents mainly with cutaneous or respiratory features. Severe anaphylactic reactions can occur, but in only a minority of patients. However, when it does occur, milk or egg anaphylaxis is often severe.

In contrast, other foods (eg apple) cause mainly oral mucosal oedema – the oral allergy syndrome, which occurs typically in patients with tree pollen rhinoconjunctivitis. Certain foods, such as apple and potato, cause reactions when uncooked but are tolerated when cooked. It is presumed that the heating denatures the proteins. The reactions caused by raw potato are unusual: scraping potatoes causes conjunctivitis and periorbital oedema or, rarely, angio-oedema of the fingers. Scraping new potatoes causes more marked symptoms than old potatoes.

☐ ASSOCIATIONS

Patients with food allergy commonly have other atopic diseases (Table 4) [3–5]. In babies and toddlers this is usually eczema, whereas asthma is more common from the age of two, and rhinitis appears mainly in children over five years old.

Patients allergic to apple usually have tree pollen allergy, which causes rhinoconjunctivitis in the spring, due to cross-reactive allergens. Similarly, in latex

Table 4 Incidence (%) of other allergies in patients with peanut and/or tree nut allergy in different series (from [3–5], with permission).

	Reference		
	3 **(n=62)**	**4** **(n=622)**	**5** **(n=122)**
Asthma	76	61	74
Rhinitis	73	62	ND
Eczema	60	49	75

ND = no data.

rubber allergy, a proportion of patients are allergic to certain fruits, including banana, kiwi and avocado.

☐ SEVERE AND FATAL REACTIONS

Peanut and nut allergy are the commonest food allergies to cause fatal or near-fatal reactions. They account for several deaths each year in the UK. Two series in the USA, each involving small numbers of subjects, found that peanut allergy accounted for half of the fatal or near-fatal food-induced reactions. In the UK, there are few specialist allergists, and in many parts of the country it is difficult to obtain good allergy advice. It is difficult to avoid nuts, which increasingly are hidden in foods where they might not be suspected. Most patients who have died were aware of their allergy, but had been unable to obtain professional advice. Even in the USA, where allergy is a major specialty, further reactions in patients who had already seen an allergist are common (55% in one series).

☐ RESOLUTION

There is no evidence to support the common belief among patients that reactions to peanuts will always get worse, and that they cannot 'grow out' of this allergy. In one study in Southampton [6], oral challenge tests in patients with mild peanut allergy found that allergy had resolved in 22%. More studies will be required, covering the full spectrum of severity and over a longer period, to determine a representative figure for resolution.

Egg and milk allergy commonly resolve, with almost 85% of children able to tolerate milk by the age of three and 80% able to tolerate egg by the age of five. Milk allergy persisting into adult life is often severe, tiny quantities of milk protein causing life-threatening reactions.

☐ DIAGNOSIS

The history is important. Tests should be made only to confirm (or refute) the suspected allergy. In acute food-induced reactions, symptoms begin quickly after ingestion of the food – often within a few mouthfuls, sometimes immediately. The majority of reactions will have begun within 5–10 minutes of ingestion. Sometimes the cause is obvious (eg a reaction within minutes of eating peanut butter on bread), but on other occasions ingredients of meals have to be checked carefully. In the latter, it is helpful if there has been more than one reaction, so that common ingredients can be looked for. It is equally important, from the history, to rule out ingredients tolerated on other occasions.

Tests for specific IgE should be used to confirm the allergic cause. Correct interpretation is essential. Many subjects have specific IgE without clinical allergy (ie are sensitised). Random measurement of food IgE may therefore give positive results which are clinically irrelevant. Specific IgE can be measured in the serum (eg by radioallergo-sorbent test or RAST, or the more sensitive CAP-RAST) or by skin-prick testing. The advantage of the skin test is that it gives an immediate result in clinic, and this is the main test used by allergists. A positive skin test in a patient with Brazil nut allergy is shown in Fig. 2. The skin test produces an immediate wheal and flare reaction, which is measured at 10–15 minutes.

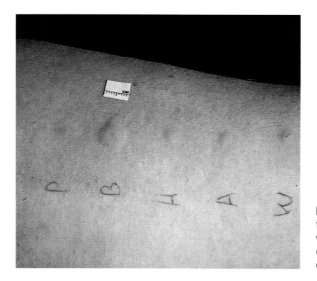

Fig. 2 A positive skin-prick test to Brazil nut showing the wheal and flare reaction and demonstrating the presence of specific immunoglobulin E.

Sampson in the USA has studied sensitivity and specificity of food-specific IgE, and found a substantial proportion of positives without associated clinical allergy – it would be misleading to describe these as false positives, as the specific IgE is present. He proposed a cut-off value which would be 95% predictive of clinical allergy, and found that this level varied greatly with the food in question but was usually quite high.

Despite the problems of interpretation, a positive skin test or RAST is of value in confirming food allergy. There are good skin test extracts or CAP-RAST assays for the commoner foods causing allergy. For other foods (eg fruits and vegetables), it can be better to perform skin tests directly through the food than to use a poor quality extract.

☐ MANAGEMENT

Acute management

The management of an acute episode depends on the severity and the presenting symptoms (Table 5). Adrenaline is the key drug for severe reactions and should be given intramuscularly (IM), using a one in 1,000 solution (1 mg/ml). The standard adult dose is 0.5 mg (0.5 ml of 1 in 1,000 strength) IM. This should be followed by chlorpheniramine 10 mg IM and hydrocortisone 100–500 mg IM or slow intravenous.

Table 5 Acute management of food-induced reactions.

Severity	Example of clinical features	Treatment
Mild	Cutaneous (pruritus, erythema, urticaria, angio-oedema)	Oral antihistamine IM antihistamine
Moderate	Most severe cutaneous Mild laryngeal oedema Mild asthma	IM chlorpheniramine IM hydrocortisone Inhaled adrenaline Inhaled salbutamol
Severe	Marked dyspnoea (laryngeal oedema and/or asthma) Hypotension	IM adrenaline IM/IV chlorpheniramine IM/IV hydrocortisone

Note: this is a general scheme for immediate drug treatment. Treatment of an individual patient will depend on exact clinical features and severity (eg additional treatment for asthma). Further measures may be required (eg oxygen, IV fluids etc).
IM = intramuscular; IV = intravenous.

Prospective management

Prospective management involves two approaches:

☐   advice on avoidance, and

☐   drugs for self-treatment of reactions following inadvertent exposure.

Avoidance

Avoidance is not easy and patients need detailed advice, best provided by an allergist. Nuts pose a particular problem as they may be hidden in foods and are increasingly used for flavouring. Patients need to learn to read labels, understand the principles of food labelling, and be aware of higher risk foods (eg restaurant meals, Indian and Chinese meals, bakery and delicatessen goods).

Emergency medication

Patients at risk of a severe reaction should carry medication, so that they can institute early treatment of reactions. This applies to those at risk of anaphylaxis. Identifying patients at risk is difficult and requires specialist experience.

Cambridge management programme

In Cambridge we have developed a management programme [7], which involves providing patients with one of three types of treatment (Table 6):

1   Oral antihistamines.

2   Oral antihistamines plus inhaled adrenaline.

3   Oral antihistamines plus intramuscular adrenaline plus an auto-injector such as EpiPen or EpiPen Junior for children (ca 15 months to 6 years, depending on weight).

Table 6 Drugs to include on emergency treatment plan for self- (or parent-) treatment by patients at risk of anaphylaxis.

- Oral antihistamine
- Inhaled adrenaline (eg Primatene Mist*)
- Adrenaline auto-injector (eg EpiPen)

* Available only on named patient basis.
Note: see text; selection of medication appropriate to risk is required; doses must be tailored to age of patient.

A written treatment plan in simple lay terms is provided, and the treatment selected depends on an assessment of severity of the allergy. It is essential to provide regular training in recognising reactions and using the medication. In the case of children, parents have to be taught. The community paediatric team needs to be involved to provide training for school staff. In a large follow-up study we have found that, with good advice on avoidance, most patients experience less severe subsequent reactions. Even if their index reaction was severe (anaphylaxis) we would expect either no further reaction or a milder one. Thus, oral antihistamines or inhaled adrenaline are the most commonly required treatment for further reactions. The fact that the EpiPen is little used does not negate the need for this; rather, it shows that avoidance measures are successful. The EpiPen is available in case avoidance fails and because, if it does occur, anaphylaxis is easier to reverse if treated early.

REFERENCES

1   Tariq SM, Stevens M, Matthews S, *et al.* Cohort study of peanut and tree nut sensitisation by age of 4 years. *Br Med J* 1996; **313**: 514–7.
2   Stewart AG, Ewan PW. The incidence, aetiology and management of anaphylaxis presenting to an Accident & Emergency department. *Q J Med* 1996; **89**: 859–64.
3   Ewan PW. Clinical study of peanut and nut allergy in 62 consecutive patients: new features and associations. *Br Med J* 1996; **312**: 1074–8.
4   Hourihane JO, Dean TP, Warner JO. Peanut allergy in relation to heredity, maternal diet, and other atopic diseases: results of a questionnaire survey, skin prick testing, and food challenges. *Br Med J* 1996; **313**: 518–21.
5   Sicherer SH, Burks AW, Sampson HA. Clinical features of acute allergic reactions to peanut and tree nuts in children. *Pediatrics* 1998; **102**: e6.

6   Hourihane JO, Roberts SA, Warner JO. Resolution of peanut allergy: case-control study. *Br Med J* 1998; **316**: 1271–5.

7   Vickers DW, Maynard L, Ewan PW. Management of children with potential anaphylactic reactions in the community: a training package and proposal for good practice. *Clin Exp Allergy* 1997; **27**: 898–903.

FURTHER READING

1   Sampson HA, Mendelson L, Rosen JP. Fatal and near-fatal anaphylactic reactions to food in children and adolescents. *N Engl J Med* 1992; **327**: 380–4.

2   Yunginger JW, Sweeney KG, Sturner WQ, *et al.* Fatal food-induced anaphylaxis. *JAMA* 1988; **260**: 1450–2.

3   Ewan PW. Treatment of anaphylactic reactions. *Prescribers' J* 1997; **37**: 125–32.

4   Ewan PW (co-author), and Project Team of The Resuscitation Council (UK). The emergency medical treatment of anaphylactic reactions. *J Accid Emerg Med* 1999; **16**: 243–7.

☐ SELF ASSESSMENT QUESTIONS

1   Type I allergic reactions:
   (a) Require the presence of immunoglobulin (Ig) G antibody
   (b) Require the presence of IgE antibody
   (c) Require the presence of specific allergen
   (d) Are usually slow in onset, over several hours
   (e) Increased capillary permeability occurs

2   Peanut and nut allergy:
   (a) Has a prevalence of 5–10%
   (b) Is one of the commoner foods to cause allergic reactions
   (c) Mainly affects adults
   (d) Always causes anaphylaxis
   (e) This diagnosis warrants further investigation, preferably by an allergist

3   The following are clinical features of nut allergy:
   (a) Urticaria
   (b) Tightening of the throat
   (c) Severe dyspnoea
   (d) Asthma
   (e) Vomiting

4   In the management of anaphylaxis:
   (a) Adrenaline is the first-line drug
   (b) The preferred route of administration for adrenaline is intravenously
   (c) Chlorpheniramine and hydrocortisone injections should be given
   (d) Monitor respiratory status
   (e) Measure blood pressure

5   In peanut allergy:
   (a) Skin-prick testing to peanuts is a valuable test

(b) Testing for peanut-specific IgE in serum (eg RAST) is not useful
(c) Measure peak expiratory flow rate
(d) Patients should be given advice and training if prescribed adrenaline auto injectors (EpiPen)
(e) Other allergies including asthma are common

ANSWERS

1a False	2a False	3a True	4a True	5a True
b True	b True	b True	b False	b False
c True	c False	c True	c True	c True
d False	d False	d True	d True	d True
e True	e True	e True	e True	e True

Bronchial disease

Robert Stockley

Chronic obstructive pulmonary disease (COPD) is a group of conditions that together are a major cause of mortality and morbidity. By the year 2020 it is predicted that COPD will be the third most important cause of mortality and lost years worldwide [1].

The common feature of COPD is the presence of fixed airflow obstruction, usually defined by a reduction in the forced expired volume in 1 second (FEV_1) and the ratio of FEV_1 to forced vital capacity or slow vital capacity. Some patients retain a degree of reversibility of the airflow obstruction acutely following inhaled β_2-agonists. These physiological differences probably reflect separate components of the COPD syndrome. For instance, COPD includes chronic bronchitis with cough and sputum expectoration, pathological changes of emphysema, abnormality of the small airways or long-standing asthma, where most of the reversible component of airflow obstruction has been lost.

To date, therapy has remained largely empirical. This includes the use of β_2-agonists and inhaled steroids in order to reverse any 'asthmatic' component, together with steroids, antibiotics and bronchodilators for exacerbations.

With the development of animal models reflecting different components of COPD, there has been an expanding research interest in the pathogenesis of the conditions. This, in turn, has led to an interest in the development of specific therapies and a more rational understanding of the application of some therapies.

☐ CHRONIC BRONCHIAL DISEASE

The normal human airway is usually sterile despite the daily inhalation of large numbers of irritant particles and microorganisms. This is achieved by the presence of a sophisticated system of lung defences that includes maintenance of the integrity of the epithelial surface, mucociliary clearance, the presence of a variety of antibacterial proteins in lung secretions, and resident airway phagocytes.

In patients with chronic bronchial disease there is major impairment of this primary defence system. Many patients have chronic bronchitis due to excess mucus production associated with inflammation in the airway wall, mucus gland hyperplasia, loss of ciliated epithelium and a reduction in mucociliary clearance, often associated with persistent bacterial colonisation by organisms of relatively low pathogenicity. In addition, repeated exacerbations add to the morbidity and reduction in health status of these patients.

Pathogenesis

The rapid development of animal models that mimic many of the features of COPD was based on the observation in 1963 that subjects with inherited deficiency of α-1-antitrypsin (the major serum inhibitor of proteolytic enzymes) suffered from early onset of severe emphysema and bronchitis [2]. This observation led workers to explore the possibility that proteolytic enzymes, normally inhibited by α-1-antitrypsin, were the major cause of the pathological changes. Instillation of human neutrophil elastase into the airway of experimental animals produces protein exudation, epithelial damage and mucus secretion within 20 minutes [3]. With time, the experimental model develops 'emphysematous-like' lesions as well as goblet cell metaplasia and loss of ciliated epithelium. Other studies *in vitro* have demonstrated that elastase can destroy the integrity of the epithelium. It is the most potent secretagogue identified to date, and has a major effect on ciliary beat frequency and, by implication, on mucociliary clearance.

These observations have led to the general concept that the recruitment of neutrophils to the airway as part of the chronic bronchitis syndrome can cause pathological changes and the development of a vicious circle which perpetuates bronchial disease and leads to its progression. This concept is outlined diagrammatically in Fig. 1. The inflammatory process begins with the inhalation of

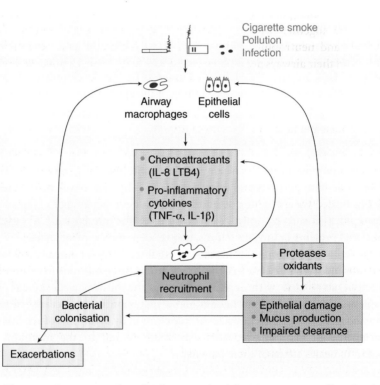

Fig. 1 Diagrammatic representation of self-perpetuating inflammatory process (IL = interleukin; LTB = leukotriene B; TNF = tumour necrosis factor).

cigarette smoke or pollutants, or with an acute infection. These processes stimulate local airway macrophages or epithelial cells to release chemoattractant cytokines such as interleukin (IL)-8 and leukotriene (LTB) 4. In addition, other pro-inflammatory cytokines such as tumour necrosis factor (TNF)-α and IL-1β are also released and, among their other properties, upregulate adhesion molecules on the endothelial surface. This, together with the chemoattractants, leads to neutrophil recruitment and activation in the airway and results in further release of the chemoattractants IL-8 and LTB4. In addition, the activated neutrophils release a variety of proteolytic enzymes and reactive oxygen species which can damage epithelial cells. The enzymes give rise to mucus gland hyperplasia and hypersecretion, whilst impairing mucociliary clearance. This process then dramatically impairs lung defences, followed by bacterial colonisation, which in its own right also stimulates inflammatory cell recruitment. The resulting circle of events can become self-perpetuating and is likely to play a key role in the progression and morbidity of bronchial disease.

Many of these concepts are supported by studies in man with particular reference to the bronchial secretions. These can be harvested in patients with chronic bronchitis following spontaneous expectoration and, more recently, using the technique of sputum induction where individuals inhale hyper-tonic saline resulting in expectoration of a mixture of the saline and mucus from the larger airways. These studies have confirmed the presence of inflammatory cells (particularly neutrophils) in the airway secretions of patients with COPD together with pro-inflammatory cytokines, neutrophil chemo-attractants and neutrophil products. Mucociliary clearance in these patients is reduced and their airways are often colonised by bacteria even in the stable clinical state [4].

Factors influencing bronchial inflammation

Cigarette smoking is associated with greater concentrations of pro-inflammatory cytokines in airway secretions. Once disease is established, cessation of smoking partially reverses the process, leading to a fall in the concentration of the neutrophil chemoattractant IL-8 and myeloperoxidase (MPO) (a marker of neutrophil recruitment and activation). Corticosteroids exert an anti-inflammatory action; although some workers have failed to demonstrate an effect of inhaled steroids [5], others have shown that they reduce neutrophil numbers in the airway and protein leakage, and influence the chemotactic activity of secretions as well as increasing protection against proteolytic enzymes [6]. These differences in the published literature may reflect not only the patients studied but also the method of sampling.

Bacterial colonisation is associated with an increase in inflammation which depends on the size of the colonising bacterial load. As the load increases, so do the concentrations of the chemoattractants IL-8 and LTB4 (Fig. 2). This is associated with greater neutrophil recruitment, as indicated by an increase in MPO concentration.

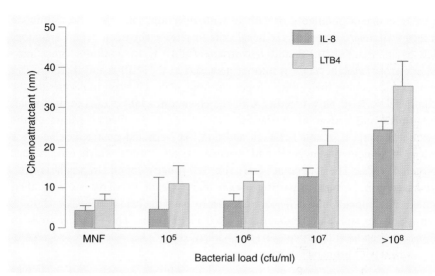

Fig. 2 Relationship of neutrophil chemoattractants to microbial load in the airway. Results are shown for samples containing small numbers of mixed normal flora (MNF) or where the culture of a single organism yielded more than 10^5 colony forming units/ml (IL = interleukin; LTB = leukotriene B (figure derived, with permission, from data to be published in the *American Journal of Medicine* [7]).

α-1-antitrypsin deficiency is also related to the degree of inflammation in the airway. A low concentration of this inhibitor will reduce the protection of the airway from the effects of elastase released by neutrophils which will, in turn, facilitate the vicious circle (Fig. 1) and lead to a greater degree of protein leakage, generation of chemoattractants and persistence of free elastase activity in the airway [8].

Sputum assessment

MPO is stored within the azurophil granule of the neutrophil. This protein is yellow/green in colour and accounts for the typical colouration of purulent fluids. This makes it possible to assess objectively the MPO concentration of airway secretions. This objective measure is clearly related to the colour of the secretions, as determined by matching to a specific colour chart (Fig. 3). Furthermore, the colour is also related (as would be expected) to the number of neutrophils present in the secretions (Fig. 4). The simple assignment of a sputum colour relates well with the degree of airway inflammation. For instance, sample-assigned colours 0–2 show little inflammation with low concentrations of neutrophil chemoattractants, protein leakage and neutrophil products. As the samples become macroscopically purulent (nos. 3–8) the concentration of the chemoattractants, protein leakage and neutrophil products rises progressively. Furthermore, the degree of inflammation relates clearly to the size of the colonising bacterial load within the airway (Fig. 5). Thus, simple assessment of sputum colour indicates the degree of inflammation in the bronchial tree.

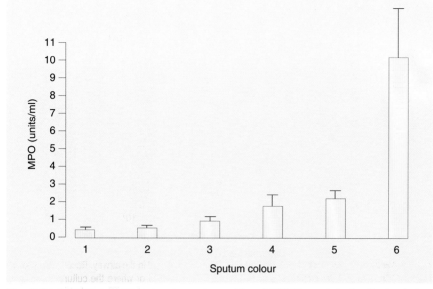

Fig. 3 Relationship of sputum colour to myeloperoxidase (MPO) (figure derived, with permission, from data to be published in the *American Journal of Medicine* [7]).

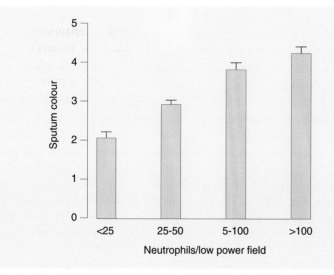

Fig. 4 Relationship of sputum colour to secretion neutrophils. Neutrophil numbers for a low power field of sputum smear are grouped as shown (data reproduced, with permission, from [9]).

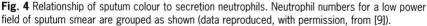

☐ PRACTICAL CONSIDERATIONS

Exacerbations

Exacerbations of COPD are episodes in which patients note a worsening of their symptoms. These include an increase in breathlessness, more sputum and a change in sputum purulence. In addition, patients may develop new chest pain, fatigue or

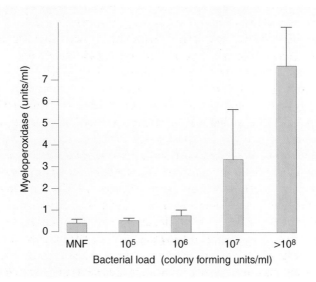

Fig. 5 Concentration of myeloperoxidase in sputum samples shown as a mean histogram plus standard error related to the bacterial load in the samples (figure derived, with permission, from data to be published in the *American Journal of Medicine* [7]) (MNF = mixed normal flora).

pyrexia. The management of these exacerbations remains empirical. Conventional therapy includes antibiotics, steroids and inhaled bronchodilator therapy. Whether such therapies are needed in individual cases remains a matter of clinical judgement in association with evidence-based guidelines.

Antibiotics undoubtedly have a place in acute exacerbations. Meta-analysis has shown an advantage for such therapy [10]. Anthonisen and colleagues [11] showed a statistical advantage of antibiotic therapy when all three major symptoms of an exacerbation were present: increased breathlessness, sputum volume and sputum purulence (Table 1). If only one or two of these symptoms were present, antibiotic therapy had no demonstrable advantage. However, despite this finding, published guidelines suggest that antibiotic therapy should be given to all patients with two or more of the three major symptoms.

Table 1 Symptoms of exacerbation.

Major symptoms	↑ Breathlessness
	↑ Sputum volume
	↑ Sputum purulence
Minor symptoms	Chest pain/tightness
	Fatigue
	Wheeze
	↑ Cough
	Pyrexia

The role of steroids in the exacerbation has also been uncertain, but two recent studies have indicated that they have an advantage over placebo [12,13] and patients on long-term inhaled steroids appear to have fewer exacerbations than those on placebo. These clinical studies, although showing a significant advantage of different therapies, do not clearly define their role in an individual patient.

In view of rising incidental bacterial resistance to commonly prescribed antibiotics, it is becoming increasingly important to use these agents rationally. An understanding of the interaction between bacteria and the lung defences may help in decision making, as it is to be expected that antibiotic therapy would have an advantage only in the presence of a new bacterial infection. Many patients have bacterial colonisation of the airway even in the stable clinical state which makes the interpretation of sputum microbiology difficult in COPD. However, the development of a new bacterial infection or an increase in the colonising bacterial load above that in the stable state changes the degree of inflammation in the airway. This can be detected by a change in sputum colour as the number of neutrophils recruited in response to the bacterial infection increases (Fig. 6). Purulent exacerbations are also associated with a clear rise in serum C-reactive protein, indicating a systemic effect of the episode (Fig. 7).

On the other hand, in subjects who present with mucoid sputum during their exacerbation, the bacterial load isolated from their sputum samples is no greater than in the stable state, and airway inflammation remains unaltered. This provides strong evidence to support withholding antibiotic therapy in such patients, but the nature and management of these episodes remain to be clarified.

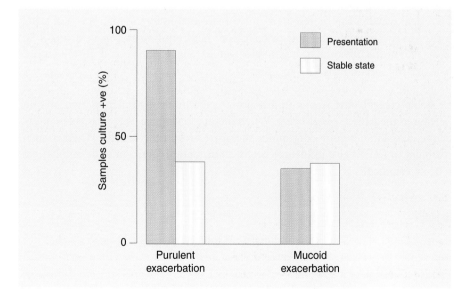

Fig. 6 Proportion of samples culture positive ($>10^5$ colony forming units/ml) for a single identified pathogen. (Repeated measure) data are shown for patients with chronic obstructive pulmonary disease who presented with a purulent or mucoid exacerbation (data reproduced, with permission, from [9]).

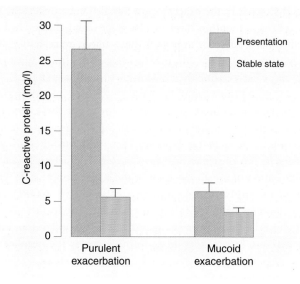

Fig. 7 Average serum C-reactive protein in patients with chronic obstructive pulmonary disease who presented with a purulent or mucoid exacerbation of their condition (data reproduced, with permission, from [9]).

Stable clinical state

Some patients' airways remain colonised by bacteria even when clinically stable. Increasing bacterial isolation is associated with worsening lung function, although it is not clear whether this represents a cause or effect. However, as high bacterial loads in the airway stimulate the host defences and neutrophil recruitment, it might be expected that the inflammation generated would damage the lung in the long term. Whether this situation is also an indication for antimicrobial therapy is currently uncertain; however, in patients with purulent bronchiectasis, antibiotic therapy in the stable clinical state results in a major change in airway inflammation and an increase in the patient's well-being. When therapy is stopped, these patients rapidly relapse, and some require continuous therapy to retain the benefit. Whether such treatment in COPD also influences health status and progression of disease has yet to be determined.

Steroids

Many patients with COPD are on long-term inhaled steroids, although this has not been shown to prevent progression of disease [14]. It has, however, long been clinical practice to give patients with a diagnostic label of COPD a trial of steroid therapy, and some patients do improve both clinically and physiologically. Recent studies with induced sputum have suggested that patients who have a significant number of eosinophils in the airway secretions are most likely to be those who benefit from steroid therapy. This clearly identifies a subset of patients who respond to steroids and it may be that these patients represent a more 'asthmatic' phenotype of COPD. It is important to note that other workers have identified an increase in eosinophils during some exacerbations, even though neutrophils still predominate; it is possible that this represents a further subset of patients in whom steroid therapy is most effective during the exacerbation. Eosinophil peroxidase, secreted by eosinophils, is also yellow in colour and a big increase in these cell numbers in the airway could, in some individuals, change the colour of the sputum. Thus, specific management of exacerbations of COPD could, in future, be determined not only by the sputum colour but also by microscopic assessment of sputum to determine its cellular content and the presence of bacteria on Gram stain. Purulent exacerbations in which neutrophils are predominant and there is little eosinophilia would require antibiotic therapy, whereas those with a significant eosinophil content may benefit from steroid therapy with or without antibiotics. Further work needs to be carried out to determine the appropriate rational therapy for such episodes. In the meantime, it seems appropriate to withhold antibiotic therapy from all exacerbations in which the sputum is mucoid, irrespective of the results of bacterial culture.

☐ FUTURE APPROACHES

As our understanding of the processes involved in airway inflammation in patients with bronchial disease increases it will be possible to develop specifically targeted therapeutic options. For instance, a reduction in neutrophil recruitment to the lung would be expected to reduce tissue damage as a cellular byproduct of this process. This could include approaches that reduce production of the chemoattractants, block their neutrophil receptors, reduce the ability of the neutrophil to respond to the chemoattractant, or block or decrease endothelial binding of the neutrophil to the relevant adhesion molecules (a critical process in cell migration).

Alternatively, it may be possible to reduce the destructive potential of the neutrophil whilst still promoting its recruitment and activation. For instance, inhibition of elastase within the cell could lead to less damage as the cell migrates, whereas supplementation of the anti-elastase defence of the lung by the oral or inhaled route may protect the lung tissues and prevent perpetuation and progression of the vicious circle indicated in Fig. 1. Finally, if bacteria play a key role in the pathogenesis of COPD and bronchial disease in general, understanding the interactions between the bacteria and the host that lead to inflammation may also result in the development of alternative (non-antibiotic) effective antibacterial strategies.

REFERENCES

1   Murray CJL, Lopez AD. Evidence-based health policy – lessons from the Global Burden of Disease Study. *Science* 1996; **274**: 740–3.

2   Eriksson S. Studies in α-1-antitrypsin deficiency. *Acta Med Scand* 1965; **177**: S1–85.

3   Suzuki T, Wang W, Linn J-T, *et al.* Aerosolised human neutrophil elastase induces airways constriction and hyperresponsiveness with protection by intravenous pre-treatment with half-length secretory protease inhibitor. *Am J Respir Crit Care Med* 1996; **153**: 1405–11.

4   Monso E, Ruiz J, Rosell A. Bacterial infection in chronic obstructive pulmonary disease: a study of stable and exacerbated outpatients using the protected specimen brush. *Am J Respir Crit Care Med* 1995; 152: 1316–20.

5   Culpitt SV, Maziak W, Loukidis S, *et al.* Effect of high dose inhaled steroid on cells, cytokines and proteases in induced sputum in chronic obstructive pulmonary disease. *Am J Respir Crit Care Med* 1999; 160: 1635–9.

6   Llewellyn-Jones CG, Harris TAJ, Stockley RA. Effect of fluticasone propionate on sputum of patients with chronic bronchitis and emphysema. *Am J Respir Crit Care Med* 1996; 153: 616–21.

7   Hill AJ, Campbell EJ, Hill SL, *et al.* Airway bacterial load in stable chronic bronchitis: a potent stimulus for airway inflammation. *Am J Med* 2000 (in press).

8   Hubbard RC, Fells G, Gadek J, *et al.* Neutrophil accumulation in the lung in alpha-1-antitrypsin deficiency; spontaneous release of leukotriene B4 by alveolar macrophages. *J Clin Invest* 1991; 88: 891–7.

9   Stockley RA, O'Brien C, Pye A, Hill SL. Relationship of sputum color to nature and patient management of acute exacerbations of COPD. *Chest* 2000; 117: 1638–45.

10 Saint S, Bent S, Vittinghoff E, Gradey D. Antibiotics in chronic obstructive pulmonary disease exacerbations, a meta-analysis. *JAMA* 1995; 273: 957–60.

11 Anthonisen NR, Manfreda J, Warren CP, *et al.* Antibiotic therapy in exacerbations of chronic obstructive pulmonary disease. *Ann Intern Med* 1987; 106: 196–204.

12 Thompson WH, Nielson CP, Carvalho P, *et al.* Controlled trial of oral prednisolone in outpatients with acute COPD exacerbation. *Am J Respir Crit Care Med* 1996; 154: 407–12.

13 Niewoehner DE, Erbland ML, Deupree RH, *et al.* Effective systemic glucocorticoids on exacerbations of chronic obstructive pulmonary disease. *N Engl J Med* 1999; 340: 1941–7.

14 Pauwels RA, Lofdahl C-D, Laitinen LA, *et al.* Long-term treatment with inhaled budesonide in persons with mild chronic obstructive pulmonary disease who continue smoking. *N Engl J Med* 1999; 340: 1948–53.

☐ SELF ASSESSMENT QUESTIONS

1   Neutrophil elastase has been shown to:
   (a) Produce bronchitis
   (b) Produce emphysema
   (c) Interfere with bacterial culture
   (d) Turn sputum green
   (e) Inactivate cilia

2   Bacterial culture of sputum chronic obstructive pulmonary disease (COPD):
   (a) Is rarely helpful
   (b) Is important only during exacerbations
   (c) Differentiates patients who need antibiotics
   (d) Supports the decision to prescribe steroids
   (e) Is rarely positive in the stable state

3   In acute exacerbations of COPD:
   (a) Steroids are shown to be of benefit
   (b) Antibiotics rarely help
   (c) Breathlessness is an indication for antibiotic therapy

(d) Raised C-reactive protein is associated with a need for antibiotic therapy
(e) Monitoring neutrophil recruitment guides antibiotic prescribing

4   Important symptoms to determine antibiotic therapy for acute exacerbations of COPD include:
(a) Chest pain
(b) Breathlessness
(c) Increased sputum volume
(d) Lethargy
(e) Any three of the above

5   The following are features of purulent sputum in COPD:
(a) High eosinophil numbers
(b) High neutrophil numbers
(c) Positive bacterial culture
(d) Increased concentration of leukotriene B4
(e) Raised myeloperoxidase activity

ANSWERS

1a True	2a False	3a True	4a False	5a False
b True	b False	b False	b False	b True
c False	c False	c False	c False	c True
d False	d False	d True	d False	d True
e True	e False	e True	e False	e True

The Lumleian Lecture
Gene-environment interactions in the pathogenesis of asthma

Stephen T Holgate

☐ INTRODUCTION

Asthma is a chronic inflammatory disorder involving a range of effector cells that include activated mast cells, eosinophils and macrophages. Through the release of inflammatory mediators, cytokines and growth factors, the airways become dysfunctional and exhibit enhanced responsiveness to a wide variety of direct (eg inhaled methacholine) and indirect (eg exercise) stimuli (bronchial hyper-responsiveness (BHR)) [1]. An additional important series of pathophysiological processes that characterise chronic asthma is restructuring of the conducting airways, with damage to the epithelium, increase in epithelial goblet cells, deposition of sub-basement membrane collagen, submucosal swelling with increased and altered matrix, proliferation of microvessels and nerves, and hypertrophy and hyperplasia of the spiral smooth muscle [2]. These changes, which represent 'remodelling', alter the way the airways respond to external stimuli and may be linked to the chronic decline in pulmonary function seen in asthmatics at a population level [3] and in asthma that is relatively refractory to the anti-inflammatory actions of corticosteroids.

☐ PATHOPHYSIOLOGY OF AIRWAY INFLAMMATION

When expressed as the population attributable risk, atopy (the propensity to generate immunoglobulin (Ig)E against common environmental allergens) accounts for up to 40% of the asthma phenotype in both adults and children [4]. This figure is somewhat lower than that given by those who cite the epidemiological literature selectively and takes account of individuals in the population who are atopic but not asthmatic. In the UK and other developed countries the incidence of atopy is as high as 50% of the population and yet asthma, while still fairly common, has a prevalence of 7–10%. Based on these statistics, it is difficult to attribute a direct relationship between atopy and asthma, otherwise all people who were atopic and were exposed to the relevant aero-allergens would express lower airways disease. Atopy, however, still remains the greatest risk factor for developing childhood asthma, especially if it is expressed at a young age [5]. Within a family, atopy compared to non-atopy in siblings increases the risk of asthma 11–20 fold. Bronchoalveolar lavage and limited mucosal studies indicate that the acquisition of childhood asthma (as distinct from recurrent virus-induced wheezing) is accompanied by an increase in activated mast cells and eosinophils and the presence of subepithelial fibrosis [6,7]. The 20–60 fold inter-country difference in the prevalence of atopic diseases (including asthma) in 7–9 and 11–13 year old children, as revealed by the International Study of Asthma and Allergies in Children (ISAAC) conducted in 56 countries [8], provides strong evidence for important genetic and environmental influences over the disease origins (Fig. 1). The rising trends of atopic

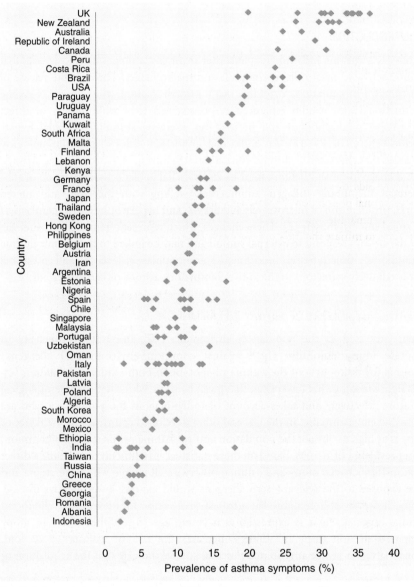

Fig. 1 Self-reported asthma symptoms of 12-month prevalence from written questionnaires (the International Study of Asthma and Allergies in Children, reproduced with permission from [8]).

disorders and asthma over the past three decades in many of these countries [9] provide further evidence for the importance of environmental factors.

Irrespective of whether asthma is accompanied by atopy, almost all forms of the disease are characterised by mast cell and eosinophil infiltration linked to the co-ordinate upregulation of a small cluster of cytokine genes encoded on the chromosome 5q31–33. These include interleukins (IL)-3, -4, -5, -9, -13 and granulocyte-macrophage colony stimulating factor (GM-CSF) [10]. These cytokines are responsible for initiating isotype switching of B cells from IgM to IgE, the growth and maturation of mast cells, basophils and eosinophils, as well as prolonging the survival of these cells by inhibiting apoptosis [10,11] (Fig. 2). IL-4 and -13 also have important functions in upregulating vascular cell adhesion molecule-1 involved in the recruitment of eosinophils, basophils and T helper (Th)-2 cells from the circulation into the airways and for inducing goblet cell formation and subepithelial fibrosis [12,13].

In non-atopic (late onset) 'intrinsic' and occupational asthma, cytokines of the IL-4 gene cluster are generated by activated T lymphocytes usually, although not exclusively, of the CD4 (helper) subtype. The increased airway population of Th-2 cells is offset by a reduced number of T cells expressing interferon (IFN)-γ and IL-2 (Th-1 cells). When asthma or atopic disease is successfully treated with corticosteroids or allergen-specific immunotherapy, the imbalance between these two functional populations of T cells is restored. This has given rise to the hypothesis that in asthma the imbalance between the T cell subsets provides the cytokine repertoire to initiate the inflammatory responses [14].

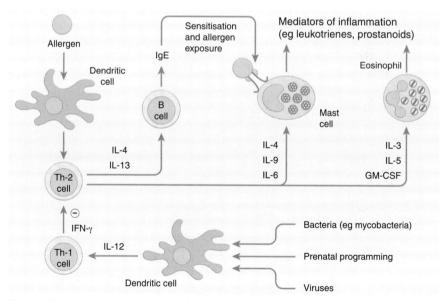

Fig. 2 Schematic representation of the cytokine pathways underlying the T helper (TH)-2 lymphocyte. Mediated inflammatory response in allergic asthma (GM-CSF = granulocyte-macrophage colony stimulating factor; IFN = interferon; Ig = immunoglobulin; IL = interleukin).

In asthma provoked by exposure to known allergens, the T cell response is driven by the presentation of selected allergen peptides by professional antigen presenting cells (APCs) (especially dendritic cells) to naïve T cells in local lymphoid collections. Effective responses require that the allergen peptide is presented in the cleft of major histocompatibility class (MHC) II molecules on the surface of APCs, to the T cell receptor, simultaneous co-stimulation employing additional signalling molecules (CD80 or CD86 (B7-1 or B7-2) on APCs and CD28 on T cells [15]), and an appropriate cytokine microenvironment (IL-12 and IL-18 for Th-1, and IL-4 and IL-10 for Th-2 polarisation [14]) (Fig. 3). On contact with allergen, and in the presence of GM-CSF, dendritic cells in the epithelium and submucosa migrate under the influence of GM-CSF to the local lymphoid collections where effective antigen presentation occurs.

Migration of dendritic cells and T cells involves the expression of selective homing molecules, some of which are receptors for specific chemoattractant molecules, the chemokines. Chemokines are also fundamental to the recruitment of inflammatory cells into the asthmatic airways. Among the ever increasing list of chemokines and their receptors, the CCR-3 receptor, which responds to the CXC chemokines RANTES, monocyte chemoattractant proteins (MCP)-1, -3 and -4 and the eotaxins (Eot)-1, -2 and -3, is particularly relevant [16]. It seems that these chemokines are intimately involved not only in the recruitment of eosinophils, basophils and Th-2 T cells and their precursors from the circulation, but also synergise with IL-3, IL-5 and GM-CSF in mobilising eosinophils from the bone marrow into the circulation in preparation for their recruitment into the airways. Whether derived from the circulation or from CD34+ precursors present in the

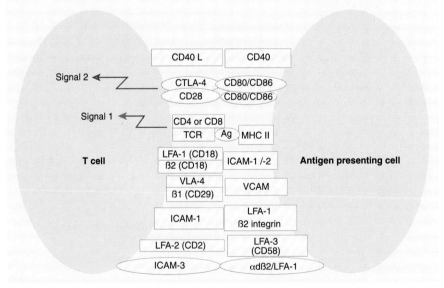

Fig. 3 Cognate interaction between antigen presenting cell accessory molecules and their ligands on T lymphocytes (Ag = antigen; MHC = major histocompatibility complex; LFA = lymphocyte function associated antigen; ICAM = intercellular adhesion molecule; TCR = T cell receptor; VCAM = vascular cell adhesion molecule; VLA = very late antigen).

airways themselves, activated mast cells, eosinophils, basophils and macrophages are the source of a wide range of autacoid mediators, enzymes, proteoglycans and cytokines that interact with the formed elements of the airways to cause dysfunction and symptoms of asthma [17]. Prominent amongst these are:

- □ the cysteinyl leukotrienes (LTs) (slow reacting substance (SRS-A); LTC_4, LTD_4 and LTE_4) which have potent effects on cysteinyl LT_1 receptors that contract airway smooth muscle, increase microvascular leakage and enhance eosinophil recruitment [18]

- □ mast cell proteases (especially tryptase) that mediate some of their effects via protease activated receptors to enhance inflammation and promote remodelling [19], and

- □ a range of Th-2 cytokines, chemokines and growth factors.

□ THERAPEUTIC INTERVENTIONS BASED ON PATHOPHYSIOLOGY

Inhaled corticosteroids have revolutionised the clinical management of asthma by interacting with many of the inflammatory pathways, especially those controlling and controlled by Th-2 cytokines. Their predominant mode of action is via corticosteroid receptors that, when activated, block the interactions of pro-inflammatory nuclear transcription factors such as NF-κB, activator protein (AP-1) and STAT-1, with nuclear histones and gene promoters linked to the induction of pro-inflammatory molecules such as adhesion molecules, inducible enzymes, chemokines and cytokines [20].

On the other hand, the β_2-adrenoceptor agonists interact with the formed airway elements, especially the smooth muscle, to produce bronchodilatation and functional antagonism against contractile mediators such as the cysteinyl LTs. Thus, in patients requiring more than a moderate dose of an inhaled corticosteroid, recent guidelines support the addition of a long-acting inhaled β_2-agonist, such as salmeterol or formoterol, in preference to progressively increasing the dose of inhaled corticosteroid. This approach is supported by the flat dose-response curve of corticosteroids and the possibility that long-acting β_2-agonists may have additional effects on components of the airway inflammation beyond that achieved with corticosteroids alone [21].

Following the structural elucidation of SRS-A as three cysteinyl LTs and the subsequent discovery of the cyst LT_1-receptor that mediates their pro-inflammatory and contractile effects, selective antagonists have been developed that include montelukast, zafirlukast and pranlukast. These LT receptor antagonists (LTRAs) are efficacious in asthma and offer the advantages of a once or twice daily oral medication without the attendant systemic effects of corticosteroids [22]. However, it seems that not all asthmatic patients are equally responsive [23]. We have recently reported that good responders to this drug class have enhanced LTC_4 production and increased expression of the terminal LT-forming enzyme, LTC_4 synthase, which is also encoded on chromosome 5q but some distance from the IL-4 gene cluster [24].

The identification of a polymorphism (-444A→C) in the promoter of LTC$_4$ synthase produces an extra transcriptional binding site to upregulate the activity of this enzyme. The same polymorphism has also been described to have a strong association with aspirin intolerant asthma [25], a form of asthma that is especially responsive to LTRAs and inhibitors of the LT generating enzyme 5-lipoxygenase (5-LO), and is a form of asthma that is accompanied by greatly enhanced cysteinyl LT production [26]. In selectively targeting this mediator pathway to reduce LT effects, it is highly likely that other gene polymorphisms will be discovered that will help explain more of the asthmatic population's response to this drug class and possibly form the basis of a pre-treatment screening test.

The importance of IgE as a sensing and effector molecule in allergen induced asthma and other diseases linked to atopy has provided the basis for developing a novel therapeutic IgE blocking antibody, Mab E25 [27]. This fully 'humanised' IgG has been raised against an epitope expressed on that part of the IgE molecule that binds with high affinity to the α-chain of the trimeric high affinity IgE receptor (Fc$_\varepsilon$R$_1$) and also to the low affinity IgE receptor Fc$_\varepsilon$R$_2$ (CD23). Thus, when IgE is bound to mast cells, basophils, dendritic cells or any other cell where it serves as an allergen-directed signalling molecule, Mab E25 is unable to bind because the relevant epitope is hidden through its interaction with Fc$_\varepsilon$R$_1$ or Fc$_\varepsilon$R$_2$ (Fig. 4). In functional terms, this renders Mab E25 non-anaphylactogenic and unable to activate mast cells or basophils for mediator secretion. When administered to atopic subjects Mab E25 results in a rapid clearance of free IgE from the blood and then from tissues by forming hexameric complexes that are effectively cleared by the reticulo-endothelial system. When administered at two-weekly intervals over nine weeks to mild atopic asthmatics, Mab E25 greatly attenuated both the early and late phase bronchoconstrictor responses to inhaled allergen, reduced the allergen acquired

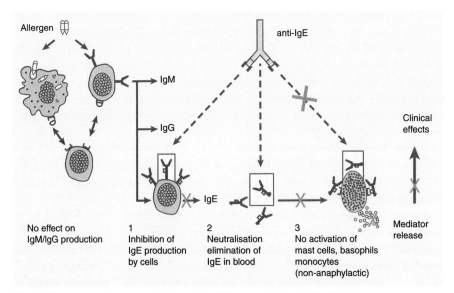

Fig. 4 The concept of non-anaphylactogenic anti-immunoglobulin (Ig)E antibodies.

increase in BHR and inhibited the accompanying sputum eosinophilia [27]. Three 12-week clinical trials of Mab E25 in moderate-to-severe asthma, one in children and two in adults [28–30], have revealed clear efficacy in measures of lung function, requirement for inhaled and oral corticosteroids, symptom scores, requirement for short acting β_2-agonists and quality of life. However, as with the LTRAs, not all patients responded equally well despite falls in circulating free IgE by over 98%, suggesting that IgE-triggered pathways are of central importance in only a proportion of patients. One particular finding which has an important bearing on the efficacy of Mab E25 is the marked (ca 1,000-fold) reduction in the number and function of $Fc_\varepsilon R_1$ receptors on circulating basophils after several weeks of treatment [31]. If this is paralleled by a similar reduction in $Fc_\varepsilon R_1$ on effector cells in affected tissues, it could in part explain the overall efficacy that this novel treatment produces – because not only is $Fc_\varepsilon R_1$ involved in triggering mediator release but it also enhances allergen uptake by tissue dendritic cells [32]. The effective, albeit temporary, removal of IgE using Mab E25 opens up new therapeutic opportunities for highly allergic patients in whom allergen specific immunotherapy is either not possible or is too dangerous because of the risk of provoking anaphylaxis. Another possibility is its use to enable allergen immunotherapy to be undertaken more safely since, as currently used, immunotherapy has the capacity to cause anaphylaxis via IgE triggering of mast cells and basophils. Examples of 'protected' anti-IgE immunotherapy might include extreme allergy to wasp and bee stings, ingested nuts, soya bean and contact with latex.

The eosinophil has been regarded as one of the principal effector cells of the chronic allergic response and asthma in particular. However, it should be stated that its role has been established by association rather than by *selective* interventions. For example, because inhaled or oral corticosteroids or LTRAs reduce blood tissue and sputum eosinophilia in parallel with their beneficial clinical effects does not necessarily mean that their efficacy is a consequence of this eosinophil reduction. IL-5 has been regarded as a pivotal cytokine involved in eosinophil maturation, recruitment, activation and survival [12] and, as such, has become a central focus for the development of a novel selective therapeutic intervention. While it has proven difficult to generate IL-5R antagonists, fully humanised blocking Mabs directed to IL-5 itself have been produced [33]. In animal models, blocking antibodies or deletion of the IL-5 gene have marked effects in inhibiting pulmonary antigen-provoked late phase responses, BHR and eosinophil infiltration. For example, in guinea-pigs and monkeys, anti-IL-5 Mabs, such as TRFK-5 and SB240563 respectively inhibit both blood and lung eosinophilia as well as BHR in sensitised animals [34,35]. Fully humanised IgG anti-IL-5 Mabs have a prolonged half-life in the circulation with effects that persist up to four months after a single administration.

Based on these encouraging results, the anti-IL-5 Mab SB240563 (mepolizumab) has been administered to atopic asthmatic subjects as a single intravenous injection, and efficacy followed as the peripheral blood and sputum eosinophil levels before and after allergen challenge, the asthmatic early and late responses, and BHR measured by inhaled methacholine provocation [36]. Mepolizumab at both 2.5 mg/kg and 10 mg/kg produced a progressive decrease in circulating eosinophils which, in the case of the higher dose, was by over 98%; this persisted to 16 weeks while, at the same time point for the lower dose, eosinophil numbers had returned to baseline. The high dose treatment also reduced sputum eosinophils post-allergen by more than 70% and blocked the increase in circulating eosinophils seen 24 hours following allergen challenge before treatment and with placebo. Despite these encouraging effects on eosinophils, mepolizumab had no effect on the early or late responses or on BHR. Clinical trials with both mepolizumab and a similar blocking Mab, SCH55700, when administered as single or multiple doses over 3–6 months, have shown little or no evidence of efficacy when assessed by standard asthma outcome measures [37]. These surprising findings cast some doubt over the previously held view that eosinophils are the mediator secreting cells in asthma, and might place the mast cell and tissue macrophage higher up the order of mediator secreting cells in this disease. One exception may be aspirin intolerant asthma where there occurs selective expression of LTC_4 synthase in eosinophils [38].

☐ THE GENETIC BASIS OF ATOPY AND ASTHMA: OPPORTUNITIES FOR NEW THERAPEUTICS

Asthma and related atopic disorders cluster in families. Clear differences have been shown in the prevalence of these disorders in monozygotic and dizygotic twins, in strong favour of the former [39]. Estimates for heritability are as high as 70% for atopy and 30–40% for BHR [39]. Whole genome screens using microsatellite markers evenly spaced across the whole genome have identified strong regions of linkage to asthma phenotypes on chromosomes 5, 6, 11, 12, 13 and 16. A meta-analysis of pooled published data from different genome screens has strengthened the confidence of linkage to these regions and helped in narrowing down the chromosomal locations [40]. Examples of the candidate genes located in these regions are shown in Table 1.

Apart from chromosome 6p containing the *MHC* and *TNF* gene clusters, and 5q31–33 containing the *IL-4* gene cluster, special interest has focused on chromosome 16p since maximum linkage overlies the *IL-4R* gene [40]. Twelve polymorphisms have been identified in this gene, of which six encode amino acid substitutions [41]. Association studies have convincingly demonstrated functional links of this gene to atopy and asthma. Several of the polymorphisms increase or decrease the ability of the IL-4R to interact with its transcription factors STAT-6 and the intracellular signalling molecules, insulin receptor substrate (IRS) 1/2 [42].

Based on these findings and the important role that IL-4 has in directing Th-2-mediated inflammation and interacting with the epithelium, endothelium and fibroblasts to alter their functions [42], IL-4 has become a new target against which to direct a novel therapy. The production of a soluble decoy in the form of human recombinant soluble IL-4R (sIL-4R; Nuvance) has provided an opportunity for intervening in this pathway [43]. When sIL-4R is administered by inhalation to mice it has powerful inhibitory effects on the antigen-induced lung eosinophilia and BHR, as well as preventing the goblet cell metaplasia that occurs with chronic inhaled antigen exposure. When administered as a single inhalation of 1.5 mg once

Table 1 Candidate genes and chromosome locations in asthma.

Candidate	Chromosome location	Function
IL-3	5q31-33	Eosinophil and basophil growth factor
IL-4	5q31-33	IgE switching, Th-2 polarisation, upregulation of VCAM-1, induction of mucus genes
IL-9	5q31-33	Mast cell growth factor
β_2-adrenoceptor	5q31-33	cAMP-dependent signalling
LTC$_4$ synthase	5q35	Cysteinyl LT generation
MHC class II	6p21.3-23	Antigen recognition
TNF-α	6p21.3-23	Pleiotropic cytokine
5-LO	10q11.2	LT synthesis
FC$_\varepsilon$R$_{1\beta}$ chain	11q13	Regulation of IgE signalling
CC16 (CC10, uteroglobulin)	11q12-13	Lung anti-inflammatory protein
NOS-1	12q24.3	Neural NO production
TCR-α chain	14q11.2	Antigen-driven immune responses
IL-4Rα	16p12	IL-4 signalling
TGF-β_1	19q13.1-13.3	↑IgE synthesis, profibrotic cytokine

cAMP = cyclic adenosine monophosphate; Ig = immunoglobulin; IL = interleukin; LO = lipoxygenase; LT = leukotriene; MHC = major histocompatibility complex; NO = nitric oxide; NOS = nitric oxide synthase; TCR = T cell receptor; TGF = transforming growth factor; Th = T helper; TNF = tumour necrosis factor; VCAM = vascular cell adhesion molecule.

weekly, sIL-4R enabled corticosteroids to be reduced and stopped in a high proportion of patients, without increase in symptoms or increased β_2-agonist use, or deterioration of lung function [44]. A further similar clinical trial in asthma has confirmed this efficacy. What is so remarkable is that efficacy becomes apparent despite the infrequency of administration, presumably due to the protein being a normal body constituent and therefore not treated as a chemical to be rapidly eliminated. Also, its 1–2 week onset of action suggests that sIL-4R is intervening in components of asthma that are not wholly dependent on Th-2 T cells, possibly epithelial cells on which the agent is directly delivered.

IL-13 shows 40% homology with IL-4 and, while it can interact with one of the IL-4 receptors (IL-13α_1), it also binds to a second receptor (IL-13α_2) for which no clear function has yet been found [13,42]. It is possible that this receptor acts as a decoy itself for the large amount of IL-13 secreted by asthmatic airways and renders the tissue more depending on IL-4. Both genetic variants of IL-13 or the IL-13α_1 receptor encoded on chromosome Xq13 are strongly associated with asthma [45]. Thus, the variant Gln 110 Arg which decreases the ability of this cytokine to bind to its receptors is associated with asthma rather than IgE levels, while the polymorphism of the α_1 chain of the IL-13α_1 RA1398G is associated with elevated IgE levels rather than asthma. Substitution of two amino acids on IL-4 creates an antagonist (double mutein) which is effective at both the IL-4 and the IL-13 receptors. Again, this and a selective IL-13 inhibitor have efficacy in a mouse model of allergic airway inflammation and trials will soon start in human asthma [46].

☐ THE ROLE OF THE ENVIRONMENT IN ATOPY AND ASTHMA

The wide geographical differences and the rising trends in disease prevalence point to important environmental factors initiating asthma and related atopic disorders in genetically susceptible subjects (Fig. 5). In many countries both atopy and asthma have increased in parallel with Westernisation of their populations [47]. It was anticipated that, on account of poorer air quality in Central and Eastern Europe prior to unification of Germany, the incidence of asthma and atopic disorders would be greater than in their Western neighbours. However, quite the reverse was found [52]. What is even more surprising is that, since unification, atopy has almost caught up to the levels in the West, but notably asthma has not [53]. A similar disparity between the prevalence of atopy and asthma has been noted in Africa where the prevalence of positive skin-prick tests to common allergens has increased from 10–12% twenty years ago to 30–45% currently. However, in the Gambia, Nigeria and Ethiopia this increase in atopy has not been paralleled by a similar increase in asthma or BHR [54].

Taken together, these findings suggest that environmental factors driving atopy and asthma may differ. Factors increasing the relative risk for atopy include increased allergen exposure, dysnutrition in pregnancy (associated with an increased head circumference), reduced δ13-polyunsaturated fatty acids in the diet, absence of breast feeding and reduced exposure to bacterial products such as endotoxins and unmethylated CG in DNA [55,56]. Thus, being brought up on a farm with livestock is strongly protective against atopy, possibly due to high exposure to animal faecal bacterial products early in life [56]. The interesting observations, that babies born of atopic mothers who later develop atopy have impaired production of IFN-γ by their circulating T cells at birth [57], and that those destined to develop atopy have impaired Th-1 mediated delayed hypersensitivity reactions to mycobacteria [58], suggest that reduced Th-1 rather than enhanced Th-2 polarisation of the T cell

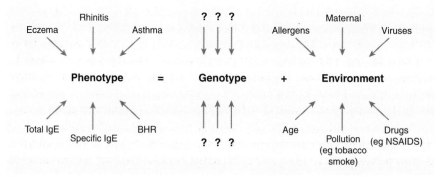

Fig. 5 Interactions between multiple genetic and environmental factors in the pathogenesis of atopy and asthma (BHR = bronchial hyperresponsiveness; Ig = immunoglobulin; NSAID = non-steroidal anti-inflammatory drug).

repertoire is primary (Fig. 2). It has recently been suggested that this is the result of reduced IL-12 receptor signalling, partly due to genetic deletion and polymorphisms of IL-12Rβ [59]. This fits with the hygiene hypothesis for atopy, which states that deprivation of appropriate bacterial stimulation of the immune system early in life predisposes to atopy in those children whose IFN-γ production is already impaired at birth [60]. A second recent suggestion is that alteration of the bowel flora consequent upon a Westernised lifestyle rather than reduced respiratory infections provides a more plausible explanation for the increase in atopy linked to a Western lifestyle. Animals raised in a sterile environment exhibit increased Th-2 responses and reduced immunological tolerance [60]. The absence of breast feeding, the premature introduction of a solid diet in weaning and excessive use of antibiotics can all change the intestinal flora to alter T cell programming. Environmental factors linked to asthma include maternal tobacco smoking, increased respiratory virus infections in childcare centres used by infants and toddlers, reduced anti-oxidant status, reduced intake of fish oils and increased intake of trans-fatty acids, impaired airway development accompanying prematurity [61] and an increased body mass index, especially in women [62].

These findings form a basis for preventive or therapeutic intervention studies. To date, very few allergen and dietary intervention studies have aimed to prevent atopy or asthma. Reduced maternal and early childhood exposure to dust mite and cat allergens, prolonged breast feeding and avoidance of early introduction of egg or cow's milk reduced the acquisition of atopy in a birth cohort of children on the Isle of Wight selected on the basis of one or more atopic parents. The 50% reduction in atopy seen at age 2, 5 and 7 years was not accompanied by a similar reduction in asthma [63,64]. This adds to the view that atopy and asthma are not equivalent and are dependent on separate but interacting gene-environment interactions [11,41,65].

There remains considerable controversy on the potential role of outdoor air pollution in asthma. While there is little doubt over the role of vehicle derived pollutants, ozone, oxides of nitrogen, sulphur dioxide and particles (PM_{10}) in exacerbating already established asthma [66], there is little evidence to support the view that increased exposure to these pollutants leads to the development of new asthma. However, particulates, especially those derived from diesel combustion, can enhance the capacity of B cells to generate IgE both *in vitro* and *in vivo* [67], and may synergise with IL-4 and IL-13 responses on other immune cells as well as on structural airway cells. The situation is even less clear with indoor air pollutants. Exposure to cigarette smoke actively or passively enhances sensitisation to occupational or domestic allergens [68,69]. The proteolytic activity of some allergens, such as those derived from house-dust mites (*Der p1* – cysteine protease, *Der p9* – serine protease), cats (*Fel d1*) or fungi, confers an advantage on certain proteins becoming allergenic by their capacity to disrupt epithelial tight junctions and enhance penetration into the airway tissue [68,69]. Blockade of this enzymic activity markedly reduces allergenicity in animal models of respiratory sensitisation.

Attempts are being made to harness the known environmental risk factors for atopy and asthma to develop new preventive or therapeutic interventions. For example, administration of intradermal *Mycobacterium vaccae* to atopic asthmatics is accompanied by a 30% reduction in the asthmatic late response with allergen challenge and a time-dependent reduction in IL-5 production by allergen-challenged peripheral blood mononuclear cells [70]. However, inhalation of IFN-γ, while reducing circulating eosinophils in a group of corticosteroid dependent asthmatics, had little effect on asthma outcome measures. Recently, we have systematically administered human recombinant (rh) IL-12 in four incremental doses of 0.1, 0.25, 0.5 and 0.5 µg/kg at weekly intervals and monitored eosinophil and asthma variables [71]. As with the anti-IL-5 Mabs, rhIL-12 resulted in a stepwise decrease in circulating eosinophils and an approximately 60% reduction in sputum eosinophils post allergen but, in common with the anti-IL-5 intervention, this was not accompanied by any change in the early or late response or in BHR. The rhIL-12 caused transient fever and flu-like symptoms including headache. These negative findings strengthen the concern over whether the eosinophil is fundamental to disordered airway functioning in asthma.

☐ ASTHMA: A NEW PARADIGM OF INFLAMMATION AND REPAIR

The failure of reducing eosinophil numbers by targeted therapies to affect asthma outcome measures, and the interdependence of atopy and asthma in epidemiological studies, raise the possibility that additional important pathways beyond Th-2-driven inflammation are needed to express the disease. The presence of epithelial stress and injury, the deposition of interstitial collagens in the lamina reticularis beneath the epithelial basement membrane, which occurs in all types of asthma irrespective of atopy and proliferation of myofibroblasts in the submucosa, suggest that the epithelial-mesenchymal trophic unit, which is fundamental for fetal branching morphogenesis and involves reciprocal signalling by epidermal growth factors and transforming growth factors (TGF)-β_1 and -β_2 (Fig. 6), becomes inactivated in asthma [65]. The same growth factor pathways are over-expressed in chronic asthma and we suggest that this underpins the airway wall remodelling response (Fig. 7) [73]. Reactivation of the trophic unit in asthma is explained by the impaired ability of the asthmatic epithelium to restitute itself following injury by viruses, pollutants or inflammatory events [73]. When the epithelium is impaired in its ability to proliferate, as evidenced by increased expression of the cell cycle inhibitor p21[WAF] and reduced expression of proliferating cell nuclear antigen [74], it produces profibrogenic growth factors [75] such as TGF-βs which further inhibit epithelial repair and activate remodelling responses including the conversion of fibroblasts to more active myofibroblasts [76] (Fig. 8). The altered asthmatic epithelium is also an important source of GM-CSF with its capacity to initiate dendritic cell migration and enhance Th-2 responses [77]. Thus, the finding that both inflammatory and epithelial changes are present in the airways of children up to four years before they develop asthma [7] provides support for the view that this disease is primarily a disease of the epithelium, with both inflammatory and remodelling responses occurring in parallel rather than sequentially (Fig. 9). This hypothesis can accommodate the separate susceptibility genes for atopy and asthma, the differential influence of environmental factors and the variable clinical phenotype (Fig. 10).

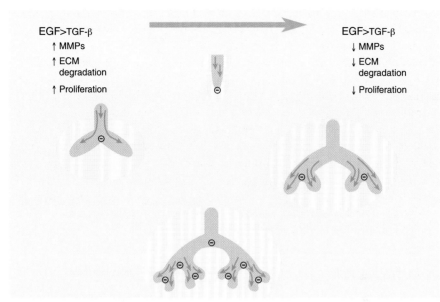

Fig. 6 Regulation of fetal branching morphogenesis of the lung by epidermal growth factor (EGF) and transforming growth factor (TGF)-β (ECM = extracellular matrix; MMP = matrix metalloproteinase).

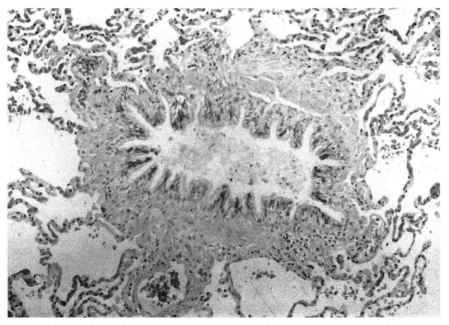

Fig. 7 A 'remodelled' asthmatic small airway showing submucosal collagen thickening, smooth muscle hyperplasia and goblet cell metaplasia with hypersecretion of mucus but little inflammation. Note the normal alveolar architecture.

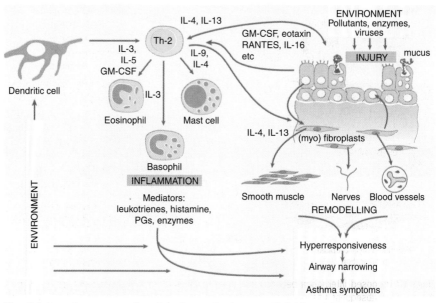

Fig. 8 Schematic representation of the interaction between Th-2-driven inflammation and inactive epithelial-mesenchymal trophic unit in asthma to generate both airway inflammatory and remodelling events linked to abnormal airway function (GM-CSF = granulocyte-macrophage colony stimulating factor; IL = interleukin; PG = prostaglandin; Th = T helper).

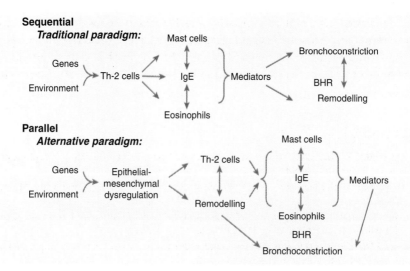

Fig. 9 Traditional 'linear' and proposed 'parallel' pathways linking airway inflammation and remodelling in asthma. In the parallel model, it is suggested that the airway microenvironment is initially disturbed and this is then host to a chronic inflammatory response (BHR = bronchial hyperreactivity; Ig = immunoglobulin; Th = T helper).

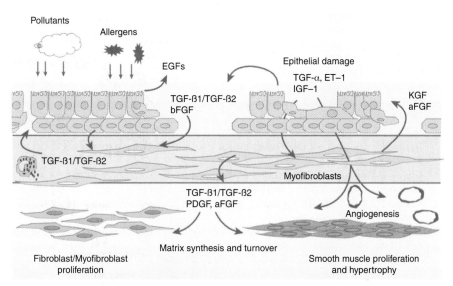

Fig. 10 Proposed interaction between inhaled environmental stimuli, epithelial injury but delayed repair and subsequent tissue remodelling involving myofibroblasts that propagate growth factor signals to airway structural cells (aFGF = acidic fibroblast growth factor; bFGF = basic fibroblast growth factor; EGF = epidermal growth factor; ET = endothelin; IGF = insulin-like growth factor; KGF = keratinocyte growth factor; PDGF = platelet-derived growth factor; TGF = transforming growth factor).

A parallel rather than a linear model that encompasses Th-2 mediated inflammation and remodelling also explains the variable phenotype of asthma and why, in most cases, the disease is not progressive.

If an altered set point at which the trophic unit responds to the external environment turns out to be fundamental to the development of asthma, it opens up new opportunities for preventing and treating the disorder based upon increasing the resistance to the inhaled environment and restoring the epithelial repair response (Fig. 10).

REFERENCES

1   Djukanovic R, Roche WR, Wilson JW, *et al.* Mucosal inflammation in asthma. State of the art. *Am Rev Respir Dis* 1990; **142**: 434–57.

2   Holgate ST. The cellular and mediator basis of asthma in relation to natural history. *Lancet* 1997; **350**: 5–9.

3   Lange P, Parner J, Vestbo J, *et al.* A 15 year follow up study of ventilatory function in adults with asthma. *N Engl J Med* 1998; **339**: 1194–200.

4   Pearce N, Pekkanen J, Beasley R. How much asthma is really attributable to atopy? *Thorax* 1999; **54**: 268–72.

5   Custovic A, Smith A, Woodcock A. Indoor allergens are a primary cause of asthma. *Eur Respir J* 1998; **53**: 155–8.

6   Stevenson EC, Turner G, Heaney LG, *et al.* Bronchoalveolar lavage findings suggest two different forms of childhood asthma. *Clin Exp Allergy* 1997; **27**: 1027–35.

7   Warner JO, Marguet C, Rao R, *et al.* Inflammatory mechanisms in childhood asthma. *Clin Exp Allergy* 1998; **28** (Suppl 5): 71–5.

8   Beasley R, Keil U, von Mutius E, Pearce N. ISAAC Steering Committee: worldwide variation in prevalence of symptoms of asthma, allergic rhinoconjunctivitis and atopic eczema symptoms: ISAAC. *Lancet* 1998; **35**: 1225–32.

9   von Mutius E. The rising trends in asthma and allergic disease. *Clin Exp Allergy* 1998; **28**: 45–9.

10   O'Byrne PM, Postma DS. The many faces of airway inflammation. *Am J Respir Crit Care Med* 1999; **159**: S41–66.

11   Holgate ST. The epidemic of allergy and asthma. *Nature* 1999; **402**: B2–4.

12   Drazen JM, Arm JP, Austen KF. Sorting out the cytokines of asthma (commentary). *J Exp Med* 1996; **183**: 1–5.

13   Grunig G, Warnock M, Wakil AE, *et al.* Requirement for IL-13 independently of IL-4 in experimental asthma. *Science* 1998; **282**: 2261–3.

14   Umetsu DT, De Krugff RH. T$_{H1}$ and T$_{H2}$ CD4+ cells in human allergic diseases. *J Allergy Clin Immunol* 1997; **100**: 1–6.

15   Jaffar ZH, Stanciu L, Pandit A, *et al.* Essential role for both CD80 and CD86 costimulation, but not CD40 interactions, in allergen-induced Th2 cytokine production from asthmatic bronchial tissue: role for αβ, but not γδ, T cells. *J Immunol* 1999; **163**: 6283–91.

16   Ying S, Meng Q, Zeibecoglou K, *et al.* Eosinophil chemotactic chemokines (eotaxin, eotaxin-2, RANTES, monocyte chemotactic protein-3 (MCP-3) and MCP-4) and CC chemokine receptor 3 expression in bronchial biopsies from atopic and non-atopic (intrinsic) asthmatics. *J Immunol* 1999; **163**: 6321–9.

17   Shute JK, Hidi R. Chemotaxis and mechanisms of cell migration. In: Holgate ST, Busse WW (eds). *Inflammation Mechanisms in Asthma.* Series: Lenfant C (ed). *Lung Biology in Health and Disease,* vol. 117. New York: Marcel Dekker Inc, 1998: 755–81.

18   Lynch KR, O'Neill GP, Liu Q, *et al.* Characterisation of the human cysteinyl leukotriene Cys LT1 receptor. *Nature* 1999; **399**: 789–93.

19   Holgate ST, Lackie PM, Davies DE, *et al.* The bronchial epithelium as a key regulator of airway inflammation and remodelling in asthma. *Clin Exp Allergy* 1999; **29**: S90–5.

20   Hart L, Lim S, Adcock I, *et al.* Effects of inhaled corticosteroid therapy on expression and DNA-binding activity of nuclear factor KB in asthma. *Am J Respir Crit Care Med* 2000; **161**: 224–31.

21   Wallin A, Sandström T, Söderberg M, *et al.* Comparative study of the effects of formoterol and budesonide on symptoms, airway responsiveness and inflammation in asthma. *Am J Resp Crit Care Med* 1999; **159**: 79–86.

22   Sampson A, Holgate S. Leukotriene modifiers in the treatment of asthma. *Br Med J* 1998; **316**: 1257–8.

23   Laitinen LA, Naya IP, Binks S, Harris A. Comparison of efficacy of zafirlukast and low dose steroids in asthmatics on prn β$_2$ agonists. *Eur Respir J* 1997; **10**: S419.

24   Sampson AP, Siddiqui S, Cowburn AS, *et al.* Variant LTC$_4$ synthase allele modifies cysteinyl-leukotriene synthesis in eosinophils and predicts clinical response to zafirlukast. *Thorax* (in press).

25   Sanak M, Simon HU, Szczeklik A. Leukotriene C$_4$ synthase promoter polymorphism and risk of aspirin-induced asthma. *Lancet* 1997; **350**: 1599–600.

26   Nasser SMS, Lee TH. Inflammatory mechanisms of aspirin-sensitive asthma. In: Holgate ST, Busse WW (eds). *Inflammation Mechanisms in Asthma.* Series: Lenfant C (ed) *Lung Biology in Health and Disease,* vol. 117. New York: Marcel Dekker Inc, 1998: 823–44.

27   Holgate ST, Corne J, Jardieu P, *et al.* Treatment of allergic disease with anti-IgE. *Allergy* 1998; **53**: S83–8.

28   Milgrom H, Fick RB, Su JQ, *et al.* Treatment of allergic asthma with monoclonal anti-IgE antibody. *N Engl J Med* 1999; **341**: 1966–73.

29   Nayak A, Milgrom H, Berger W, *et al.* Rhumab-E25 improves quality of life (QOL) in children with allergic asthma. *Am J Respir Crit Care Med* 2000; **161**: A504.

30 Metzger WJ, Fick RB. E-25 Study Group Investigators. Corticosteroid (cs) withdrawal in a study of recombinant humanised monoclonal antibody to IgE (rhu mAB E25). *J Allergy Clin Immunol* 1998; **101**: S231.

31 MacGlashan DW, Bochner BS, Adelman DC, *et al.* Down regulation of $Fc_\epsilon R_1$ expression on human basophils during *in vivo* treatment of atopic patients with anti-IgE antibody. *J Immunol* 1997; **158**: 1438–45.

32 Tunon-de-Lara JM, Redington AE, Bradding P, *et al.* Dendritic cells in normal and asthmatic airways: expression of the α subunit of the high affinity immunoglobulin E receptor ($FC_\epsilon RI$-α). *Clin Exp Allergy* 1996; **26**: 648–55.

33 Cuss FM. Therapeutic effects of antibodies to interleukin-5. *Allergy* 1998; **45**: S97–100.

34 Mauser PJ, Pitman A, Witt A, *et al.* Inhibitory effect of TRFK-5 anti-IL-5 antibody in a guinea pig model of asthma. *Am Rev Respir Dis* 1993; **148**: 1623–7.

35 Egan RW, Umland SP, Cuss FM, Chapman RW. Biology of interleukin-5 and its relevance to allergic disease. *Allergy* 1996; **51**: 71–81.

36 Leckie MJ, Ten Brinke A, Khan J, *et al.* Effects of an interleukin-5 blocking monoclonal antibody on eosinophils, airway hyperresponsiveness and the response to allergen in patients with asthma. *Lancet* (in press).

37 Kips JC, O'Connor BJ, Langley SJ, *et al.* Results of a phase I trial with SCH 55700, a humanised anti-IL-5 antibody in severe persistent asthma. *Am J Respir Crit Care Med* 2000; **161**: A505.

38 Cowburn AS, Sladek K, Adamek L, *et al.* Over expression of leukotriene C4 synthase on bronchial biopsies of aspirin intolerant asthmatics. *J Clin Invest* 1998; **101**: 834–46.

39 Skadhenge LR, Christensen K, Kyrik KO, Sigsgaard T. Genetic and environmental influence on asthma: a population based study of 11,688 Danish twin pairs. *Eur Respir J* 1999; **13**: 8–14.

40 Lonjou C, Collins A, Ennis S, *et al.* Meta-analysis and retrospective collaboration: two methods to map oligogenes for atopy and asthma. *Clin Exp Allergy* 1999; **29**: S57–9.

41 Holgate ST. Genetic and environmental interactions in allergy and asthma. *J Allergy Clin Immunol* 1999; **104**: 1139–46.

42 Shirakawa T, Deichman KA, Izuhara K, *et al.* Atopy and asthma: genetic variants of IL-4 and IL-13 signalling. *Immunol Today* 2000; **21**: 60–4.

43 Maliszewski CR. Soluble IL-4 receptor inhibits airway inflammation following allergen challenge in a mouse model of asthma. *J Immunol* 200; **164**: 1086–95.

44 Borish LC, Nelson HS, Lanz MJ, *et al.* Interleukin-4 receptor in moderate atopic asthma: a phase I/II randomised, placebo-controlled trial. *Am J Respir Crit Care Med* 1999; **160**: 1816–23.

45 Heinzmann A, Mao X-Q, Akaiwa M, *et al.* Genetic variants of IL-13 signalling and human asthma and atopy. *Hum Mol Genet* 2000; **9**: 549–59.

46 White N, Innes C. Interleukin-4 receptor – a breath of fresh air for asthmatics. In: *Pharma* 2000 No. 1231: 7–8.

47 Beasley R, Crane J, Lai KW, Pearce N. Epidemiology and genetics of asthma: prevalence and aetiology of asthma. *J Allergy Clin Immunol* 2000; **105**: S466–72.

48 Yunginger JW, Reed CE, O'Connell EJ, *et al.* A community based study of the epidemiology of asthma. Incidence rates 1964–1983. *Am Rev Respir Dis* 1992; **146**: 823–4.

49 Huovinen E, Kaprio J, Laitinen LA, Koskenvuo M. Incidence and prevalence of asthma among adult Finnish men and women of the Finnish twin cohort from 1975 to 1990 and their relation to hay fever and chronic bronchitis. *Chest* 1999; **115**: 928–36.

50 Strachan DP, Butland BK, Anderson HR. Incidence and prognosis of asthma and wheezing illness from early childhood to age 33 in a national British cohort. *Br Med J* 1996; **312**: 1195–9.

51 Christie GL, Helms PJ, Godden DJ, *et al.* Asthma, wheezy bronchitis and atopy across two generations. *Am J Respir Crit Care Med* 1999; **159**: 125–9.

52 von Mutius E, Martinez FD, Fritzsch C, *et al.* Prevalence of asthma and atopy in two areas of West and East Germany. *Am J Respir Crit Care Med* 1994; **149**: 358–64.

53 von Mutius E, Weiland SK, Fritzsch C, *et al.* Increasing prevalence of hay fever and atopy among children in Leipzig, East Germany. *Lancet* 1998; **251**: 862–6.

54   Scrivener S, BrittonJ. Immunoglobulin E and allergic disease in Africa. *Clin Exp Allergy* 2000; **30**: 304–7.

55   Woolcock AJ, Peat JK, Trevillion LM. Is the increase in asthma prevalence linked to increase in allergen load? *Allergy* 1995; **50**: 935–40.

56   Kilpeläinen E, Terho EO, Helenius H, Koskenvuo M. Farm environment in childhood prevents the development of allergies. *Clin Exp Allergy* 2000; **30**: 201–8.

57   Tang MLK, Kemp AS, Thorburn J, Hill DJ. Reduced interferon-gamma secretion in neonates and subsequent atopy. *Lancet* 1994; **344**: 983–6.

58   Shirakawa T, Enomoto T, Shimazu S, Hopkin J. The inverse association between tuberculin responses and atopic disorder. *Science* 1997; **275**: 77–9.

59   Holt PG. Regulation of immune responses at mucosal surfaces: allergic respiratory disease as a paradigm. *Immunol Cell Biol* 1998; **76**: 119–24.

60   Holt PG. Key factors in the development of asthma: atopy. *Am J Respir Crit Care Med* 2000; **161**: S172–5.

61   Peat JK, Ki J. Reversing the trend: reducing the prevalence of asthma. *J Allergy Clin Immunol* 1999; **103**: 1–10.

62   Shaheen S, Sterne MJ, Montgomery S, Azima H. Birth weight, body mass index and asthma in young adults. *Thorax* 1999; **54**: 396–402.

63   Hide DW, Matthews S, Tariq S, Arshad SH. Allergen avoidance in infancy and allergy at 4 years of age. *Allergy* 1996; **51**: 89–93.

64   Kurukulaaratchy R, Fenn M, Matthews S, Arshad SH. Wheezing from infancy to age 10 years and its relationship to bronchial responsiveness and atopy. *Am J Respir Crit Care Med* 2000; **161**: A704.

65   Holgate ST, Davies DE, Lackie PM, *et al.* Epithelial-mesenchymal interactions in the pathogenesis of asthma. *J Allergy Clin Immunol* 2000; **105**: 193–204.

66   Salvi S, Frew AJ, Holgate ST. Is diesel a cause for increasing allergies? *Clin Exp Allergy* 1999; **29**: 4–8.

67   Diaz-Sanchez D, Dotson AR, Takenaka H, Saxon A. Diesel exhaust particles induce local IgE *in vivo* and alter the pattern of IgE mRNA isoform. *J Clin Invest* 1994; **94**: 1417–25.

68   Stein RT, Holberg CJ, Sherrill D, *et al.* Influence of parental smoking on respiratory symptoms during the first decade of life: the Tucson Children's Respiratory Study. *Am J Epidemiol* 1999; **149**: 1030–7.

69   Upton MN, Watt GCM, Smith GD, *et al.* Permanent effects of maternal smoking on offsprings' lung function. *Lancet* 1998; **352**: 453.

70   Camporota L, Corkhill A, Long H, *et al.* Effects of intradermal injection of SRL-172 (killed *Mycobacterium vaccae* suspension) on allergen-induced airway responses and IL-5 generation by PMBC in asthma. *Am J Respir Crit Care Med* 2000; **161**: A477.

71   Bryan SA, Kanabar V, Matti S, *et al.* Effects of recombinant human interleukin-12 on eosinophils, airway hyperreactivity and the late asthmatic response. *Lancet* 2000 (in press).

72   Evans MJ, van Winkle LS, Fanucchi MV, Plopper CG. The attenuated fibroblast sheath of the respiratory tract epithelial-mesenchymal trophic unit. *Am J Respir Cell Mol Biol* 1999; **21**: 655–7.

73   Puddicombe SM, Polosa R, Richter A, *et al.* The involvement of the epidermal growth factor receptor in epithelial repair in asthma. *FASEB J* 2000; **14**: 1362–74.

74   Torres-Lozano C, Puddicombe SM, Howarth PH, *et al.* Expression of the cell cycle inhibitor p21^{waf} is increased in the bronchial epithelium of severe asthmatic subjects. *Am J Respir Crit Care Med* 2000; **161**: A260.

75   Zhang S, Smartt H, Holgate ST, Roche WR. Growth factors secreted by bronchial epithelial cells control myofibroblast proliferation: an *in vitro* co-culture model of airway remodelling in asthma. *J Lab Invest* 1999; **79**: 395–405.

76   Puddicombe SM, Richter A, Djukanovic R, *et al.* The epithelial-mesenchymal trophic unit in asthma. *Am J Respir Crit Care Med* 2000; **161**: A259.

77   Chung KF, Barnes PF. Cytokines in asthma. *Thorax* 1999; **54**: 825–57.

Advances in treatment for acute stroke

Martin M Brown

Stroke caused over 4.3 million deaths worldwide in 1990, according to the World Health Organization (WHO) global burden of disease study, second only to ischaemic heart disease as the major cause of mortality throughout the world [1]. However, the burden of the disease is much more than just mortality since half of the two-thirds of patients who survive their first stroke remain disabled. About one in six people will have a stroke at some time in their life. Stroke has been neglected until recently, despite its importance, but several advances are now transforming the approach to acute stroke management in forward-looking units, and have been instrumental in the development of the new and exciting discipline of stroke medicine.

This chapter will concentrate on the treatment of acute ischaemic stroke, including antiplatelet therapy, anticoagulation, thrombolysis, neuroprotection and early rehabilitation (the principles of which apply equally to haemorrhagic stroke). 'Stroke' is not a diagnosis, but a description of the clinical presentation of the patient with the sudden onset of a focal neurological deficit, likely to be of vascular origin. To guide appropriate treatment, it is essential to establish the underlying pathology (infarction or haemorrhage), the site of the lesion (anatomy) and the mechanism of stroke (aetiology). A variety of processes may lead to ischaemic stroke (Table 1), and it would be naïve to think that a single drug treatment will be appropriate whatever the cause of stroke. For example, thrombolysis is unlikely to be effective if the vessel is occluded by atheromatous debris, while neuroprotective agents, designed to inhibit excitotoxicity in the cortex, are unlikely to help a lacunar infarct in the deep white matter or brainstem. There is a huge difference between a

Table 1 Pathophysiological mechanisms of acute ischaemic stroke.

Pathophysiological mechanism		
Embolism	*Materials*	*Sources*
	Thrombus	Cardiac
	Calcific debris	Aorta
	Atheromatous debris	Cervical vessels
Intracranial large vessel occlusion		
Small vessel occlusion (lacunar stroke)		
Haemodynamic stroke		

large wedge of infarction secondary to middle cerebral artery occlusion and a small lacunar infarct a few millimetres across in the internal capsule, although the motor deficit may appear identical. Lacunar infarcts account for 30–40% of stroke, yet the pathological evidence suggests that atherothrombosis may not necessarily play an important part in the underlying pathology.

Despite these differences, almost all recent clinical trials have treated acute stroke as a single condition, assuming an underlying mechanism of athero-thrombosis analogous to myocardial infarction. In this model, stroke is seen to be the end product of the ulceration or rupture of atheromatous plaque. The exposure of the underlying lipid core to the circulating blood acts as a potent precipitant of platelet aggregation and then thrombosis, leading to ischaemia and the symptoms of stroke (Fig. 1). Control of vascular risk factors therefore has an important role in the management of stroke. Extracranial vessel stenosis may promote platelet aggregation, but leads to stroke by embolism and not usually by reduction in flow. Thus, recent drug trials have concentrated on antiplatelet therapy, anticoagulants, thrombolysis and neuroprotection. Surgery or angioplasty and stenting have an important role in prevention, but not in the acute treatment of stroke.

☐ ANTIPLATELET THERAPY

Aspirin

It has been recognised for many years that aspirin prevents recurrent stroke and other vascular events in patients who have recovered from a previous transient

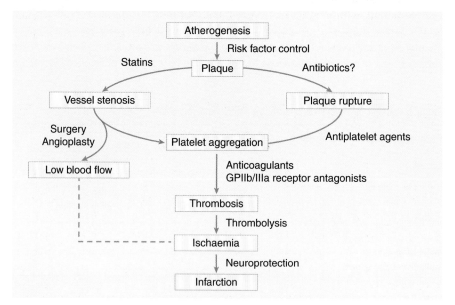

Fig. 1 Mechanisms of atherothrombotic stroke and potential targets for therapy (GP = glycoprotein).

ischaemic attack or minor stroke. Until recently, there was doubt about using aspirin in acute stroke because of concern about the risks of promoting haemorrhagic transformation of an infarct in ischaemic stroke. However, aspirin might have benefit in preventing thrombus propagation, new platelet aggregation, deep vein thrombosis and pulmonary embolism. There is now good evidence about its benefits from two large randomised trials, the International Stroke Trial (IST) [2] and the Chinese Acute Stroke Trial (CAST) [3] (Table 2). Both trials showed a small, but significant reduction in recurrent ischaemic stroke in about 1% of treated patients. Encouragingly, this was not accompanied by a significant increase in haemorrhagic stroke. Analysis at the end of the study (IST, 6 months; CAST, 4 weeks) showed a small, not statistically significant reduction in death and dependency. However, when the two trials were combined in a meta-analysis together with a small amount of data from another trial, the reduction in death and dependency associated with aspirin use became highly significant. The number needing to be treated to prevent one patient from dying or being disabled was approximately 100 [3]. This benefit may seem small, but in fact translates into a substantial cost benefit, given that stroke is common and aspirin costs little. For example, if every patient with acute ischaemic stroke in the UK was given aspirin (300 mg od) within 48 hours of onset, 1,000 patients would be saved from death or disability every year.

Although there are trials suggesting that alternative antiplatelet agents or combination antiplatelet therapy may be more effective than aspirin alone in the prevention of stroke, no other antiplatelet regimen has been tested extensively in acute stroke. One small study suggests that a glycoprotein IIb/IIIa receptor antagonist may be safe in stroke [4], but larger trials are needed. It can therefore be concluded that all ischaemic strokes should be treated with aspirin, unless contraindicated, within 48 hours of onset. It is, however, desirable that all patients should have a computed tomography (CT) or magnetic resonance (MR) scan before starting aspirin to exclude haemorrhage or non-stroke pathology.

Table 2 Summary of the results of the International Stroke Trial (IST) [2] and the Chinese Acute Stroke Trial (CAST) [3].

	CAST		IST		IST	
	Aspirin	**Control**	**Aspirin**	**Control**	**Heparin**	**Control**
No. randomised	10,335	10,320	9,719	9,714	9,717	9,718
Deaths in 28/14 days (%)†	3.3*	3.9	9.0	9.4	9.0	9.3
Recurrent ischaemic stroke (%)	1.6**	2.1	2.8**	3.9	2.9*	3.8
Haemorrhagic stroke (%)	1.1	0.9	0.9	0.8	1.2**	0.4
Death or dependency at 28 days/6 months (%)†	30.5	31.6	61.2	63.5	62.9	62.9

* $p < 0.01$, ** $p < 0.001$
† Outcomes were assessed at 28 days in CAST, and at 14 days and 6 months in IST.

□ ANTICOAGULATION

Intravenous heparin

If aspirin is effective in stroke, it might be thought that anticoagulation would be more effective.

Although intravenous (IV) heparin is widely used in many countries as a first-line treatment for stroke, almost all the randomised trial evidence is against routine anticoagulation being beneficial. The largest trial, the IST [2], showed no overall benefit of subcutaneous heparin, with virtually identical death and dependency rates at six months (Table 2). There was a reduction in the rate of recurrent ischaemic stroke in about one in 100 patients treated (similar to that of aspirin) but, in contrast to aspirin, the rate of haemorrhagic stroke after treatment was significantly increased. This risk of haemorrhagic transformation was almost identical to the rate of reduction of recurrent stroke, balancing out the benefit.

Low-molecular weight heparin

There have been several trials of low-molecular weight heparin. Considerable excitement was first generated by a trial of fraxiparine in 312 patients with acute stroke in Hong Kong which appeared to show a striking benefit [5], but this was not confirmed in a much larger trial of the same agent. This latter trial has never been published in full, illustrating the potential danger of basing treatment decisions on a single small trial. Several other trials of alternative low-molecular weight heparins have been equally disappointing, with no evidence of a significant overall benefit.

Heparin in acute stroke

It can therefore be concluded that there is no place for the routine use of heparin in acute stroke. However, the low-dose subcutaneous heparin (5,000 units bd) arm in IST was neutral [2], and therefore many stroke physicians continue to recommend prophylactic low-dose subcutaneous heparin in patients thought to be at high risk of deep vein thrombosis. I would also use IV heparin in patients at high risk of early recurrence, for example patients with an obvious cardiac source, and those with acute vertebral or carotid artery dissection or occlusion, provided that they do not have a large infarct (ie more than one-third of the middle cerebral artery territory). The latter recommendations are based on consensus practice, not randomised evidence.

□ ISCHAEMIC PENUMBRA

The concept of the ischaemic penumbra is essential to understanding the potential for acute stroke treatment [6]. Extensive animal studies have demonstrated that the fate of neuronal tissue in the brain depends vitally on the degree of reduction in local cerebral blood flow and the duration of the ischaemia. If blood flow in the cortex is reduced from the normal of about 50 ml/100 g/min to below 10 ml/100 g/min, membrane electrolyte exchange mechanisms fail rapidly, potassium leaks out of the cell and the neurone dies within 10 minutes. This reduction in blood flow corresponds to the infarct core supplied by an occluded blood vessel. The cells die so rapidly that it is unlikely it will ever be possible to do much about the infarct core unless high risk patients are pretreated with a neuroprotective agent, for example prior to carotid surgery. The brain tolerates ischaemia with intact neuronal function between the normal blood flow of 50 ml/100 g/min and about 20 ml/100 g/min because of increased oxygen extraction. A blood flow reduction of 10–20 ml/100 g/min results in neurones stopping working (ie they are electrically silent), but the membranes remain intact and there is no leakage of potassium into the extracellular space. If blood flow is restored to normal, the cells recover electrical and functional activity. In ischaemic stroke, reductions of 10–20 ml/100 g/min can be expected at the edge of the ischaemic area where there is some collateral flow from adjacent patent blood vessels (Fig. 2).

This area of intermediate blood flow, known as the penumbra, therefore represents an area of salvageable brain. In clinical terms, the patient may have a focal deficit (eg hemiparesis) because of electrical failure of the neurones in the penumbra, but rapid recovery can occur if blood flow is restored. Unfortunately, animal studies show that neurones in the ischaemic penumbra survive only up to 2–3 hours, at most, before irreversible cell death occurs. The duration of the viability of the ischaemic penumbra in humans is uncertain, but evidence from clinical studies suggests that it is unlikely to be much longer than the three hours found in animal studies.

The current challenge is therefore to treat patients with stroke within three hours of onset to preserve neurones in the ischaemic penumbra. Two approaches have been tried:

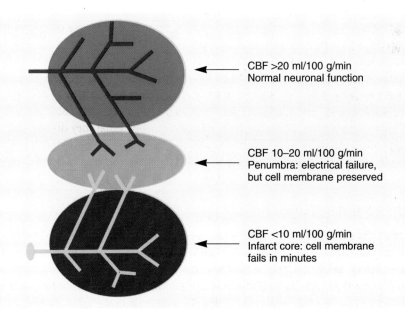

CBF >20 ml/100 g/min
Normal neuronal function

CBF 10–20 ml/100 g/min
Penumbra: electrical failure,
but cell membrane preserved

CBF <10 ml/100 g/min
Infarct core: cell membrane
fails in minutes

Fig. 2 The concept of the ischaemic penumbra (CBF = cerebral blood flow).

1   To restore blood flow by thrombolysis.

2   To use neuroprotective agents to preserve cells in the ischaemic penumbra from the cascade of biochemical events which leads to cell death.

☐ THROMBOLYSIS

Streptokinase

The first thrombolytic agent to be tried in acute stroke was streptokinase. Three trials, the Multicentre Acute Stroke Trial (MAST) in Italy [7], MAST in Europe [8] and the Australian Streptokinase Trial (ASK) [9], all showed a significantly worse outcome in streptokinase treated patients. Each of the trials gave IV streptokinase within six hours of onset. The worse outcome in the streptokinase treated patients was almost entirely caused by a significant excess of cerebral haemorrhage, which resulted in approximately twice as many deaths at 10 days in treated patients compared to controls (Table 3). Despite the early excess of mortality, it is interesting to note that there was little difference in the death and dependency rate at the six-months' follow-up in the MAST trials. This suggests that streptokinase had some benefit in those patients who did not succumb to haemorrhage. Nevertheless, the high rate of haemorrhage has led to the abandonment of streptokinase as a potential treatment for stroke.

Table 3 Summary of the results of trials of thrombolysis using intravenous streptokinase in acute stroke, including the Multicentre Acute Stroke Trial (MAST)-Italy [7], MAST-Europe [8] and the Australian Streptokinase Trial (ASK) [9].

	MAST-Italy		MAST-Europe		ASK	
	SK	Control	SK	Control	SK	Control
No. randomised	622		310		228	
Death within 10 days (%)	26.5*	11.7	34.0*	18.2	46.0*	22.0
Intracranial haemorrhage (%)	6.0	0.6*	21.2*	2.6		
Death or dependency at 6 months (%)	62.6	64.7	79.5	81.8		

* $p < 0.001$
SK = streptokinase.

Alteplase

Intravenous thrombolysis with alteplase

In contrast, our approach to stroke was transformed by the results of the first trial of IV thrombolysis using alteplase, a recombinant tissue plasminogen activator. The National Institute of Neurological Diseases and Stroke Study (NINDS) randomised 624 patients in two groups within three hours of onset of stroke in 48 hospitals in the USA [10]. All the patients had neurological assessment and CT scan before randomisation to alteplase, 0.9 mg/kg over one hour, or placebo. It is notable that the blood pressure was carefully controlled in all patients, with IV agents if necessary – emphasising the intensive approach required for the successful treatment of acute stroke.

The results were exciting. The patients treated with alteplase had a significantly better outcome in terms of good recovery, whatever outcome measure was used. However, as expected, there was a significant incidence (6%) of symptomatic intracranial haemorrhage in treated patients compared to 1% in the placebo group, but this did not translate into an excess of deaths which were similar in both groups (Table 4).

The positive results of the NINDS alteplase trial led to the licensing and widespread adoption in America and Canada of IV thrombolysis within three hours of stroke onset. However, two consecutive trials in Europe, the European Co-operative Acute Stroke Studies (ECASS I and ECASS II) [11,12], failed to show a significant benefit with alteplase on an intention-to-treat primary analysis, which examined the patients making an almost complete recovery (Rankin scale 0 or 1) (Table 4). There were a number of differences between the ECASS and NINDS trials. Both ECASS trials used a longer time window (up to six hours) after onset, during which treatment could be started. ECASS I also used a slightly higher dose. This study had the problem that a significant proportion of the patients entered had exclusion criteria, particularly subtle changes on the pre-randomisation CT, indicating that more than one-third of the middle cerebral artery territory was already severely ischaemic. These patients appear not to benefit from thrombolysis and have a high risk of haemorrhagic transformation. *Post hoc* analysis of the 'target' population in ECASS I on only those patients without exclusion criteria showed that the alteplase-treated patients had a significantly better outcome than those on placebo.

This trial demonstrated the difficulty for inexperienced centres in interpreting the CT changes of early infarction, which can be quite subtle. The investigators therefore carried out a second trial of IV alteplase, ECASS II, this time training up the centres to read CTs beforehand [12]. Disappointingly, ECASS II also failed to show a significant benefit in the primary analysis of those patients who made an almost complete recovery to Rankin grade 0 or 1. However, a *post hoc* analysis examining the number of patients who recovered without serious disability (Rankin grades 0, 1 or 2), the more usual dichotomy used in clinical trials, showed a significant benefit for alteplase.

The ECASS trials thus individually suggested a benefit for thrombolysis given within six hours of stroke onset, but were not convincingly positive given the failure of the primary analysis to reach statistical significance.

The main difference between the convincingly positive NINDS trial and the less convincing ECASS trials is the longer time window in the European studies. It is also noticeable that the mortality rate in the placebo group of the NINDS trial was higher than in that group in ECASS I and double that of the placebo group in ECASS II. This probably represents the randomisation of more severely affected patients in NINDS, which is confirmed by a comparison of the baseline NIH Stroke Scale scores (Table 4). This may reflect the fact that patients with severe deficits are more likely

Table 4 Summary of the results of thrombolysis in acute stroke using intravenous alteplase, including the National Institute of Neurological Disorders Stroke Study (NINDS) [10], the European Co-operative Acute Stroke Studies (ECASS I and II) [11,12] and Alteplase Thrombolysis for Acute Noninterventional Therapy in Ischemic Stroke Study (ATLANTIS) [14].

	NINDS		ECASS I		ECASS II		ATLANTIS	
	Alteplase	Placebo	Alteplase	Placebo	Alteplase	Placebo	Alteplase	Placebo
No. randomised	624		620		800		613	
Dose (mg/kg)	0.9		1.1		0.9		0.9	
Time window (hours)	0–3		0–6		0–6		3–5	
Baseline NIHSS	14	15	12	13	11	11	11	11
Rankin grade 0/1 (%)	39*	26	36	29	40	37	42	41
Symptomatic ICH (%)	6*	1	NR	NR	9*	3	7*	1
Mortality (%)	17	21	22	16	11	11	11	7

* statistically significant
ICH = intracranial haemorrhage; NIHSS = National Institutes of Health Stroke Scale; NR = not recorded.

to reach hospital within three hours. It is therefore relevant to examine the benefit in the ECASS trials in the patients who were randomised under three hours after stroke onset (Fig. 3). In these patients, there was a strong trend in ECASS I and a weaker trend in ECASS II to positive outcomes in patients treated with thrombolysis. This does not individually reach statistical significance because of the small numbers of patients randomised under three hours, and therefore wide confidence intervals. However, when all patients treated with thrombolysis within three hours of onset in the three trials are combined in a meta-analysis, the benefits of thrombolysis are highly significant, with a reduction in unfavourable outcomes (Rankin score ≥ 3) [13]. In contrast, a meta-analysis of the patients treated in the ECASS trials at 3–6 hours showed only a non-significant trend towards favourable outcomes when combined with the recently published Alteplase Thrombolysis for Acute Noninterventional Therapy in Ischemic Stroke Study (ATLANTIS) of alteplase in acute stroke [14], which randomised patients at 3–5 hours after onset and had a neutral result (G Ford; personal communication).

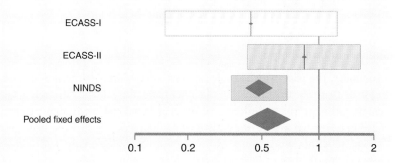

Fig. 3 Meta-analysis of the effects of thrombolysis within three hours of stroke onset using intravenous alteplase (from [13]) (ECASS = European Co-operative Acute Stroke Study; NINDS = National Institute of Neurological Diseases and Stroke Study).

Intra-arterial thrombolysis with prourokinase

The trials discussed above have all examined the benefits of IV thrombolysis. There has also been one positive randomised trial of intra-arterial thrombolysis using prourokinase, the Prolyse in Acute Cerebral Thromboembolism Trial (PROACT) II [15]. Intra-arterial thrombolysis has the advantage that the agent can be infused exactly where it is needed, partly avoiding systemic effects. In addition, the site of occlusion can be confirmed, excluding patients who have already undergone spontaneous thrombolysis. This study showed a significant benefit of intra-arterial thrombolysis given within six hours of onset of symptoms (Table 5) but, because of the requirement to scan the patients and perform cerebral angiography within the time window, only a few patients were eligible for the study. In fact, to randomise 180 patients, an extraordinary 12,323 acute stroke patients were screened and 474 angiograms performed. The median time to randomisation was 4.7 hours,

Table 5 The results of the Prolyse in Acute Cerebral Thromboembolism Trial (PROACT II) trial of thrombolysis with intra-arterial prourokinase (from [15]).

	PROACT II	
	Prourokinase	**Placebo**
No. randomised	180	
Dose (mg in 2 hours)	9	
Time window (hours)	0–6	
Baseline NIHSS	17	17
Rankin grade 0/1 (%)	40*	25
Symptomatic ICH (%)	10**	2
Mortality (%)	25	27

* $p = 0.04$; ** $p = 0.06$
ICH = intracranial haemorrhage; NIHSS = National Institutes of Health Stroke Scale..

demonstrating that in patients with favourable angiographic features arterial thrombolysis can still be beneficial even beyond three hours.

Summary of thrombolysis

In summary, the trial evidence suggests that streptokinase is hazardous and has no place in acute stroke treatment. On the other hand, the evidence strongly suggests that alteplase given within three hours of onset is beneficial, with about eight patients needed to be treated to save one patient being disabled. A licence has been granted for IV alteplase within three hours of onset of stroke in Germany, and is likely to be granted within the rest of Europe shortly. A small number of specialist centres in the UK and other European countries are already using alteplase in selected patients. Patients and carers need to be warned that thrombolysis provides a chance of benefit, but also a risk of harm from cerebral haemorrhage. It is essential that centres contemplating thrombolysis for stroke should adhere strictly to the NINDS and ECASS protocols and audit their results. Those that still have doubts about thrombolysis should consider joining the third IST (IST-3) which plans to investigate further the benefits and risks of alteplase.

Thrombolysis will never be suitable for all stroke patients, particularly since many patients will not reach hospital within three hours of onset. In the NINDS study centres, only 6% of patients with acute stroke were entered into the trial. It might be thought that even fewer patients would reach hospital in time in the UK. However, a recent audit of stroke in accident and emergency (A&E) departments at 14 district general hospitals in the UK showed that a surprising 24% of patients actually reached the A&E department within three hours of onset of symptoms (Fig. 4) [16]. Most of these have dialled 999 rather than calling a general practitioner which delays admission. Unfortunately, few of these patients were seen by a doctor immediately after they arrived in hospital, and a change in attitudes is needed so that acute stroke is dealt with as an emergency equivalent to an acute myocardial infarct.

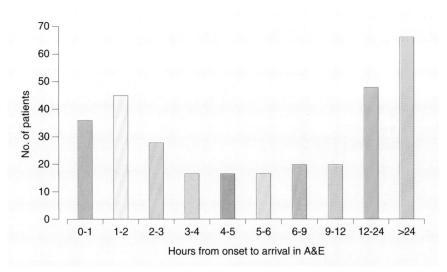

Fig. 4 Bar graph showing the time of arrival in the accident and emergency (A&E) department after the onset of stroke in 14 centres in the UK in 1998 (from the Acute Stroke Intervention Study (ASIST) [16]).

One way of shortening the time taken for the patient to reach specialised services is to arrange with the ambulance service for patients with symptoms suggesting stroke to be taken directly to an acute stroke unit, bypassing the A&E department. This has been successfully trialled in Newcastle, and has substantially increased the number of patients treated with thrombolysis and benefiting from early stroke assessment.

☐ NEUROPROTECTION

The biochemical processes which lead to cell death have been extensively investigated in animal models of stroke. Some of the main processes are outlined in Fig. 5. Provided that the appropriate neuroprotective drug is given before or soon after ischaemia, blocking almost any of these stages in the pathway results in a significant reduction in infarct size in animal models. Numerous neuroprotective agents have been tried in human stroke, with disappointing results. No agent has yet been shown to be beneficial, despite the promise from animal studies [17].

A number of possible reasons may explain the failure to translate benefits in animals to humans. First, no human study has included only patients presenting within three hours of onset, many including patients presenting up to 12 hours or later. Secondly, no attempt has usually been made to select outpatients with stroke types likely to benefit from neuroprotection, or those with persisting penumbra. In particular, most neuroprotective agents will protect only the cortex, so no reduction in the size of subcortical or lacunar infarction could be expected. Finally, in some studies there have been problems with tolerability, and doses may have been used which failed to replicate sufficiently high intracerebral concentrations of the neuroprotective agent. Nevertheless, a number of agents are still undergoing clinical trials and it is likely that, given better trial design, an appropriate neuroprotective

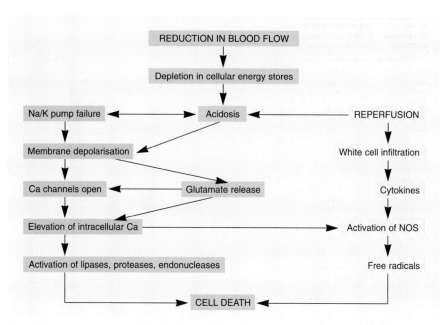

Fig. 5 Chart showing some of the features of the ischaemic cascade, a sequence of biochemical events which leads to cell death after neuronal ischaemia (Ca = calcium; K = potassium; Na = sodium; NOS = nitric oxide synthase).

agent will eventually be found to benefit human stroke. In particular, there is considerable evidence that reperfusion may exacerbate cell toxicity after ischaemia (Fig. 5). It would therefore make sense in the future to combine thrombolysis with a neuroprotective agent to gain maximum benefit.

☐ EARLY REHABILITATION

Although thrombolysis is applicable to only a proportion of acute stroke, and neuroprotection is only on the horizon, early rehabilitation via a specialist multidisciplinary stroke team benefits all patients. The Stroke Unit Trialists Collaboration has demonstrated a highly significant benefit of care by a dedicated stroke unit compared with care in a general medical ward in a meta-analysis of 18 trials (Fig. 6) [18]. Meta-analysis of subgroups strongly suggests that all types of patients benefit from stroke unit care, irrespective of gender, age or severity of stroke. On average, the mortality is reduced from 27% on general medical wards to 22% on a stroke unit. There is a similar reduction in the combined outcome measure of death and dependency from 68% to 61%. This benefit, with the number needed to treat of about 14, is achieved despite an average reduction in the length of stay and without necessarily increasing resource use.

The benefits of stroke unit care are achieved not simply by gathering the patients together in a single location labelled 'stroke unit', but by the development of a specialised multidisciplinary team. The characteristics of stroke unit care that contribute to the benefit include:

Review	Organised inpatient (stroke unit) care for stroke					
Comparison:	Organised stroke unit care vs conventional care					
Outcome:	Death or dependency by the end of scheduled follow-up					
Study	Expt n/N	Ctrl n/N	Peto OR (95%CI Fixed)	Weight (%)	Peto OR (95%CI Fixed)
Akershus	103/271	110/279		18.1	0.94 (0.67 , 1.33)
Birmingham	8/29	9/23		1.6	0.60 (0.19 , 1.90)
Dover	65/116	79/117		7.7	0.62 (0.36 , 1.04)
Edinburgh	93/155	94/156		10.4	0.99 (0.63 , 1.56)
Helsinki	47/121	65/122		8.4	0.56 (0.34 , 0.93)
Illinois	20/56	17/35		2.9	0.59 (0.25 , 1.39)
Kuopio	31/50	31/45		3.0	0.74 (0.32 , 1.72)
Montreal	58/65	60/65		1.5	0.69 (0.21 , 2.27)
New York	23/42	23/40		2.8	0.90 (0.38 , 2.13)
Newcastle	26/34	28/33		1.5	0.59 (0.18 , 1.96)
Nottingham	123/176	100/139		8.9	0.91 (0.56 , 1.48)
Orpington 1993	101/124	108/121		4.3	0.54 (0.27 , 1.09)
x Orpington 1995	36/36	37/37		0.0	Not estimable
Perth	10/29	14/30		2.0	0.61 (0.22 , 1.71)
Tampere	53/98	55/113		7.3	1.24 (0.72 , 2.13)
Trondheim	54/110	81/110		7.3	0.36 (0.21 , 0.61)
Umea	52/110	102/183		9.5	0.71 (0.44 , 1.14)
Uppsala	45/60	41/52		2.8	0.81 (0.34 , 1.94)
Total (95%CI)	948/1682	1054/1700		100.0	0.75 (0.65 , 0.87)
Chi-square 17.95 (df=16) Z=3.89			.1 .2 1 5 10		

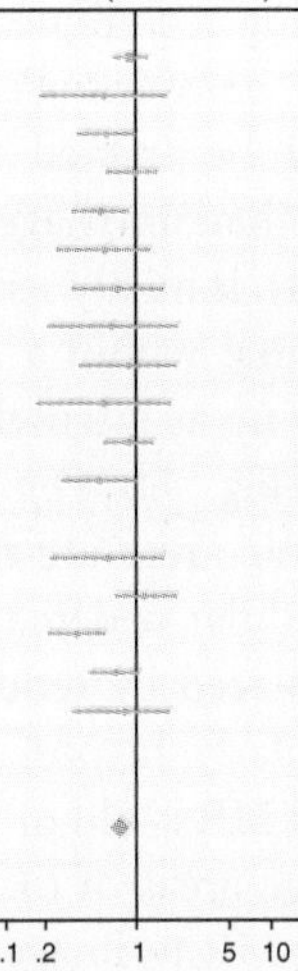

Fig. 6 Meta-analysis of the benefits of organised stroke care (from Stroke Unit Trialists Collaboration [18]) (CI = confidence interval; ctrl = control; df = degrees of freedom; Expt = experimental; OR = odds ratio; Z = Z score).

☐ nurses interested in stroke

☐ a physician interested in stroke

☐ multidisciplinary team meetings

☐ regular staff training

☐ the involvement of carers, and

☐ the early onset of rehabilitation.

Specialised nursing is particularly important because nurses can practise the principles of active rehabilitation 24 hours of the day. Aspects of stroke care facilitated by stroke units are listed in Table 6.

Table 6 Processes involved in stroke unit care.

• Positioning	• Blood pressure control
• Early mobilisation	• Antibiotics for infection
• Early rehabilitation	• Full investigation
• Swallowing assessment	• Psychological support
• Early hydration and feeding	• Informed advice to patient and carers
• Neurological observations	• Knowledge and enthusiasm
• Specialised nursing	

☐ ADVANCES IN ACUTE IMAGING

The need rapidly to diagnose and treat acute stroke has been a stimulus to the development of new MR scanning techniques [19]. CT is often normal in acute stroke, or the early changes may be overlooked, leading to diagnostic uncertainty and the risk that patients will be treated with thrombolysis inappropriately, unnecessarily causing a cerebral haemorrhage. Fortunately, a new MR sequence, diffusion weighted imaging (DWI), is highly sensitive to the early changes of cerebral ischaemia. DWI becomes abnormal within a few minutes of the onset of critical ischaemia, and the changes show up as intensely bright increases in signal intensity on the scan ('lightbulb sign') (Fig. 7). The diagnosis of acute stroke and the identification of severely ischaemic areas are therefore made easy. The increase in signal on DWI is the result of cellular oedema; these changes reverse within about two weeks after onset, to be replaced by reduction in signal intensity in chronic infarction. DWI can be particularly helpful in identifying whether an area of infarction on CT or conventional MR is old or new.

MR can also be used to image areas of local reduction in cerebral blood flow, using the technique of perfusion MR to image the distribution and transit time of contrast medium injected intravenously. In some cases, perfusion imaging may show a much larger area of reduction in blood flow than is shown by DWI [20]. This mismatch between a large area of perfusion and a smaller area of cell swelling indicated by the abnormal DWI signal may indicate the presence of a salvageable penumbra. Areas of abnormal DWI signal are usually destined to infarct permanently, but thrombolysis with early reperfusion may prevent the area of infarction extending throughout the territory shown to be ischaemic on perfusion imaging (Fig 7). DWI and perfusion imaging can be combined with intracranial MR angiography (multimodal MR), enabling the pathophysiology to be elucidated.

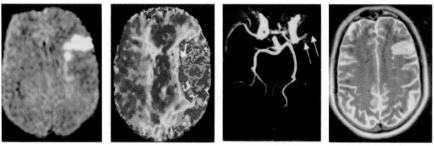

| (a) DWI | (b) Perfusion weighted Image | (c) MR angiogram | (d) Conventional T2 weighted MR scan at 5 days |

Fig. 7 Magnetic resonance (MR) scans showing perfusion-diffusion mismatch in a patient with an acute middle cerebral artery (MCA) occlusion: **(a)** diffusion weighted image (DWI) 2.5 hours after onset of stroke showing a bright signal in the right frontal area, indicating early cell swelling in the areas of severe ischaemia; **(b)** perfusion weighted imaging showing a reduction in blood flow in a much larger area of the MCA territory; **(c)** MR angiogram showing absent flow in the left MCA (arrows); **(d)** conventional T2-weighted MR image on day 5 after successful thrombolysis with recanalisation of the MCA, showing only a small left frontal infarct in the area of previous DWI abnormality (from [20]).

At present, these techniques are not widely available, but may in the future help to select the appropriate patients for thrombolysis or neuroprotection, and may allow the time window for treatment to be extended, for example by identifying patients who have both a persisting vessel occlusion and a perfusion-diffusion mismatch indicating the presence of salvageable penumbra.

☐ CONCLUSIONS

The approach to stroke should change from passive indifference to an active management policy, where stroke is seen as an emergency 'brain attack', not a cerebrovascular accident for which little can be done. Although stroke units in the past have taken patients up to a week or more after admission to hospital, it is likely that the benefits of stroke unit care will be even greater if patients are admitted directly to the stroke unit rather than to a general medical ward. The advent of thrombolysis requires that patients should be fast-tracked directly to the stroke unit for consideration of thrombolysis, and early multidisciplinary assessment if they are not suitable. Unfortunately, less than 50% of patients in the UK are admitted to a stroke unit, and even fewer see a physician particularly interested in stroke. There is a need for hospitals without stroke units to reorganise their services and for more doctors to become interested in stroke. In the future, patients with acute stroke will have sophisticated MR imaging, when available, to make the diagnosis, identify ischaemic penumbra and to select patients for thrombolysis. It can be anticipated that it will not be long before we have further active treatments for acute stroke, including new antiplatelet therapies, thrombolytic agents and neuroprotective agents.

REFERENCES

1   Murray CJL, Lopez AD. Global burden of disease study. *Lancet* 1997; **349**: 269–76.

2   International Stroke Trial Collaborative Group. The International Stroke Trial (IST): a randomised trial of aspirin, subcutaneous heparin, both or neither among 19,435 patients with acute ischaemic stroke. *Lancet* 1997; **349**: 1569–81.

3   CAST (Chinese Acute Stroke Trial) Collaborative Group. CAST: randomised placebo-controlled trial of early aspirin use in 20,000 patients with acute ischaemic stroke. *Lancet* 1997; **349**: 1641–9.

4   The Abaximab in Ischemic Stroke Investigators. Abaximab in acute ischemic stroke: a randomized, double-blind, placebo-controlled, dose-escalation study. *Stroke* 2000; **31**: 601–9.

5   Kay R, Wong KS, Yu YL, *et al*. Low-molecular weight heparin for the treatment of acute ischemic stroke. *N Engl J Med* 1995; **333**: 1588–93.

6   Hakim AM. Ischemic penumbra: the therapeutic window. *Neurology* 1998; **51**(Suppl 3): S44–6.

7   Candelise L, Aritzu E, Ciccone A, *et al*. Multicentre Acute Stroke Trial-Italy (MAST-I) Group. Randomised controlled trial of streptokinase, aspirin, and combination of both in treatment of acute ischaemic stroke. *Lancet* 1995; **346**: 1509–14.

8   Hommel M, Cornu C, Boutitie F, Boissel JP. The Multicentre Acute Stroke Trial-Europe Study Group. Thrombolytic therapy with streptokinase in acute ischemic stroke. *N Engl J Med* 1996; **335**: 145–50.

9   Donnan GA, Davis SM, Chambers BR, *et al*. Trials of streptokinase in severe acute ischaemic stroke. *Lancet* 1995; **345**: 578–9.

10 Tissue plasminogen activator for acute ischemic stroke. The National Institute of Neurological Disorders and Stroke rt-PA Stroke Study Group. *N Engl J Med* 1995; **333**: 1581–7.

11 Hacke W, Kaste M, Fieshchi C, *et al* for the ECASS Study Group. Intravenous thrombolysis with recombinant tissue plasminogen activator for acute hemispheric stroke. *JAMA* 1995; **274**: 1017–25.

12 Hacke W, Kaste M, Fieschi C, *et al.* Randomised double-blind placebo-controlled trial of thrombolytic therapy with intravenous alteplase in acute ischaemic stroke (ECASS-II). Second European–Australasian Acute Stroke Study Investigators. *Lancet* 1998; **352**: 1245–51.

13 Ford G, Freemantle N. ECASS-II: intravenous alteplase in acute ischaemic stroke. European Co-operative Acute Stroke Study-II. *Lancet* 1999; **353**: 65; discussion 67–8.

14 Clark WM, Wissman S, Albers GW, *et al.* Recombinant tissue-type plasminogen activator (Alteplase) for ischemic stroke 3 to 5 hours after symptom onset. The ATLANTIS Study: a randomized controlled trial. Alteplase Thrombolysis for Acute Noninterventional Therapy in Ischemic Stroke. *JAMA* 1999; **282**: 2019–26.

15 Furlan A, Higashida R, Wechsler L, *et al.* Intra-arterial prourokinase for acute ischemic stroke. The PROACT II Study: a randomized controlled trial. Prolyse in Acute Cerebral Thromboembolism. *JAMA* 1999; **28**: 2003–11.

16 Gregson JM, Baldwin N, Brown MM, *et al.* How many patients are suitable for thrombolysis in the United Kingdom? The Acute Stroke Intervention Study (ASIST) (submitted for publication).

17 Dyker AG, Lees KR. Duration of neuroprotective treatment for ischemic stroke. Review. *Stroke* 1998; **29**: 535–42.

18 Stroke Unit Trialists Collaboration. Organised inpatient (stroke unit) care for stroke (Cochrane Review). In: *The Cochrane Library*, Issue 2. Oxford: Update Software, 2000.

19 Beauchamp N Jr, Barker PB, Wang PW, vanZijl PC. Imaging of acute cerebral ischemia. Review. *Radiology* 1999; **212**: 307–24.

20 Jansen O, Schellinger P, Fiebach J, *et al.* Early recanalisation in acute ischaemic stroke saves tissue at risk defined by MRI. *Lancet* 1999; **353**: 2036–7.

☐ SELF ASSESSMENT QUESTIONS

1   In acute ischaemic stroke:
  (a) All patients should receive aspirin 300 mg within 48 hours of onset (unless contraindicated)
  (b) Intravenous (IV) heparin prevents progression of stroke if given within 48 hours of onset
  (c) Low molecular weight heparin is more effective than unfractionated heparin in acute stroke
  (d) All patients should have computed tomography (CT) or magnetic resonance (MR) imaging before starting aspirin therapy
  (e) Aspirin therapy could save 1,000 patients a year from death or disability after stroke in the UK

2   Concerning thrombolysis in acute ischaemic stroke:
  (a) Streptokinase and alteplase are equally beneficial
  (b) Benefit has been demonstrated for IV thrombolytic therapy only within three hours of onset of symptoms
  (c) Subtle CT changes in more than one-third of the middle cerebral artery territory are a contraindication to thrombolysis

(d) The risk of intracerebral haemorrhage after IV thrombolysis is less than 6%

(e) Thrombolysis should be administered only by experienced teams

3   Concerning stroke unit care after stroke:
(a) There is a reduction in dependency, but no reduction in mortality
(b) Length of stay is greater on stroke units than on general medical wards
(c) Multidisciplinary team meetings play an important role
(d) Only patients with moderate, but not severe, disabilities benefit
(e) Neuroprotective drug treatments contribute to the improvement in outcome

4   The following play an important part in the care of the patient on a stroke unit:
(a) Early mobilisation
(b) Therapy to increase blood pressure
(c) Assessment of swallowing
(d) Full investigation
(e) Early hydration and tube feeding

5   After acute ischaemic stroke:
(a) Reperfusion inhibits nitric oxide synthase
(b) Diffusion weighted imaging (DWI) is not helpful until at least six hours after onset
(c) DWI can distinguish between recent and old infarcts
(d) MR angiography can be used to identify intracranial occlusion
(e) A larger area of perfusion deficit than seen as abnormal on DWI may indicate ischaemic penumbra

ANSWERS

1a True	2a False	3a False	4a True	5a False
b False	b True	b False	b False	b False
c False	c True	c True	c True	c True
d True	d False	d False	d True	d True
e True	e True	e False	e True	e True

Disorders of the basal ganglia and their modern management

Anette Schrag and Niall Quinn

☐ PARKINSON'S DISEASE

Epidemiology and genetic aspects

Parkinson's disease (PD) is a common disorder, particularly among the elderly, with a prevalence of 100–200 per 100,000 in the general population [1]. In most patients, PD is sporadic, but rare genetic forms exist. Causative mutations have recently been identified on the α-synuclein gene on chromosome 4, responsible for Lewy body-positive, autosomal dominant PD, and the parkin gene on chromosome 6, responsible for Lewy body-negative autosomal recessive juvenile parkinsonism. An increased familial risk for PD has also been shown in monozygotic as opposed to dizygotic twins when onset is below the age of 50 [2].

Diagnosis

Clinically, PD is characterised by the classical triad of bradykinesia, rigidity and frequently tremor, but with advancing disease postural instability and other features become evident. The diagnosis is clinical, based on these criteria and on the exclusion of other atypical features such as dementia at onset, cerebellar or pyramidal signs.

Treatment

Figure 1 is a simplified illustration of the major neuronal pathways within the basal ganglia in a normal individual. The principal pathological correlate of the motor disorder of PD is degeneration of the dopaminergic nigrostriatal neurons leading to impaired dopaminergic neurotransmission in the basal ganglia. The treatment of PD therefore concentrates on replacing dopamine, on dopaminergic stimulation in the striatum or on surgically inactivating certain deep brain structures (Table 1).

Antiparkinsonian drugs

Levodopa preparations. The mainstay, and still the 'gold standard', of anti-parkinsonian treatment in terms of efficacy, remains levodopa, given together with

[Updated from *J R Coll Physicians Lond* 1999;**33**:323–7.]
163

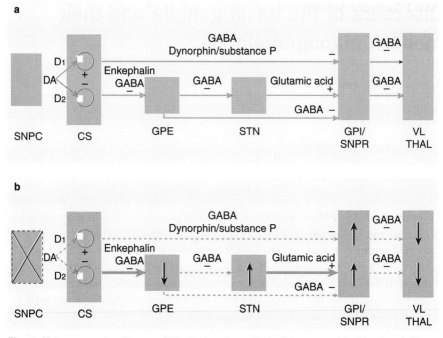

Fig. 1 Major neuronal pathways within the basal ganglia in (a) a normal individual and (b) an individual with Parkinson's disease (much simplified illustrations). In crude terms, the substantia nigra pars compacta (SNPC) may be regarded as an 'accelerator' for movement, and the subthalamic nucleus (STN) and internal pallidum (GPI)/substantia nigra pars reticulata (SNPR) as 'brakes'. The consequence of nigral cell loss in Parkinson's disease is to 'remove the foot from the accelerator' which, along the line in the outflow pathways, results in 'braking' of the ventrolateral thalamus (VL THAL) and hence of the motor cortex (CS = corpus striatum (putamen and caudate); DA = dopamine; D_1 and D_2 = dopamine receptors; GABA = gamma-aminobutyric acid; GPE = external pallidum; + = excitation; — = inhibition; green = inhibitory pathways; mauve = excitatory pathways (adapted from [3]).

a peripheral decarboxylase inhibitor to reduce peripheral side effects and enhance efficacy. However, long-term treatment with levodopa is, sooner or later, complicated by the development of fluctuations in motor response and abnormal involuntary movements. Controlled-release (CR) levodopa preparations are absorbed more slowly than standard preparations (delaying onset of action), but give a longer 'tail' of plasma concentration (delaying offset of action). Their relative bioavailability is only 70% of that of standard preparations, so some patients are often inadvertently underdosed after switching to CR preparations. They can also worsen dyskinesias and give a less predictable response in some patients. Two large multicentre trials [4,5] of CR versus standard preparations of Sinemet and Madopar as *de novo* treatment have failed to show any clinically significant delay or reduction in the development of fluctuations or dyskinesias in the CR groups. CR preparations are most consistently helpful when given at bedtime for night-time immobility. A more rapid onset of action can sometimes be achieved with dispersible levodopa – particularly useful to 'kick in' in the morning.

Table 1 The medical and surgical treatment of Parkinson's disease.

Indication	Treatment
No functional impairment	No symptomatic treatment
	Neuroprotective role of selegiline unproven
Early functional impairment:	
old (>70 years)	Start with levodopa preparation
young (<50 years)	Try to delay levodopa if possible by using:
	anticholinergics
	dopamine agonists
	selegiline
	amantadine
	When levodopa is needed, consider combination with an
	agonist
intermediate (50–70 years)	Optimal approach uncertain
Fluctuations and dyskinesias:	
Medical	Attempt to smooth peaks and troughs of
	dopaminergic stimulation with:
	fractionated levodopa doses
	controlled-release levodopa
	selegiline
	COMT-inhibitor
	adjunctive dopamine agonists
	amantadine
	apomorphine sc 'rescue' injections or pump
Surgical	If severe problems despite above measures:
	deep brain stimulation/lesioning of:
	thalamus* for tremor and rigidity
	pallidum* for dyskinesias>parkinsonism
	subthalamic nucleus for parkinsonism and dyskinesias

* Now largely superseded by subthalamic nucleus as target of choice in Parkinson's disease.
COMT = catechol-O-methyltransferase; sc = subcutaneous.

Dopamine agonists. Dopamine agonists, which act directly on striatal dopamine receptors and have a longer duration of action than levodopa preparations, frequently help smooth response fluctuations, and can delay their onset when used as monotherapy [6–10]. A number of different dopamine agonists are currently available, including the newly licensed long-acting cabergoline and the non-ergot derivatives ropinirole and pramipexole. It remains to be shown whether these drugs are generally superior to the older dopamine agonists bromocriptine and pergolide. The only subcutaneously applicable antiparkinsonian drug, the dopamine agonist apomorphine, can rapidly reverse off periods or, if given via a continuous pump, can smooth severe fluctuations of motor response.

Other drugs

Anticholinergics. These drugs, which are mainly effective for tremor, should be avoided in elderly patients, particularly if there is cognitive impairment, as they have a high propensity to cause psychiatric side effects, especially hallucinations and organic confusional states.

Amantadine. Amantadine is a mild antiparkinsonian drug with a complex profile comprising anticholinergic, dopamine reuptake blocking, amphetamine-like and N-methyl-D-aspartate antagonist activities, the last of which may be responsible for its recently observed efficacy in reducing dyskinesias.

Enzyme inhibitors:

☐ Monoamine oxidase inhibitors. Selegiline, which was associated with an increased mortality in one study [11] but not in others, has mild antiparkinsonian efficacy when given alone, and may improve wearing-off when added to levodopa therapy. A new buccally absorbed formulation, which does not undergo first-pass metabolism and therefore produces less selegiline metabolites, has been marketed recently.

☐ Drugs in the new category of catechol-O-methyltransferase (COMT) inhibitors, comprising tolcapone (central and peripheral COMT-inhibitor, suspended in Europe due to hepatic complications) and entacapone (peripheral COMT-inhibitor), prolong the elimination half-life, and hence the duration of action, of levodopa. As a result, doses of levodopa may need to be reduced by 20–40% [12].

Peak-dose dyskinesias and motor response fluctuations are usually managed by titrating combinations of the above medications in order to even out peaks and troughs of dopaminergic stimulation. Beginning- and end-of-dose dyskinesias, which are related to intermediate levels, are however much more difficult to treat.

Surgical treatment

Lesioning and deep brain stimulation. In addition to medical treatment of PD, stereotactic surgery, targeting the thalamus for tremor, the internal pallidum mainly for dyskinesias, and the subthalamic nucleus (STN) for all aspects of parkinsonism, has experienced a renaissance [13]. Both lesioning and deep brain stimulation (DBS) (which effectively inhibits structures stimulated at high frequency) have been successfully used in patients with advanced PD no longer satisfactorily controlled by medical treatment. DBS may carry a lower morbidity than lesioning (controlled comparative studies are needed), but is more costly and requires indefinite follow-up. Today, the optimal procedure is probably either lesioning [14] or DBS [15] of the STN; this allows major reductions in levodopa dosage, and hence improves not only parkinsonism but also dyskinesias, and off period dystonia and freezing.

Neural grafting. Transplantation of human fetal nigral neurons has been shown to have beneficial effects in several studies, but remains experimental. Most recently, implants of fetal porcine nigral cells are being investigated.

Non-motor problems in Parkinson's disease

In addition to the problems of mobility, many patients with PD, especially those with advanced disease, develop other problems which need to be addressed, such as depression, dementia, other neuropsychiatric disturbances, postural hypotension, and urinary dysfunction. Dementia with Lewy bodies may present with either parkinsonism or dementia, or both [16]. This is probably the second commonest cause of dementia after Alzheimer's disease (AD), and accounts for many cases previously labelled 'plaque only' AD.

☐ ATYPICAL PARKINSONISM

The most common causes of atypical parkinsonism are multiple system atrophy (MSA) [17] and progressive supranuclear palsy (PSP) [18]. These are two distinct disorders with more extensive characteristic pathological abnormalities involving the basal ganglia, but also involving other areas of the central nervous system which account for additional clinical features. Both are frequently misdiagnosed, and many of these patients die with an incorrect diagnosis of PD.

Diagnosis

An important characteristic in both conditions is a poor or declining response to levodopa, but some patients with MSA may, at least initially, show a good response. Other clues to the diagnosis of MSA include:

☐ cerebellar features

☐ early and prominent autonomic failure

☐ urogenital dysfunction

☐ pyramidal signs.

Features of PSP include:

☐ early impairment of postural stability with falls

☐ a vertical supranuclear gaze palsy

☐ prominent axial rigidity, often with relatively preserved limb mobility

☐ early dysarthria or dysphagia.

The diagnosis of MSA and PSP, like that of PD, is primarily clinical. However, investigations that can help support the clinical diagnosis, and exclude other symptomatic causes of parkinsonism, are magnetic resonance imaging of the brain, sphincter-electromyography (EMG), and (in MSA) autonomic function tests.

Treatment

As mentioned above, treatment is usually disappointing in these disorders due to the extent of degeneration in multiple areas. Amantadine can sometimes provide benefit when levodopa fails. However, the most important forms of help for these patients are physiotherapy, speech therapy, occupational therapy, and treatment of postural hypotension and urinary dysfunction.

☐ ESSENTIAL TREMOR

Essential tremor (ET) is characterised by a postural and/or kinetic tremor of the hands, with optional additional involvement of other body parts. Up to 4% of the population may have ET, but affected subjects are often unaware of their tremor, while those who are aware rarely consult a doctor (particularly a specialist) because of it [19]. Additionally, differentiation from dystonic or parkinsonian tremor can be difficult [20]. Inheritance is often autosomal dominant, and ET is most likely a genetically heterogeneous disorder. Linkage to regions on chromosomes 2 and 3 has already been identified in two families with an ET phenotype. The great majority of those affected do not require treatment; if treatment is required, propranolol and primidone provide some relief in 50–70% of patients. If these are not successful, intramuscular injections of botulinum toxin are occasionally helpful. In severe cases, unilateral or bilateral DBS of the ventral intermediate nucleus of the thalamus or unilateral lesioning, with or without contralateral DBS, can cause dramatic improvement [21].

☐ CHOREA

Hereditary

Huntington's disease (HD) is the archetypal cause of hereditary chorea, and is associated with dementia, psychiatric manifestations, and a relentlessly progressive course. It is an autosomal dominantly inherited CAG repeat disorder. A genetic test for the abnormal expansion in the responsible gene on chromosome 4 is now available for diagnosis and, after appropriate counselling, as a predictive test in at-risk adults. A family history may however be lacking, particularly when onset is at a late age or if the transmitting parent died young. Rarer inherited causes include dentatorubropallidoluysian atrophy, caused by a trinucleotide CAG repeat expansion on chromosome 12 and which can be tested for, and neuro-acanthocytosis. Other movement disorders also occur in HD, and juvenile cases (with longer repeat expansions) are more likely to have predominant parkinsonism and dystonia rather than chorea (Westphal variant).

Chorea may be reduced by administration of neuroleptics and/or tetrabenazine, but these drugs should be used sparingly as they often concomitantly worsen underlying parkinsonism and depression. The most disabling features of HD are usually neuropsychiatric, including personality change, psychosis and depression, which may need specific treatment. Potentially disease-modifying treatments such as fetal striatal tissue transplantation and anti-excitotoxic drug regimens are under experimental investigation.

Sporadic

The differential diagnosis of sporadic chorea includes Sydenham's chorea, pregnancy, drugs (especially levodopa in patients with Parkinson's disease, anticholinergics, anticonvulsants, the contraceptive pill and, most commonly, chronic exposure to neuroleptics), thyrotoxicosis, polycythaemia rubra vera, vascular disease (usually as hemichorea/hemiballism), systemic lupus erythematosus, the lupus anticoagulant syndrome and new variant Creuzfeldt-Jakob disease.

☐ DYSTONIA

The classification and nomenclature of the dystonias has recently been revised [22] into four main categories:

- ☐ primary dystonia (only dystonia ± tremor)
- ☐ dystonia-plus (including dopa-responsive dystonia)
- ☐ secondary dystonia (eg cerebral palsy, drug-induced)
- ☐ heredodegenerative dystonia (eg Wilson's disease (WD)).

This review will consider dystonia, mainly according to its distribution.

Generalised dystonia

Generalised primary dystonia typically starts in childhood, often first affecting a leg. Other causes must first be excluded, particularly WD, which can be treated with penicillamine, trientine or zinc. Structural causes, especially in hemidystonia must also be excluded. Although the gene for WD on chromosome 13 has been isolated and sequenced, gene-specific diagnosis is not generally possible because of the many different mutations within this very large gene. The diagnosis still depends on measuring serum caeruloplasmin and copper excretion, slit-lamp examination of the eyes for Kayser-Fleischer rings and, if doubt remains, liver biopsy copper content.

In childhood- or adolescent-onset dystonia, it is also crucial to exclude dopa-responsive dystonia (DRD) which is potentially 'curable' by lifelong administration of levodopa. It has recently been recognised that the spectrum of DRD is wider than previously thought, and that many atypical variants exist, including apparent 'athetoid cerebral palsy' with developmental delay in infants. It is a dominantly inherited disorder (with incomplete penetrance) caused by a mutation in the GTP cyclohydrolase-1 gene (*DYT 5*) on chromosome 14. Genetic testing is, however, complicated by genetic heterogeneity, with a great number of different 'private' mutations causing DRD [23]. In contrast, the dominant (and 30–40% penetrant) mutation (*DYT 1* on chromosome 9), responsible for approximately 40% of all cases of typical early limb-onset primary dystonia (Oppenheim's dystonia), has recently been identified. Diagnostic testing in conjunction with genetic counselling is recommended for patients with onset before age 26 years or those with an affected relative with onset before age 26, if the patient wishes [24].

Genetic advances will undoubtedly revolutionise our understanding of dystonia and potentially lead to new treatments. At present, the treatment of patients with dystonia is largely symptomatic [25]. When DRD has been excluded by a trial of a levodopa preparation (in the case of childhood or adolescent-onset dystonia), anticholinergics are the most successful drugs, particularly in children, who tend to tolerate them better than adults. However, anticholinergics alone do not provide satisfactory benefit in most patients. Occasional patients derive some benefit from benzodiazepines, dopamine antagonists, levodopa, carbamazepine or baclofen. In the face of severe, sometimes life-threatening, 'dystonic storms', triple therapy with tetrabenazine, a neuroleptic and an anticholinergic may, by rendering patients akinetic, tide them over a severe exacerbation. Recently, pallidotomy or pallidal stimulation has been shown to be effective in a few patients with severe generalised dystonia [26,27], and is currently under trial in some centres.

Focal dystonia

Isolated adult-onset cervical and cranial dystonias are not caused by the *DYT 1* gene. There is usually little progression or spread, and most patients with spasmodic torticollis (ST/cervical dystonia), blepharospasm, or laryngeal dystonia ('spasmodic dysphonia') respond to injections of botulinum toxin into the involved muscles. ST patients who lose an initial favourable response have often developed antibodies against botulinum toxin type A. Botulinum toxin type B will soon be available as an alternative, and other new types of botulinum toxin (C, F) are currently under trial. Posterior primary ramicectomy may also be useful and pallidal DBS is currently under investigation, with promising but, as yet, unpublished results. Other focal dystonia such as writer's cramp and task-specific dystonia (eg 'occupational cramps') may also respond to botulinum toxin, but EMG-guided identification of responsible muscles is often necessary for successful treatment.

☐ PAROXYSMAL DYSKINESIAS

Paroxysmal dyskinesias mainly comprise:

- ☐ Stereotyped, short-lived (30–60 sec), often frequent attacks precipitated by sudden movements (kinesigenic) which are virtually 'cured' by long-term treatment with carbamazepine. Most cases are idiopathic, and commonly familial, but symptomatic cases occur. The pathophysiology is unclear, but it may be an ion-channel disorder.

- ☐ Less frequent, longer lasting (minutes to hours) non-kinesigenic attacks that sometimes respond to levodopa. In two families, the gene has been linked to chromosome 2q, close to a cluster of ion-channel genes, suggesting this may also be a channelopathy.

☐ USEFUL ADDRESSES

Parkinson's Disease Society
215 Vauxhall Bridge Rd
London SW1V 1EJ
Tel: 020 7931 8080

The Progressive Supranuclear Palsy Association
The Old Rectory
Wappenham Nr Towcester
Northamptonshire NN12 85Q
Tel: 01327 860 299

Autonomic Disorders Association
Sarah Matheson Trust
Pickering Unit
St Mary's Hospital
Praed Street
London W2 1NY
Tel: 020 7886 1520

National Tremor Foundation
Harold Wood Hospital (DSC)
Gubbins Lane
Romford
Essex RM3 0BE
Tel: 01708 378 050

The Dystonia Society
46–47 Britton Street
London EC1M 5UJ
Tel: 020 7490 5671

Huntington's Disease Association
108 Battersea High Street
London SW11 3HP
Tel: 020 7223 7000

REFERENCES

1 Ben-Shlomo Y. The epidemiology of Parkinson's disease. *Baillière's Clin Neurol* 1997;6:55–68.

2 Tanner CM, Ottman R, Goldman SM, *et al.* Parkinson disease in twins: an etiologic study. *JAMA* 1999;281:341–6.

3 Chase TN, Engber TM, Mouradian MM. Pathogenetic studies of motor response complications in levodopa-treated patients with advanced Parkinson's disease. In: Rinne UK, Nagatsu T, Horowski R (eds). *Parkinson's Disease*. International Workshop Berlin. Bussum: Medicom Europe, 1991:197.

4 Block G, Liss C, Reines S, *et al.* Comparison of immediate-release and controlled release carbidopa/levodopa in Parkinson's disease. A multicenter 5-year study. The CR First Study Group. *Eur Neurol* 1997;37:23–7.

5 Dupont E, Andersen A, Boas J, *et al.* Sustained-release Madopar HBS compared with standard Madopar in the long-term treatment of de novo parkinsonian patients. *Acta Neurol Scand* 1996;93:14–20.

6 Montastruc JL, Rascol O, Senard JM, Rascol A. A randomised controlled study comparing bromocriptine to which levodopa was later added, with levodopa alone in previously untreated patients with Parkinson's disease: a five year follow up. *J Neurol Neurosurg Psychiatry* 1994;57:1034–8.

7 Rascol O, Brooks DR, Korczyn AD, *et al.* A five-year study of the incidence of dyskinesia in patients with early Parkinson's disease who were treated with ropinirole or levodopa. 056 Study Group. *N Engl J Med* 2000; 342: 1484–91.

8 Hundemer HP, Lledo A, van Laar T, *et al.* The safety of pergolide monotherapy in early-stage Parkinson's disease. One-year interim analysis of a 3-year double-blind, randomized study of pergolide versus levodopa. *Mov Disord* 2000; 15 (Suppl 3): 115.

9 Shoulson I. Pramipexole versus levodopa in early Parkinson's disease: the Randomized Controlled CALM-PD Trial. *Mov Disord* 2000; 15 (Suppl 3): 4.

10   Musch B. The Investigators Study Group. Evaluation of patients with Parkinson's disease treated with cabergoline alone in a 5-year comparative study of cabergoline versus levodopa: a subgroup analysis. *Mov Disord* 2000: **15** (Suppl 3): 121.

11   Lees AJ. Comparison of therapeutic effects and mortality data of levodopa and levodopa combined with selegiline in patients with early, mild Parkinson's disease. Parkinson's Disease Research Group of the United Kingdom. *Br Med J* 1995;**311**:1602–7.

12   Nutt JG. Catechol-O-methyltransferase inhibitors for treatment of Parkinson's disease. *Lancet* 1998;**351**:1221–2.

13   Quinn N, Bhatia K. Functional neurosurgery for Parkinson's disease. *Br Med J* 1998;**316**: 1259–60.

14   Limousin P, Krack P, Pollak P, *et al.* Electrical stimulation of the subthalamic nucleus in advanced Parkinson's disease. *N Engl J Med* 1998;**339**:1105–11.

15   Gill SS, Heywood P. Bilateral dorsolateral subthalamotomy for advanced Parkinson's disease. *Lancet* 1997;**350**:1224.

16   McKeith IG, Galasko D, Kosaka K, *et al.* Consensus guidelines for the clinical and pathologic diagnosis of dementia with Lewy bodies (DLB): report of the consortium on DLB international workshop. *Neurology* 1996;**47**:1113–24.

17   Wenning GK, Quinn NP. Multiple system atrophy. *Baillière's Clin Neurol* 1997;**6**:187–204.

18   Litvan I, Agid Y, Calne D, *et al.* Clinical research criteria for the diagnosis of progressive supranuclear palsy (Steele-Richardson-Olszewski syndrome): report of the NINDS-SPSP international workshop. *Neurology* 1996;**47**:1–9.

19   Louis ED, Ford B, Wendt KJ, Cameron G. Clinical characteristics of essential tremor: data from a community-based study. *Mov Disord* 1998;**13**:803–8.

20   Chouinard S, Louis ED, Fahn S. Agreement among movement disorder specialists on the clinical diagnosis of essential tremor. *Mov Disord* 1997;**12**:973–6.

21   Benabid AL, Benazzouz A, Hoffmann D, *et al.* Long-term electrical inhibition of deep brain targets in movement disorders. *Mov Disord* 1998;**13**:S119–25.

22   Fahn S, Bressman SB, Marsden CD. Classification of dystonia. *Adv Neurol* 1998;**78**:1–10.

23   Bandmann O, Valente EM, Holmans P, *et al.* Dopa-responsive dystonia: a clinical and molecular genetic study. *Ann Neurol* 1998;**44**:649–56.

24   Bressman SB, Sabati C, Raymond D, *et al.* The DYT1 phenotype and guidelines for diagnostic testing. *Neurology* 2000; **54**: 1746–52.

25   Jankovic J. Medical therapy and botulinum toxin in dystonia. *Adv Neurol* 1998;**78**:169–83.

26   Lang AE. Surgical treatment of dystonia. *Adv Neurol* 1998;**78**:185–9.

27   Coubes P, Roubertie A, Vayssiere N, *et al.* Treatment of DYT1-generalised dystonia by stimulation of the internal globus pallidus. *Lancet* 2000; **355**: 2220–1.

☐ SELF ASSESSMENT QUESTIONS

1   The following drugs are dopamine agonists:
(a) Ropinirole
(b) Selegiline
(c) Cabergoline
(d) Apomorphine
(e) Entacapone

2   In Parkinson's disease, continuous release preparations of levodopa:
(a) Can worsen dyskinesias and unpredictability of response
(b) Have a higher bioavailability than standard preparations
(c) Used alone *de novo* delay the development of fluctuations and dyskinesia relative to standard preparations

(d) Given at bedtime, often improve night-time immobility
(e) Work 'faster' than standard preparations

3   In a young patient with dystonia:
(a) Wilson's disease must be excluded
(b) A trial of levodopa is mandatory
(c) Anticholinergics are poorly tolerated relative to adults
(d) The dystonia usually remains focal
(e) A diagnosis of 'cerebral palsy' should always be questioned

4   Treatment of Parkinson's disease should be started:
(a) As soon as the diagnosis is made
(b) When functional impairment interferes with quality of life
(c) As late as possible
(d) Always with levodopa
(e) With anticholinergics in the elderly

5   Huntington's disease
(a) Can be confirmed by genetic testing
(b) Is due to a genetic point mutation
(c) In young patients often presents with parkinsonism
(d) Is excluded if the family history is negative
(e) Is the commonest cause of hereditary chorea

ANSWERS

1a True	2a True	3a True	4a False	5a True
b False	b False	b True	b True	b False
c True	c False	c False	c False	c True
d True	d True	d False	d False	d False
e False	e False	e True	e False	e True

Physiotherapy in neurological disease: evidence-based medicine

Mark Wiles

☐ REHABILITATION, PHYSIOTHERAPY AND GOALS

Rehabilitation means to restore or re-establish a previous condition. Originally, it referred to 'rehabilitating' the memory or good name of a person or the restoration of privileges of rank by an authoritative act or statement. Would that things were now so simple! Rehabilitation has come to refer to the processes of assisting individuals with disease or injury to realise their maximum potential, whether this be in the physical, social or vocational domains of life. In the neurological context, both single event injuries (eg stroke, head injury) and progressive diseases (eg multiple sclerosis (MS)) are susceptible to rehabilitation. How to determine the maximum potential of any person is unclear and, pragmatically, must be defined by the afflicted individuals and/or their family and carers, often advised and informed by a range of health professionals. The setting of realistic goals is one of the primary objectives of any rehabilitation plan and, in order to maintain a relevant approach, the health professional needs to try to categorise the problem at several levels: pathology, impairment, disability (activity), handicap (participation), and the patient's sense of well-being (Fig. 1). Disagreement between patient and health professional about the relative importance of different aspects of quality of life (eg physical, mental health, general vitality) is probably a common occurrence, and may have a profound effect on the goal setting process for any treatment [1]. Misunderstanding between doctors and their patients about what benefit can accrue from medical or therapy interventions can arise due to varying combinations of poor communication, ignorance and inappropriateness of goals. Time spent explaining the limitations of all treatments in the individual context of the patient, and against the background of improved understanding of the disease in question, would seem to be an important role of the medical specialist and may avoid much disappointment and, possibly, wasted resources.

Physiotherapy (from the Greek meaning 'nature therapy') refers to the employment of physical measures to restore function after disease or injury or, to quote a pragmatic view from the Chartered Society of Physiotherapy's pamphlet on stroke [2]:

> to help the patient regain mobility and relearn, as far as possible, the movements required to perform, on their own, everyday tasks such as walking and eating, and to improve their quality of life.

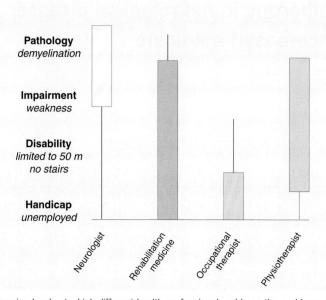

Fig. 1 Overlapping levels at which different health professionals address the problems of a multiple sclerosis patient. All have an interest in patient's sense of well-being/quality of life and level of distress (shaded rectangles = major areas of clinical activity; single lines = lesser areas of clinical activity.

Increasingly, health professionals all work as part of a multidisciplinary team. However, there is a tendency to regard all members of this team as more or less doing the same thing. This is partly because any experienced health worker can immediately recognise numerous deficiencies in information provision, facilities, home care and opportunities for many neurologically disabled patients in our healthcare system. Different healthcare workers, whilst sharing areas of clinical expertise, clearly have a distinctive potential contribution by virtue of their training and knowledge in specific skills. A neurologist may emphasise certain aspects of history and physical signs primarily relevant to making a diagnosis but without any relevance to disability as perceived by the patient. In rehabilitation medicine, impairments caused by the disease or injury must be enumerated and linked to the disability and handicap experienced by the patient in order to formulate a plan of management. A physiotherapist treating neurologically disabled patients uses a different approach based on an assessment of function that patients recognise as relevant to their disability, and which is, in part, independent of pathological diagnosis or specific impairment. When there is recovery or cure of a pathological state (eg demyelinisation) the resultant impairments and disability do not necessarily recover without some relearning of function. To a patient paralysed from Guillain-Barré syndrome it is self-evident that knowledge, assistance, guidance and teaching are required to recover function. For the patient, it is not an issue for a trial, and one could not conceive of admitting such a patient to a trial and not utilising the skills of a physiotherapist, despite a lack of formal evidence of benefit. As commented recently [3], the question as to whether rehabilitation 'works' is rather like asking if surgery or education 'works'. More focused questions are required, leading to appropriate research on specific therapeutic processes and procedures regardless of the discipline of origin. The right answers seem most likely to be found through multidisciplinary working.

☐ EVIDENCE BASE

Increasingly, there is an evidence base for many aspects of the rehabilitation process. For physiotherapy in particular, a brief survey of the Cochrane database, National Research Register and Medline revealed 22 randomised/controlled trials (RCT/CT) in neurological disorders in 1999, nine in 1998, 16 in 1997, six in 1996 and four in 1995. Research reviews and meta-analyses are starting to appear, specialist societies have regular scientific meetings, journals specifically publish these findings and, of course, the therapy professions are increasingly university based both at undergraduate and postgraduate level. Medical staff need to work and consult closely with therapist colleagues in order to bring best practice to their patients, and they have a duty to assist, by scientific clinical study, in further defining what best practice should be. This is more crucial as we move into an era of restorative neurology using pharmacological, brain grafting or brain stimulation/ablation techniques for modifying chronic progressive disease. Put simply, if such patients are not assisted and guided to renew physical and mental functions once lost, such elaborate treatments may fail to convert into improved physical activity, mental health and quality of life. Wasted quadriceps muscles due to a trophic deficiency, such as vitamin D, do not return to normal strength because the missing factor is replaced; they have to be used, and the patient may require help in developing this new usage. Furthermore, the means are available, using techniques such as real-time functional brain imaging or magnetic brain stimulation and neuropsychological evaluation, to examine the mechanisms underlying some of the nebulous phrases surrounding this area such as 'neuroplasticity', 'facilitation', 'mid-line orientation', and 'modification of postural set'.

☐ RESEARCH APPROACH

The research base is currently evolving in a 'top down' manner, largely because of accumulated and cogent evidence that people who have strokes do better if they are looked after in specialised units. There are factors (and not just human ones) at work, too many to enumerate, in 'specialised units' which make it hard to tease out the contributions (if any) of individual disciplines. An important step is reliably and systematically to record what is actually delivered to a patient in terms of therapy. Only in this way will it be possible to peer inside the 'black box' and form a clearer idea of which components of treatment actually matter [4]. A physiotherapist (like many health practitioners) targets a number of specific and non-specific issues when confronted with a clinical problem (Table 1). Though based on an analysis of function, the approach may be directed at specific impairments (eg spasticity,

Table 1 Spectrum of physiotherapy approach.

Specific approaches	Non-specific benefits
Tone	Exercise
Posture (mid-line, symmetry, stance)	Diagnostic skills
Increased movement and range	Information about disorder
Walking (avoidance of falls)	Practical issues and assistance
Sensory stimulation	Links to other agencies
Tremor (ataxia) reduction	Mood
Specific equipment	Counselling
Avoidance of injury or deficit	Going out and meeting others (outpatients)
Appropriate aids	

posture, weakness) or may take a task directed approach (eg how best to climb some stairs). The latter approach might be most effective in the patient's home, whilst the former is more appropriate to the gym. Sometimes the therapist must stop unproductive therapy and circumvent disability rather than treat it. The 'dosage' of therapy is currently based on face-to-face time – but what exactly is done in this time and how important is the experience and grade of therapist? Even if two therapists have the same therapeutic skills for a particular problem their ability to assess and set achievable goals may be different.

The mechanics of doing single case studies and RCTs of therapy do not differ from any other area of medicine in principle, but frequently there are weaknesses, often difficult to overcome, in recruitment of adequate numbers, confounders of therapy delivery, and blinding and independence of assessors. 'Non-therapy' trials are rare, and it may be difficult to exclude placebo or non-specific effects.

☐ SPECIFIC DISORDERS

Recent trials have examined the benefits of an overall package of care (eg stroke unit vs general medical ward) or attempted to dissect specific components of those processes (Tables 2 and 3). In these studies, it is striking how those employing a generic rehabilitation approach are usually strongly positive, whereas those which have carefully examined the benefits of specific techniques have, so far, often been borderline or negative. This may be due to lack of appropriate outcome measures in some of the latter studies but it seems unlikely that this is the full story. Furthermore, the practical difficulties faced by therapists undertaking randomised trials in our current health system should not be underestimated.

The issue of outcome measures sometimes seems to present an insurmountable hurdle to further progress in therapy research. There are increasing numbers of clinical outcome measures at all levels of the World Health Organization Disease Classification – impairment, disability/activity, and handicap/participation, as well as both generic and disease-specific scales [5] and quality of life measures. It often seems that designing new outcome scales with collection of related reliability and

Table 2 Some generic trials of process after stroke.

Study	Type	n	Subject	Outcome
Baskett J, et al. Clin Rehabil 1999;**13**:23–33	RCT	100	Supervised home versus outpatient based therapy	Equal benefit
Widen Holmqvist L, et al. Stroke 1998;**29**:591–7	RCT	81	Early supported home discharge	Equal benefit
Rudd AG, et al. Br Med J 1997; **315**:1039–44	RCT	331	Early discharge (specialist community rehabilitation)	Equal benefit
Dennis M, et al. Br Med J 1997; **314**:1071–6	RCT	417	Stroke family care worker	– physical /+satisfaction
Gladman JR, et al. J Neurol Neurosurg Psychiatry 1993; **56**:960–6	RCT	327	Domiciliary or hospital based rehabilitation after discharge	Equal benefit
Kalra L, et al. Stroke 1993; **24**:1462–7	RCT	245	Stroke unit or general medical ward	Benefit from stroke unit
Stroke Unit Trialists' Collaboration. Br Med J 1997;**314**:1151–9	Systematic review	2060	Organised inpatient care after stroke	Benefit from stroke unit
Rice-Oxley M, Turner-Stokes L. Clin Rehabil 1999;**13**:S7–24	Critical review		Brain injury rehabilitation	

RCT = randomised controlled trial.

validity data [6] has become a diversion away from the design of quality experimental formats needed to test new therapies. In understanding how a therapy brings benefit, in order to improve or change it, measurements at the level of impairment remain important: if the patient became more mobile, was it because of improved posture, less spasticity or improved strength and, if the last, was this due to reduced coactivation of antagonist muscles?

The perspective for a patient with an acute single event brain injury such as a stroke differs from that for someone with a progressive neurological disorder. In particular, the former often knows the worst but the latter does not – indeed, it may be impossible to tell the latter what the worst will be or when it will happen. To some extent, those with major brain injury in youth or early life (eg major brain injury, cerebral palsy) face similar difficulties because to their burden is added a progressive deterioration due to intercurrent disease and/or complications of their neurological state. Nevertheless, issues in progressive disease are being addressed in a number of such disorders by means of both RCTs and single subject trials (Table 4).

Whilst it is clear from most of the studies in Table 4 that inpatient rehabilitation and physiotherapy are of benefit to patients with secondary or primary progressive

Table 3 Some specific trials of physiotherapy techniques after stroke.

Study	Type	n	Subject	Outcome
Kwakkel G, et al. Lancet 1999;**354**:191–96	RCT	101	Intensity of arm and leg therapy after MCA stroke	Benefit
Lincoln N, et al. Stroke 1999;**30**:573–9	RCT	282	Intensity of physio-therapy treatment of arm function	No benefit
van der Lee JH, et al. Stroke 1999;**30**:2369–75	RCT	66	Forced use of paretic arm	Benefit (±)
Duncan P, et al. Stroke 1998;**29**:2055–60	RCT	20	Post-discharge home exercise programme	No benefit
Bradley L, et al. Clin Rehabil 1998;**12**:11–22	RCT	21	EMG feedback vs none for gait training	No benefit
Langhorne P, Physiother Res Int 1996;**1**:75–88	Systematic review	597	Physiotherapy after stroke. Is more better?	Benefit (±)
Sackley CM, Lincoln NB. Disabil Rehabil 1997;**19**:536–46	RCT	26	Visual feedback on stance symmetry and function	Benefit (±)
Burridge JH, et al. Clin Rehabil 1997;**11**:201–10	RCT	32	Common peroneal stimulation vs none and walking	No benefit
Young J, Forster A. J R Coll Physicians Lond 1993;**27**:252–8	RCT	124	Day hospital or home physiotherapy after discharge	Benefit
Moreland J, Thomson MA. Phys Ther 1994;**74**:534–43	Systematic review	135	EMG biofeedback vs conventional physiotherapy in arm	No benefit
Wade DT, et al. Br Med J 1992;**304**:609–13	RCT	94	Late physiotherapy intervention after stroke	Benefit (±)

± transient benefit.
MCA = middle cerebral artery; RCT = randomised controlled trial.

MS, the specific reasons are elusive. Such patients are often isolated at home, have affective and cognitive impairments and a variety of needs that may be uncatered for by the health system: for instance, they may have untreated or undiagnosed bladder symptoms, frank depression and problematic anxiety. Therefore, the non-specific benefit to be obtained from the personal contact offered by a regular home visit from any health professional with specific knowledge of their condition is likely to be substantial (Table 1). Finding an appropriate experimental control for this non-specific

Table 4 Randomised/controlled trials (RCT/CT) of rehabilitation or physiotherapy in multiple sclerosis.

Study	Type	n	Subject	Outcome
Solari A, et al. Neurology 1999;**52**:57–62	RCT	50	Inpatient therapy (3 weeks)	Benefit
Lord SE, et al. Clin Rehabil 1998;**12**:477–86	RCT	23	Facilitation vs task orientated physiotherapy in MS	= Benefit
Di Fabio RP, et al. Arch Phys Med Rehabil 1998;**79**:141–6	CT	46	Waiting list controlled – outpatient rehabilitation	? Benefit
Freeman JA, et al. Ann Neurol 1997;**42**:236–44	RCT	66	Waiting list controlled – inpatient rehabilitation	Benefit
Petajan JH, et al. Ann Neurol 1996;**39**:432–41	RCT	54	Aerobic training versus non-exercise	Benefit
Jones L, et al. Clin Rehabil 1996;**10**:277–82	RCT	37	Ataxia and tremor: physiotherapy and occupational therapy	Benefit
Fuller KJ, et al. Clin Rehabil 1996;**10**:195–204	RCT	45	Inpatient physio-therapy vs none	No benefit
Wiles CM, et al. J Neurol, Neurosurg Psychiatry 2000;**68**:259	RCXT	42	Home, hospital outpatient and no physiotherapy	Benefit
Ko Ko C. Clin Rehab 1999;**13**:S31-41	Critical review			

RCXT = randomised crossover trial.

component of benefit, so that the specific content of therapy may be investigated, is important in the development of this type of research. Furthermore, the natural history of MS provides obstacles which make randomisation an essential element of any controlled trial. The referral process to medical, rehabilitation or physiotherapy contact is likely to be triggered by subtle, often ill specified, changes in physical or mental status, which are often likely to represent relapses of disease whose natural history will be equally subtle improvement which could be mistaken for the effects of therapy if randomisation is not undertaken. Alternatively, dramatic changes in dependency resulting in referral may result from purely intercurrent conditions (eg infection) separate from the underlying disease. By contrast non-referred patients recruited with similar disability will be less likely to show spontaneous improvement. Finally, in progressive disease, prevention of deterioration from the primary or secondary effects of a condition may be as important an aim of therapy as immediate benefit.

Apart from stroke and MS, lumbosacral radicular symptoms and low back pain have been major topic areas for RCTs, helped by the fact that the conditions are common and physiotherapists have a firmly established role in their management. It

Table 5 Examples of trials of physiotherapy in disorders other than multiple sclerosis and stroke.

Study	Type	n	Subject	Outcome
Moffett JK, et al. Br Med J 1999;**319**:279–83	RCT	187	Exercise for low back pain	Benefit
Lindeman E, et al. Arch Phys Med Rehabil 1995;**76**:612–20	RCT	62	Strength training in myotonic dystrophy and HMSN	No benefit
Bower E, et al. Dev Med Child Neurol 1996;**38**:226–37	RCT	44	Intensity of physiotherapy and goal setting in cerebral palsy	Benefit
Comella CL, et al. Neurology 1994;**44**:376–8	RCXT	18	Physical therapy in Parkinson's disease	Benefit (±)
Gibberd FB, et al. Br Med J 1981;**282**:1196	RCT	24	Physiotherapy and occupational therapy in Parkinson's disease	No benefit
Coxhead CE, et al. Lancet 1981;**1**:1065–8	RCT	322	Physiotherapy for sciatic symptoms	Early benefit
Parker GB, et al. Aust N Z J Med 1978;**8**:589–93	RCT	85	Cervical manipulation for migraine chiropractor/physiotherapist	No benefit
Haigh R, Clarke AK. Clin Rehabil 1999;**13**:S63–81	Critical review	Back pain		

± transient benefit.
HMSN = hereditary motor and sensory neuropathy; RCT = randomised controlled trial; RCXT = randomised crossover trial.

remains problematic to undertake randomised trials of physiotherapy in less common neurological disorders, but nevertheless some have been achieved (Table 5).

☐ COST-EFFECTIVENESS

Cost-effectiveness of treatment is a major issue for our health service. The benefits on disability found in some trials of the new disease-modifying drugs look quite small (though for some individuals perceived as very important) and very expensive. Thus, in secondary progressive MS, the number needed to treat with beta interferon-1b for 30 months to delay wheelchair independence in one person by nine months was 18 (95% confidence interval 5–26), with six relapses also prevented in the 18 people at a cost of about £440,000 [7]. At £25 per session, 70 MS patients might be provided with two home sessions of physiotherapy per week for the same period (2.5 years) with this sum. It seems proper to ask whether provision of physiotherapy could not attain the same, much fêted, aim of reduction of disability, at considerably less cost. Ideally, combined approaches would seem to offer the best way forward, but to pour large sums into a drug budget at the expense of other potentially useful forms of treatment seems ill-advised.

☐ CONCLUSION

All aspects of disease management and rehabilitation are under scrutiny for evidence of effectiveness. Therapy services have, like medicine, moved forward considerably in this area. Collaboration between health professionals to undertake better and more effective research about the best way of achieving clearly defined goals in specific conditions seems certain to be for the good of our patients.

REFERENCES

1   Rothwell PM, McDowell Z, Wong CK, Dorman PJ. Doctors and patients don't agree: cross sectional study of patients' and doctors' perceptions and assessments of disability in multiple sclerosis. *Br Med J* 1997; **314**: 1580–3.

2   The Chartered Society of Physiotherapy. [Stroke pamphlet] (Available from CSP, 14 Bedford Row, London WC1R 4ED. Tel: 020 7242 1941).

3   Wade D. Editorial. *Clin Rehabil* 1998; **12**: 95–7.

4   Ballinger C, Ashburn A, Low J, Roderick P. Unpacking the black box of therapy – a pilot study to describe occupational therapy and physiotherapy interventions for people with stroke. *Clin Rehabil* 1999; **13**: 301–9.

5   Wade DT. *Measurement in Neurological Rehabilitation*. Oxford: Oxford Medical Publications, 1992.

6   Hobart JC, Lamping DL, Thompson AJ. Evaluating neurological outcome measures: the bare essentials [editorial]. *J Neurol Neurosurg Psychiatry* 1996; **60**: 127–30.

7   Forbes RB, Lees A, Waugh N, Swingler RJ. Population based cost utility study of interferon beta-1b in secondary progressive multiple sclerosis. *Br Med J* 1999; **319**: 1529–33.

What's new in metabolic bone disease?

Stuart H Ralston

☐ INTRODUCTION

Advances in cell biology, molecular biology and genetics have revolutionised our understanding of the mechanisms which regulate bone turnover and susceptibility to several bone diseases. This chapter reviews some recent developments in this area, with an emphasis on those that have had or will have an impact on clinical practice.

☐ CANCER-ASSOCIATED BONE DISEASE

Bone metastases and hypercalcaemia are important causes of morbidity in cancer. Hypercalcaemia causes diverse symptoms including nausea, vomiting, dehydration, malaise and neuropsychiatric deterioration, whereas the main manifestations of bone metastases are bone pain and pathological fracture. It is now established that most cases of hypercalcaemia in malignancy are due to overproduction of parathyroid hormone-related protein (PTHrP) by the tumour. PTHrP is a peptide regulatory hormone with homology to parathyroid hormone (PTH), and is normally produced in tissues such as breast, skin and lung where it acts as a local mediator of cellular activity and differentiation. In patients with tumours of these tissues, excessive amounts of PTHrP are released into the systemic circulation, which causes hypercalcaemia by mimicking the effects of PTH on bone and kidney. The only tumour that commonly causes hypercalcaemia without producing PTHrP is myeloma; here, multifocal bone resorption is stimulated by cytokines such as interleukin (IL)-1, tumour necrosis factor (TNF)-alpha and lymphotoxin [1].

Bone metastases are also a common cause of morbidity in cancer patients but the incidence differs markedly in different tumour types. Some tumours such as breast cancer, myeloma and prostate carcinoma are characterised by extensive metastatic bone involvement whereas other tumours seldom target to bone. The preferential targeting of certain tumours to bone is thought to be due to the 'seed and soil' hypothesis (Fig. 1). Tumour cells which enter the circulation appear to be preferentially attracted to sites of bone remodelling by chemotactic effects of bone resorption products. Tumour cells then become established in the marrow space, and attach to bone matrix by adhesive interactions that involve the beta 1 and beta 3 integrin receptors [2]. Substances which are produced by bone cells or are released during the process of bone resorption act as growth factors for the tumour, thereby promoting tumour cell survival and expansion in the bone marrow space. In multiple myeloma, for example, IL-6 is released by bone cells in response to

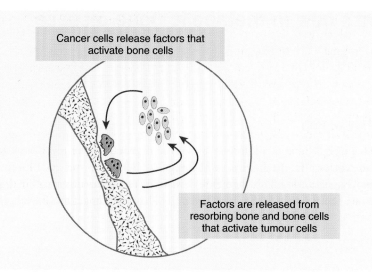

Fig. 1 'Seed and soil' hypothesis for growth of bone metastases.

cytokines such as IL-1 and TNF secreted by myeloma cells. The IL-6 then stimulates myeloma cell growth, resulting in a positive feedback loop of increased tumour growth and bone resorption [3]. In breast cancer, release of transforming growth factor (TGF)-beta during bone resorption has been postulated to set up a similar positive feedback loop in which PTHrP production is increased and bone resorption enhanced [4]. A similar situation may arise in prostate carcinoma which is associated with osteoblastic metastases. Recent studies have identified endothelin-1 as a mediator of osteoblastic metastases in prostate cancer [5] and have shown that expression of this factor is also upregulated by TGF-beta [6].

☐ TREATMENT OF BONE METASTASES WITH BISPHOSPHONATES

Advances in understanding the pathogenesis of bone metastases have been accompanied by advances in treatment. It is well established that osteoclastic bone resorption, mediated by products released by tumour cells, is the primary mechanism responsible for bone destruction in cancer. This osteoclast activation can be effectively inhibited by bisphosphonate treatment. Bisphosphonates are non-hydrolysable analogues of inorganic pyrophosphate, in which the central oxygen atom of the P-O-P structure is replaced by a carbon, giving a P-C-P structure. Like pyrophosphate, bisphosphonates have high affinity for binding hydroxyapatite and are targeted to sites of osteoclastic bone resorption. The potency of individual bisphosphonates depends on the structure of the side chains which are attached to the central carbon atom. Bisphosphonates such as clodronate, etidronate and tiludronate, which have simple side chains, have relatively low potency; they exert their inhibitory action on bone resorption by forming non-hydrolysable analogues of ATP that trigger osteoclast apoptosis. Bisphosphonates with nitrogen containing side chains are, by comparison, much more potent. Aminobisphosphonates also stimulate osteoclast apoptosis, but do so by inhibiting enzymes in the mevalonate pathway which are responsible for attaching farnesyl- and geranylgeranyl-lipid groups to small GTP binding proteins such as Rho, Ras and Rac. In the absence of lipid modification, these proteins are unable to target to the cell membrane and take part in signalling pathways which are necessary for cell survival (Fig. 2) [7]. Interestingly, HMG Co-A reductase inhibitors (statins) act at a different point on the same pathway and also have modulatory effects on bone cells *in vitro* [8].

Large-scale randomised clinical trials support the routine use of bisphosphonates such as oral clodronate and intravenous pamidronate in the secondary prevention of bone metastases due to multiple myeloma and breast carcinoma [9–11]. Some studies have also shown evidence of a survival benefit in patients treated with clodronate for breast cancer [12], raising the possibility that bisphosphonates may exert anti-tumour effects as well as an anti-bone resorptive effect.

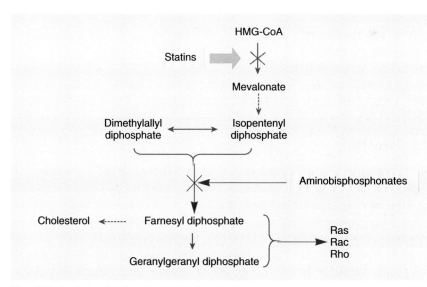

Fig. 2 Mechanisms of action of aminobisphosphonates.

☐ HYPERCALCAEMIA

The most significant advance in understanding the mechanisms of hypercalcaemia has stemmed from the molecular cloning of the calcium sensing receptor (CaSR). The CaSR is a seven transmembrane G-protein coupled transmembrane receptor, encoded by a single gene on chromosome 3q which is highly expressed in the parathyroid glands, kidneys and other tissues. Signalling through the CaSR plays an important role in regulating PTH secretion in response to circulating serum calcium concentrations. Recent work indicates that normal variation in serum calcium concentration and most cases of familial hypocalciuric hypercalcaemia (FHH) are due to sequence variations in the CaSR [13,14]. Several inactivating mutations of the CaSR have been described in affected individuals from kindreds with FHH – a rare condition inherited in an autosomal dominant manner, characterised by mild to moderate hypercalcaemia, normal or slightly elevated circulating PTH values and low urinary calcium excretion (Table 1). Most cases of FHH map to chromosome 3q, but families have been described which map to chromosomes 19q and 19p suggesting that there may be other genes in the CaSR pathway which can give the same phenotype. More subtle polymorphisms of the CaSR have also been described, related to variations in serum calcium levels in normal individuals.

Pharmacological treatments have also been developed which mimic the effects of calcium on the CaSR, opening up the possibility of developing a medical treatment for primary hyperparathyroidism.

Table 1 Clinical and biochemical features of familial hypocalciuric hypercalcaemia.

Asymptomatic hypercalcaemia
Normal/high serum magnesium
Low urinary calcium excretion
Normal/high serum parathyroid hormone values
Autosomal dominant inheritance

☐ OSTEOPOROSIS

Much interest has focused on the role of genetic factors in the pathogenesis of osteoporosis. Twin and family studies have shown that 50–85% of the variance in bone mass is genetically determined, and other factors such as bone turnover, femoral neck geometry and ultrasound properties of bone also have strong genetic components. Family history of osteoporotic fracture predicts the occurrence of fractures independent of bone mass. Taken together, these data are consistent with strong genetic influences on the pathogenesis of osteoporosis, involving variation in genes which affect not only bone density but also other aspects of fracture risk such as skeletal geometry, bone turnover and bone quality.

Linkage studies in families and sibling pairs have suggested that multiple regions of the genome regulate bone mass, with susceptibility loci on several chromosomes (Table 2) [15–17]. Association studies have similarly identified polymorphisms of several candidate genes that have been associated with bone mass, including the vitamin D receptor, oestrogen receptor, TGF-beta and collagen type I alpha 1 (COLIA1). Studies of the COLIA1 gene have identified a polymorphism which affects a Sp1 binding site that is associated with an increased risk of osteoporotic fracture by mechanisms that are partly independent of differences in bone mass [18]. This polymorphism may predispose to fracture by impairing bone strength. Although the mechanism by which this occurs is still being investigated, data so far indicate that the polymorphism increases affinity for Sp1 binding and alters the transcriptional regulation of COLIA1.

Table 2 Candidate genes and quantitative trait loci for regulation of bone mass.

Quantitative trait loci	1p36
	1q21-22
	2p23-24
	4q32-34
	5q33-35
	6p11-12
	11q12-13
Candidate genes	Vitamin D receptor
	Oestrogen receptor
	Collagen type I alpha 1
	Transforming growth factor beta
	Apolipoprotein E
	Calcitonin receptor

☐ PAGET'S DISEASE OF BONE

Paget's disease of bone is characterised by focal areas of increased and disorganised bone remodelling which predominantly affects individuals from the age of 55 years and above. It is a common disease in Caucasians, affecting about 3% of individuals over the age of 55 in the UK and 1% of individuals in the USA. Two main hypotheses have been suggested to account for the development of Paget's disease: one is that Paget's disease is due to a slow virus infection of osteoclasts with one of the paramyxoviruses, and the other is that it is primarily a genetic disease. A unifying hypothesis suggests that Paget's disease may arise as the result of a genetic predisposition to a viral infection. The viral hypothesis of Paget's disease followed the description of nuclear inclusion bodies in Pagetic osteoclasts which were thought to resemble paramyxovirus nucleocapsids. A wide variety of approaches including reverse-transcription/polymerase chain reaction, immunohistochemistry and *in situ* hybridisation have failed to detect conclusive evidence of persistent virus infection in Paget's disease (reviewed in [19]).

Several lines of evidence support a role for genetic factors in the pathogenesis of Paget's disease. Familial clustering of Paget's disease is well recognised, and it has been estimated that 14–40% of Pagetic patients have one or more affected first-degree relatives [20]. Familial expansile osteolysis (FEO) is a rare condition which has been considered to be a genetic model of Paget's disease. FEO shares many features in common with Paget's disease, but has an earlier age at onset, rarely affects the axial skeleton, and is characterised by premature deafness and loss of dentition [21]. The gene responsible for FEO was mapped to an approximately 20 cM interval on chromosome 18q21-22 in 1994. The similarities between Paget's disease and FEO led two other groups of workers to look for evidence of 18q linkage in familial Paget's disease. Both groups reported positive lod scores across the FEO critical region in families with autosomal dominant Paget's disease [22,23], although linkage was excluded in some of the families, demonstrating evidence of genetic heterogeneity [23]. Positional cloning studies localised the gene for receptor activator of nuclear factor kappa B (RANK) to the FEO/Paget's critical region. RANK is a strong candidate gene for both diseases since it plays an essential role in osteoclast differentiation and function [24]. Hughes *et al* [25] identified two heterozygous insertion mutations of the RANK signal peptide which co-segregated with the disease in several families with FEO and one family with clinical features of severe early onset Paget's disease. No evidence of RANK mutations were found in three other Pagetic families where previous studies had shown possible evidence of linkage to 18q21-22, or in a large number of sporadic cases of Paget's disease. Expression studies showed that both mutations activated NFκB signalling *in vitro*. The mutations interfere with normal processing of the receptor, possibly leading to increased self-association and activation of signalling (Fig. 3). From these data it appears that insertion mutations of RANK cause FEO, and may rarely cause severe, early onset familial Paget's disease. The genes responsible for other cases of familial Paget's disease remain to be defined, although components of the RANK signalling pathway seem likely candidates.

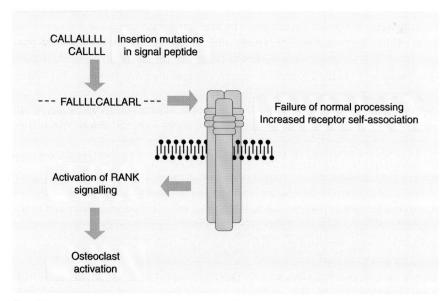

Fig. 3 Receptor activator of nuclear factor kappa B mutations in familial expansile osteolysis and severe early Paget's disease.

REFERENCES

1   Guise TA, Mundy GR. Cancer and bone. *Endocr Rev* 1998; **19**: 18–54.
2   Boissier S, Magnetto S, Frappart L, *et al.* Bisphosphonates inhibit prostate and breast carcinoma cell adhesion to unmineralized and mineralized bone extracellular matrices. *Cancer Res* 1997; **57**: 3890–4.

3 Barille S, Collette M, Bataille R, Amiot M. Myeloma cells upregulate interleukin-6 secretion in osteoblastic cells through cell-to-cell contact but downregulate osteocalcin. *Blood* 1995; **86:** 3151–9.

4 Guise TA, Yin JJ, Taylor SD, *et al.* Evidence for a causal role of parathyroid hormone-related protein in the pathogenesis of human breast cancer-mediated osteolysis. *J Clin Invest* 1996; **98:** 1544–9.

5 Nelson JB, Hedican SP, George DJ, *et al.* Identification of endothelin-1 in the pathophysiology of metastatic adenocarcinoma of the prostate. *Nat Med* 1995; **1:** 944–9.

6 Le Brun G, Aubin P, Soliman H, *et al.* Upregulation of endothelin 1 and its precursor by IL-1 beta, TNF-alpha, and TGF-beta in the PC3 human prostate cancer cell line. *Cytokine* 1999; **11:** 157–62.

7 Rogers MJ, Watts DJ, Russell RGG. Overview of bisphosphonates. *Cancer* 1997; **80:** 1652–60.

8 Rogers MJ. Statins: lower lipids and better bones? *Nat Med* 2000; **6:** 21–3.

9 Berenson JR, Lichtenstein A, Porter L, *et al.* Efficacy of pamidronate in reducing skeletal events in patients with advanced multiple myeloma. Myeloma Aredia Study Group. *N Engl J Med* 1996; **334:** 488–93.

10 Hortobagyi GN, Theriault RL, Lipton A, *et al.* Long-term prevention of skeletal complications of metastatic breast cancer with pamidronate. Protocol 19 Aredia Breast Cancer Study Group. *J Clin Oncol* 1998; **16:** 2038–44.

11 McCloskey EV, MacLennan IC, Drayson MT, *et al.* A randomized trial of the effect of clodronate on skeletal morbidity in multiple myeloma. MRC Working Party on Leukaemia in Adults. *Br J Haematol* 1998; **100:** 317–25.

12 Diel IJ, Solomayer E-F, Costa SD, *et al.* Reduction in new metastases in breast cancer with adjuvant clodronate treatment. *N Engl J Med* 1998; **339:** 357–63.

13 Pollak MR, Brown EM, Chou YH, *et al.* Mutations in the human Ca(2+)-sensing receptor gene cause familial hypocalciuric hypercalcemia and neonatal severe hyperparathyroidism. *Cell* 1993; **75:** 1297–303.

14 Cole DE, Peltekova VD, Rubin LA, *et al.* A986S polymorphism of the calcium-sensing receptor and circulating calcium concentrations. *Lancet* 1999; **353:** 112–5.

15 Devoto M, Shimoya K, Caminis J, *et al.* First-stage autosomal genome screen in extended pedigrees suggests genes predisposing to low bone mineral density on chromosomes 1p, 2p and 4q. *Eur J Hum Genet* 1998; **6:** 151–7.

16 Koller DL, Rodriguez LA, Christian JC, *et al.* Genome screen for QTLs contributing to normal variation in bone mineral density and osteoporosis. *J Bone Miner Res* 1999; **14:** S141.

17 Koller DL, Rodriguez LA, Christian JC, *et al.* Linkage of a QTL contributing to normal variation in bone mineral density to chromosome 11q12-13. *J Bone Miner Res* 1999; **13:** 1903–8.

18 Grant SFA, Reid DM, Blake G, *et al.* Reduced bone density and osteoporosis associated with a polymorphic Sp1 site in the collagen type I alpha 1 gene. *Nat Genet* 1996; **14:** 203–5.

19 Helfrich MH, Hobson RP, Cash B, *et al.* No evidence of paramyxovirus RNA in bone or bone marrow of patients with Paget's disease: a multicentre study using nested RT/PCR. *J Bone Miner Res* 1996; **11:** S164.

20 Siris ES, Ottman R, Flaster E, Kelsey JL. Familial aggregation of Paget's disease of bone. *J Bone Miner Res* 1991; **6:** 495–500.

21 Osterberg PH, Wallace RGH, Adams DA, *et al.* Familial expansile osteolysis: a new dysplasia. *J Bone Joint Surg Br* 1988; **70:** 255–60.

22 Cody JD, Singer FR, Roodman GD, *et al.* Genetic linkage of Paget's disease of the bone to chromosome 18q. *Am J Hum Genet* 1997; **61:** 1117–22.

23 Haslam SI, Van Hul W, Morales-Piga A, *et al.* Paget's disease of bone: evidence for a susceptibility locus on chromosome 18q and for genetic heterogeneity. *J Bone Miner Res* 1998; **13:** 911–7.

24 Hofbauer LC, Khosla S, Dunstan CR, *et al.* The roles of osteoprotegerin and osteoprotegerin ligand in the paracrine regulation of bone resorption. Review. *J Bone Miner Res* 2000; **15:** 2–12.

25 Hughes AE, Ralston SH, Marken J, *et al.* Mutations in the RANK signal peptide cause familial expansile osteolysis. *Nat Genet* 2000; **24:** 45–9.

☐ SELF ASSESSMENT QUESTIONS

1 Mediators of increased bone resorption in cancer include:
(a) Parathyroid hormone (PTH)
(b) PTH-related protein
(c) Calcitonin
(d) Interleukin (IL)-1
(e) IL-5

2 Bisphosphonates:
(a) Are an effective treatment for bone metastases
(b) Are concentrated in the liver
(c) Cause necrosis of osteoclasts
(d) Inhibit bone resorption by chelating calcium
(e) Are rapidly metabolised and hydrolysed by phosphatases in bone

3 Familial hypocalciuric hypercalcaemia is characterised by:
(a) Hypermagnesaemia
(b) Autosomal recessive inheritance
(c) Undetectable levels of PTH
(d) Mutations of the calcium sensing receptor
(e) Renal stone disease

4 The following are true about osteoporosis:
(a) Poor diet and lack of exercise are the main factors in pathogenesis
(b) The genetic contribution is usually monogenic
(c) Family history is an important clinical risk factor
(d) Polymorphisms of the angiotensin-converting enzyme gene have been implicated in pathogenesis
(e) The vitamin D receptor is a candidate gene

5 Familial expansile osteolysis is characterised by:
(a) Paget's disease-like bone lesions
(b) Deafness
(c) Autosomal recessive inheritance
(d) Mutations in the receptor activator of nuclear factor kappa B gene
(e) Involvement of the axial skeleton

ANSWERS

1a False	2a True	3a True	4a False	5a True
b True	b False	b False	b False	b True
c False	c False	c False	c True	c False
d True	d False	d True	d False	d True
e False	e False	e False	e True	e False

Osteoporosis: how and who to treat

Juliet Compston

☐ INTRODUCTION

In recent years there have been significant advances in the management of osteoporosis and a number of treatment options are now available (Table 1) [1,2]. For historical reasons, the level of evidence on which the registration of these interventions is based varies widely. Thus, adequately powered randomised controlled trials (RCTs) with fracture as the primary end-point exist only for alendronate, raloxifene, risedronate and combined calcium and vitamin D, whereas, in the case of hormone replacement therapy (HRT), evidence for anti-fracture efficacy is based almost solely on observational data which are subject to bias and likely to overestimate beneficial effects.

Table 1 Agents licensed for the prevention and treatment of postmenopausal osteoporosis.

Hormone replacement therapy
Bisphosphonates (alendronate, risedronate and cyclic etidronate)
Raloxifene
Calcitriol
Calcitonin
Nandrolone (use not recommended)
Calcium and vitamin D (adjunct)

Fracture is the only important clinical outcome of osteoporosis and the primary aim of an intervention is therefore to reduce fracture risk. There is increasing evidence that therapeutically induced increases in bone mineral density (BMD) do not reliably predict accompanying reductions in fracture rate, and demonstration of anti-fracture efficacy is therefore a mandatory requirement for registration. For regulatory purposes, a distinction is made between prevention and treatment of osteoporosis, but this is not useful in clinical practice nor is it logical since all interventions currently used act by reducing bone turnover. Furthermore, there is increasing evidence that relatively short-term intervention with anti-resorptive agents, even in elderly women with established osteoporosis, produces a significant reduction in fracture rate. It is therefore more useful to consider the indication for therapeutic intervention as prevention of osteoporotic fracture, whether or not fragility fracture has already occurred.

Table 2 Factors influencing the positioning of agents in postmenopausal osteoporosis.

Anti-fracture efficacy
Site-specificity
Rate of onset and offset of treatment effect
Adverse effects
Long-term extraskeletal risks and benefits
  (hormone replacement therapy and raloxifene)
Cost

☐ POSITIONING OF INTERVENTIONS: GENERAL CONSIDERATIONS

Issues relevant to the positioning of treatment in osteoporosis are shown in Table 2. The magnitude of anti-fracture efficacy is an important theoretical consideration; however, it is not possible to compare directly results for different interventions because of differences in the trial designs, the populations studied and the criteria used to define vertebral deformity.

The rate of onset and offset of treatment effect is also important and has particular implications for the timing and duration of therapy. Site-specificity may also affect the positioning of agents; since fracture at any site is an independent risk factor for fragility fracture elsewhere, an intervention will ideally be effective at all common fracture sites. The adverse effect profile clearly may affect choice of treatment, as may any extraskeletal risks and benefits of long-term treatment. Finally, cost is an increasingly important consideration which has to be set against the risks and benefits of the particular therapy.

☐ INTERVENTIONS

Hormone replacement therapy

The beneficial effects of oestrogen replacement on bone mass at and after the menopause are well established and observational data indicate that there is also significant protection against fracture at the hip, spine and wrist. Oral, transdermal and parenteral formulations of oestrogen are effective, and unopposed oestrogen and combined oestrogen/progestogen replacement appear to have similar effects.

There is growing evidence for attenuation of the beneficial effects of HRT on the skeleton following withdrawal of therapy. In a recent population-based case-control study from Sweden of women with hip fracture [1], greater protection against fracture was seen in current as opposed to past users, and five years after cessation of HRT the risk of hip fracture in former users had reverted to that of non-users. These observations have two major implications:

1   Life-long treatment after the menopause is required to maintain fracture protection.

2   Strategies which target high risk women for treatment are likely to be most cost-effective.

Short-term side effects of HRT include breast tenderness and withdrawal bleeding. Although continuous combined 'no-bleed' preparations are now available, some vaginal bleeding is experienced by up to 30% of women during the first few months of such therapy. The major concern with long-term use is an increase in the risk of breast cancer; after 5–10 years' use, the relative risk increases by 30%, which is highly significant in terms of absolute risk. Other adverse extraskeletal side effects include a two to three-fold increase in risk of venous thromboembolism and a small increase in the risk of endometrial cancer, even in those women taking combined formulations.

HRT also has important short- and long-term benefits. It is effective in alleviating vasomotor and other menopausal symptoms and may also have beneficial effects on postural stability. Observational data indicate a significant reduction in morbidity and mortality attributable to coronary heart disease (CHD); however, in a recent study of the effects of combined HRT in older women with CHD more deaths due to heart disease occurred during the first year in treated women than in controls. Other potential, but as yet unproven, benefits of long-term HRT include improved cognitive function, protection against Alzheimer's disease and a reduction in risk of colon cancer (Table 3).

Table 3 Potential long-term risks and benefits of hormone replacement therapy.

Risks	Benefits
Endometrial cancer	Prevention of osteoporosis
Breast cancer	Protection against coronary heart disease
Venous thromboembolism	Protection against colon cancer
	Improved cognitive function
	Reduced risk of Alzheimer's disease

Bisphosphonates

The bisphosphonates are synthetic analogues of the naturally occurring compound pyrophosphate. Three bisphosphonates are currently licensed for use in osteoporosis. Etidronate is administered cyclically and intermittently, the three-month cycle consisting of etidronate 400 mg daily for two weeks followed by calcium alone for 76 days. In contrast, alendronate and risedronate are given as single daily doses of 10 mg and calcium is not included in the formulation.

All three bisphosphonates prevent bone loss in the spine and hip, both in healthy perimenopausal women and in more elderly women with osteoporosis. In the Fracture Intervention Trial (FIT), treatment with alendronate for nearly three years was associated with a reduction of approximately 50% in vertebral and non-vertebral fractures in postmenopausal women with established spinal osteoporosis [3], although in women with low BMD (at the hip) and no prevalent fracture, a significant reduction only in vertebral fracture rate was seen [4]. In the case of cyclic etidronate therapy, the clinical trials were not adequately powered to demonstrate fracture reduction but favourable trends for vertebral fracture were observed after three years treatment, and observational data also indicate protective effects against hip and other non-vertebral fractures. Because of the different designs of the clinical trials for these two bisphosphonates, it is not possible directly to compare anti-fracture efficacy; however, there is no reason to believe that they should not be comparable in this respect.

Recently, the results of an RCT of the effects of risedronate have been published [5]. Administration of 5 mg daily for three years to postmenopausal women with established vertebral osteoporosis was associated with a 41% and 39% reduction in risk of new vertebral and non-vertebral fractures, respectively.

Bisphosphonates are generally well tolerated. Gastrointestinal side effects may occur, especially with aminobisphosphonates and a small number of cases of erosive oesophagitis have been reported with alendronate. Because of this potential problem, it is important that patients take the drug according to the instructions (ie in the morning with a full glass of water, 30 minutes before food, drink or other medications and remain upright for 30 minutes after the dose). Alendronate is contraindicated in patients with oesophageal abnormalities or disease and should be withdrawn immediately if dyspepsia or dysphagia develop during therapy.

The rate of onset and offset of the effects of bisphosphonates requires further study. However, there is evidence for both alendronate and risedronate that significant reduction in fracture rate may be achieved after only one year of therapy. Despite their high skeletal retention, preliminary indications are that bone loss resumes soon after treatment is discontinued although further studies are required in this area. There are theoretical concerns that prolonged suppression of bone turnover may have adverse effects on bone strength and, at present, treatment is usually given for a period of 3–5 years.

Raloxifene

Raloxifene is a selective oestrogen receptor modulator (SERM), exerting a range of agonist and antagonist actions in different tissues. The mechanisms underlying its tissue specificity have not been precisely defined but possible factors are shown in Table 4.

In a large RCT of postmenopausal women with osteoporosis, three years' treatment with raloxifene 60 mg daily was shown to reduce vertebral fracture rate by 30%, and there were significant treatment benefits on BMD in the spine, proximal femur and total body [6]. The absence of a demonstrable reduction in non-vertebral fractures in this study may be attributable to the consistent supplementation with

Table 4 Mechanisms by which selective oestrogen receptor modulators may achieve tissue specificity.

- Ligand-specific conformational changes in ligand binding domain of oestrogen receptor
- Differential tissue distribution and gene modulating effects of oestrogen receptor subtypes (and their isoforms)
- Involvement of different response elements in oestrogen signalling pathway
- Involvement of cell- and gene-specific co-repressors and co-activators required for formation of a transcriptionally competent ligand/receptor complex

calcium and vitamin D across treatment and placebo groups, the withdrawal from the study of women who sustained a fracture or exhibited high rates of bone loss, and the relatively young age of the cohort as compared to women at highest risk of hip fracture. Another possible explanation is the lower anti-resorptive potency of raloxifene. Raloxifene has also been shown to prevent bone loss at multiple skeletal sites in healthy perimenopausal women.

Unlike HRT, raloxifene does not stimulate the endometrium and thus its use is not associated with vaginal bleeding. In addition, a highly significant protective effect against breast cancer has emerged, with a 76% reduction in new cases of invasive breast cancer during a median of 40 months' follow-up [7]. Effects on CHD have not been established but potentially beneficial effects on serum lipid profile have been demonstrated. Raloxifene does not alleviate, and may exacerbate, vasomotor symptoms associated with the menopause and is therefore contraindicated in perimenopausal women with active symptoms. Other minor side effects include leg oedema and leg cramps; finally, as with HRT, there is an approximately three-fold increase in the relative risk of venous thromboembolism. Potential advantages and disadvantages of raloxifene versus HRT are shown in Table 5.

Table 5 Potential advantages and disadvantages of raloxifene versus hormone replacement therapy.

Advantages	Disadvantages	Unknown
Lack of endometrial stimulation	Lack of effect on vasomotor menopausal symptoms	Effect on coronary heart disease
Protection against breast cancer	Possibly weaker effect on bone	Effect on cognitive function

Vitamin D and calcium

Vitamin D deficiency is common in many elderly populations and there is increasing evidence that vitamin D and calcium supplementation protects against non-vertebral fractures. In an RCT of vitamin D and calcium in daily doses of 800 IU and 1.2 g, respectively, a significant reduction in hip and other non-vertebral fractures was seen after 12–18 months' treatment in a cohort of elderly women (mean age 84 years) living in sheltered accommodation [8]. Subsequently, a significant reduction in non-vertebral fractures was reported after three years in community-dwelling men and women aged over 65 years in an RCT of 700 IU vitamin D and 500 mg calcium daily [9]. It is not possible from these studies to deduce the relative contribution of vitamin D and calcium to the observed benefits; vitamin D without calcium has been shown in some studies to reduce non-vertebral fracture rate in the elderly, but this finding has not been universal. The important question of whether vitamin D alone reduces hip fracture thus remains unanswered at present.

Vitamin D metabolites and analogues

Both calcitriol (1,25-dihydroxyvitamin D, the active metabolite of vitamin D) and alfacalcidol (1α-hydroxyvitamin D3, a synthetic analogue of calcitriol) have been reported to reduce vertebral fracture rate; but this effect has not been demonstrated in all studies. Preservation of BMD at the spine and hip has been demonstrated for both agents, and in one study calcitriol therapy was associated with a reduction in non-vertebral fractures [10]. The dosages of calcitriol and alfacalcidol are generally between 0.5 and 1.0 μg daily; hypercalciuria and hypercalcaemia may occur and serum calcium levels should be regularly monitored.

Calcitonin

Calcitonin acts directly on osteoclasts, with inhibitory effects on bone resorption. It may be administered parenterally or intranasally; both forms of treatment have been shown to prevent spinal bone loss in postmenopausal women, but treatment benefits at other sites such as the proximal femur and radius have not been clearly demonstrated.

The effects of calcitonin therapy on fracture are controversial. Small prospective studies have claimed significant reduction in vertebral fracture rate and retrospective data have been used to support protection against hip fracture. In a recent RCT of intranasal calcitonin on vertebral fracture rate in women with postmenopausal osteoporosis, a significant reduction in vertebral fracture was observed in women treated with 200 IU daily but not in those receiving 100 IU or 400 IU daily. However, because of the high drop-out rate in this study (nearly 50%) and the lack of significant treatment benefits on spinal BMD, the results of this study should be interpreted with caution.

Adverse effects with intranasal calcitonin are rare. Nausea and flushing may occur shortly after parenteral administration of calcitonin, and vomiting and diarrhoea also sometimes occur. These symptoms are usually transient but may persist for some hours after injection.

Calcium

Beneficial effects of calcium on BMD have been documented in children and adults, particularly at appendicular skeletal sites. In the spine, these effects are generally less evident and may be transient; the benefits of calcium are also less marked in perimenopausal women, presumably because of the dominant effects of oestrogen deficiency. Although several small studies have reported a reduction in vertebral fracture rate in calcium supplemented individuals, evidence from adequately powered studies is not available and calcium should be regarded as an adjunct to treatment rather than definitive therapy.

☐ CONCLUSIONS

There is currently insufficient evidence upon which to base firm statements about the positioning of drugs in the prevention of osteoporotic fracture. The anti-fracture efficacy of the available interventions at the spine and non-vertebral sites is summarised in Table 6 but it must be emphasised that the level of evidence for these evaluations is variable. Furthermore, the potentially important but as yet un-quantified extraskeletal risks and benefits of long-term HRT and raloxifene add further complexity to decision making.

Selection of patients for treatment is currently based on a case-finding approach in individuals with strong risk factors, using bone densitometry in the majority of cases to determine the need for treatment. The increasing recognition that there may be a relatively rapid onset and offset of treatment effect and that, even in women with established osteoporosis, relatively short-term intervention produces significant reduction in fracture risk has stimulated a move away from long-term prevention towards strategies which target individuals with a high absolute risk of fracture. These could be defined as those with a BMD T score below −2.5, a previous fragility fracture or other strong risk factors such as high-dose glucocorticoid therapy. Future strategies may include population-based screening of elderly women (for example those aged 65–70 years) using a combination of bone densitometry and risk factors; in addition, a strong case can be made for universal treatment of the very elderly with calcium and vitamin D in view of the evidence for protection against non-vertebral fracture and the safety of this medication.

Table 6 Summary of evidence for anti-fracture efficacy of interventions used in the prevention of osteoporotic fractures in postmenopausal women.

Agent	Spine	All non-vertebral	Hip
Hormone replacement therapy	+	+	+*
Raloxifene	+	−	−
Alendronate	+	+	+
Cyclic etidronate	+[1]	+*	+*
Risedronate	+	+	+
Calcitonin	+	−	−
Calcitriol	+	+	−
Vitamin D + calcium	−	+	+[2]

*evidence based on observational data.
[1] insufficiently powered clinical trial but favourable trends observed.
[2] reduction in hip fracture shown only in elderly living in sheltered accommodation.

REFERENCES

1   Compston JE. Prevention and management of osteoporosis: current trends and future prospects. Review. *Drugs* 1997; **53**: 727–35.

2   Eastell R. Treatment of postmenopausal osteoporosis. *N Engl J Med* 1998; **338**: 736–46.

3   Black DM, Cummings SR, Karpf DB, *et al.* Randomised trial of effect of alendronate on risk of fracture in women with existing vertebral fractures. *Lancet* 1996; **348**: 1535–41.

4   Cummings SR, Black DM, Thompson DE, *et al.* Effect of alendronate on risk of fracture in women with low bone density but without vertebral fractures: results from the Fracture Intervention Trial. *JAMA* 1998; **280**: 2077–82.

5 Harris ST, Watts NB, Genant HK, *et al*. Effects of risedronate treatment on vertebral and non-vertebral fractures in women with postmenopausal osteoporosis. A randomized controlled trial. *JAMA* 1999; **282**: 1344–52.

6 Ettinger B, Black DM, Mitlak BH, *et al*. Reduction of vertebral fracture risk in postmenopausal women with osteoporosis treated with raloxifene: results from a 3-year randomized clinical trial. *JAMA* 1999; **282**: 637–45.

7 Cummings SR, Eckert S, Krueger KA, *et al*. The effect of raloxifene on risk of breast cancer in postmenopausal women: results from the MORE randomized trial. Multiple Outcomes of Raloxifene Evaluation. *JAMA* 1999; **281**: 2189–97.

8 Chapuy MC, Arlot ME, Delmas PD, *et al*. Effect of calcium and cholecalciferol treatment for three years on hip fractures in elderly women. *Br Med J* 1994; **308**: 1081–2.

9 Dawson-Hughes B, Harris SS, Krall EA, *et al*. Effect of calcium and vitamin D supplementation on bone density in men and women 65 years of age and older. *N Engl J Med* 1997; **337**: 670–6.

10 Tilyard MW, Spears GFS, Thomson J, *et al*. Treatment of postmenopausal osteoporosis with calcitriol or calcium. *N Engl J Med* 1992; **326**: 357–62.

□ SELF ASSESSMENT QUESTIONS

1 Long-term hormone replacement therapy (HRT):
   (a) Is effective in the secondary prevention of coronary heart disease
   (b) Increases the risk of venous thromboembolism
   (c) Reduces fracture risk at vertebral and non-vertebral sites
   (d) Is associated with a 30% increase in the relative risk of breast cancer after five years
   (e) Is associated with a 10% increase in the relative risk of breast cancer after five years

2 The selective oestrogen receptor modulator, raloxifene:
   (a) Has anti-oestrogenic effects on the skeleton
   (b) Increases breast cancer risk
   (c) Increases the risk of thromboembolism
   (d) Causes endometrial hyperplasia
   (e) Exacerbates menopausal hot flushes

3 The following interventions have been shown to reduce vertebral fracture risk in women with postmenopausal osteoporosis:
   (a) HRT
   (b) Calcium
   (c) Calcitriol
   (d) Vitamin D
   (e) Raloxifene

4 The following interventions have been shown to reduce non-vertebral fracture risk in women with postmenopausal osteoporosis:
   (a) Raloxifene
   (b) Calcium and vitamin D

(c) Calcitonin
(d) Risedronate
(e) Alendronate

ANSWERS

1a False	2a False	3a True	3a False
b True	b False	b False	b True
c True	c True	c True	c False
d True	d False	d False	d True
e False	e True	e True	d True

Autoimmune Hepatitis

Margaret F Bassendine

Autoimmune hepatitis (AIH) is a syndrome that encompasses diverse clinical and immunological manifestations. It is a chronic necroinflammatory liver disease of unknown origin that, untreated, carries a three-year mortality rate of up to 50%. The introduction in the 1970s of corticosteroid-based immunosuppressive regimens, with or without azathioprine as a steroid-sparing agent, dramatically improved quality and duration of life. The disease is characterised by histological features of interface (periportal or periseptal) hepatitis (Fig. 1), by hyper-gammaglobulinaemia and, in the majority of patients, by the presence of autoantibodies in the serum [1]. Diagnosis is based on a combination of clinical, biochemical and histological features together with careful exclusion of other causes of liver disease. A scoring system has been devised and revised [2], which allows patients to be classified as definite or probable AIH, but its relative complexity and inadequate specificity make it of limited value in routine clinical practice.

☐ AUTOANTIBODIES

AIH can be classified into at least three serologically distinct subgroups on the basis of different autoantibody specificities. The clinical utility of this subclassification is uncertain, but it is widely used and may help in understanding the immunopathogenesis of the disease [3]. The different autoantibodies found in AIH may be regarded as biological probes that could ultimately provide insight into the nature of an important triggering antigen.

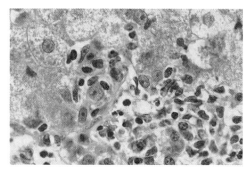

Fig. 1 Interface hepatitis: lymphocytes and plasma cells surround periportal hepatocytes (H & E stain) (courtesy of Professor AD Burt).

Type 1 autoimmune hepatitis

Antinuclear antibodies (ANA) characterise AIH type 1, the classical disease, previously termed 'lupoid' chronic active hepatitis. ANA are directed to components in the cell nucleus such as DNA, RNA or DNA-binding proteins (histone and non-histone protein). There is considerable heterogeneity of ANA in AIH, possibly reflecting different environmental triggers to the autoimmune reaction. For example, antibodies to single-stranded (anti-ssDNA) and double-stranded DNA (anti-dsDNA) have been found in 85% and 34%, respectively, of ANA positive AIH type 1, and it has been suggested that patients with anti-dsDNA have a poorer immediate response to corticosteroid therapy. In AIH type 1, smooth muscle antibodies (SMA) are also frequently detectable and heterogeneous, directed against actin and non-actin components (Table 1). Anti-actin antibodies have been advocated by some as a better marker for AIH than SMA, but a recent study showed that routine screening for antibodies to actin may miss patients with AIH type 1, and that the conventional determination of SMA by routine immunofluorescence is preferable [4].

Table 1 Immunoglobulin G antibodies to cytoskeleton proteins (smooth muscle antibodies) in autoimmune hepatitis type 1.

Antibody to:	Frequency (%)
Actin	82
Myosin	19
Actomyosin	41
Tropomyosin	38
Vimentin	46
Tubulin	41
Desmin	32
Cytokeratin-8	32
Cytokeratin-16	30

Type 2 autoimmune hepatitis

AIH type 2 is characterised serologically by liver and kidney microsomal (LKM) antibodies. The term 'microsome' was created for small vesicles made up of endoplasmic reticulum disrupted during centrifugation and re-associated into round particles. Several LKM (endoplasmic reticulum) antigens have been identified (Table 2). Antibodies to LKM1 react with cytochrome P4502D6 (previously known as CYP450db1). These autoantibodies, which recognise a short linear sequence on the CYP4502D6 molecule and inhibit the enzyme activity *in vitro*, are the main serological marker of AIH type 2. Antibodies to another LKM are found in AIH induced by the diuretic drug tienilic acid (now withdrawn) and react with CYP4502C9. This is the enzyme that catalyses hepatic metabolism of tienilic acid to

Table 2 Anti-endoplasmic reticulum antibodies.

| Antibody | Antigen | | Disorder | Prevalence (%) |
	Name	MW kDa		
Anti-LKM1	CYP4502D6	50	AIH type 2	84
			Hepatitis C virus infection	3
Anti-LKM2	CYP4502C9	52	Tienilic acid-induced hepatitis	>95
Anti-LKM	CYP4502A6	51	APS1	27
Anti-LM	CYP4501A2	52	Dihydralazine-induced hepatitis	>95
			APS1	9

AIH = autoimmune hepatitis; APS = autoimmune polyendocrine syndrome; CY = cytochrome; LKM = liver and kidney microsome; LM = liver microsome; MW = molecular weight.

its reactive, short-lived metabolite which has been found to bind covalently to CYP2C9, resulting in neoantigen formation. This neoantigen triggers the autoimmune reaction in susceptible individuals [5]. A similar process may be involved in AIH induced by dihydralazine which is characterised by antibodies to CYP4501A2 (CYP1A2). Interestingly, antibodies to both CYP1A2 and CYP2A6 are serological markers of chronic hepatitis which is found in 10–18% of autoimmune polyendocrine syndrome type 1 (APS1) (see below).

Type 3 autoimmune hepatitis

A third subgroup of patients (up to 20%) are negative for ANA, SMA and LKM autoantibodies, but frequently have antibodies to soluble liver antigen (SLA) or liver-pancreas antigen. These antigens are identical [6] and highly specific for AIH. In a recent study of AIH, anti-SLA and ANA/SMA positive patients were found to share most clinical, biochemical, histological and prognostic features [7]. However, diagnosis of AIH type 3 has often been delayed (a mean of 68 months from first elevation of transaminases) since testing for anti-SLA autoantibodies is currently not generally available. Recent cloning of the SLA antigen [6] will allow a generally available diagnostic assay to be established in the near future.

☐ AETIOPATHOGENESIS

Although the aetiology of the disease is largely unknown, the current concept assumes that the autoimmune reaction is triggered by various environmental agents in genetically predisposed individuals.

Environmental triggers

Various environmental agents (viruses, bacteria, drugs or chemicals) can trigger AIH. In rare cases of AIH type 2 the disease is drug-induced (tienilic acid, dihydralazine) and characterised by specific anti-LKM autoantibodies. Another drug that induces idiosyncratic necroinflammatory liver injury with strong autoimmune characteristics is minocycline [8]. AIH induced by minocycline is characterised by ANA, but SMA is absent (Fig. 2). Most patients recover on drug withdrawal, but corticosteroids have been given to a few individuals and a liver-related death has been reported. Viruses are the other favoured triggering agents, and there are reports of onset of AIH after acute infection with hepatitis A and C viruses, Epstein-Barr virus, measles virus and herpes simplex virus 1. The likelihood that a number of different environmental factors can trigger the syndrome underlines its heterogeneity.

Immunogenetics

Like other autoimmune diseases, AIH is a 'polygenic' disorder programmed by genes with small and additive effects. No single gene is thought to be either necessary for the development of AIH or sufficient to cause it, so these disease genes are referred to as 'encoding susceptibility'. All the published data on genetic predisposition to AIH have been obtained from association studies, based on comparing the frequency of an allele in unrelated affected and unaffected individuals from a population. However, many of these studies have examined only small numbers.

Major histocompatibility complex associations

Evidence from several different populations supports a role for the human leukocyte antigens (HLAs) which form part of the major histocompatibility complex (MHC)

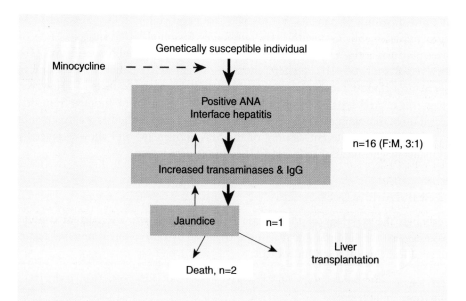

Fig. 2 Putative natural history of minocycline-induced autoimmune hepatitis (ANA = antinuclear antibody; F = female; IgG = immunoglobulin G; M = male).

on chromosome 6p21.3. Early studies in AIH type 1 identified strong associations with HLA A1, B8 and later with DR3 (60–70% of patients were found to be B8 or DR3 positive compared to 20–30% of controls). In the 1990s, these studies were superseded by more accurate molecular genotyping, which showed that haplotypes containing DRB1*0301 with DRB3*0101 (coding for DR3 and DR52a, respectively) are the principal risk factor in Caucasoid patients of Northern European extraction (Table 3), while haplotypes containing DRB1*1501 (DR2) are associated with protection against the disease [9]. An independent risk factor in this population is the DRB1*0401 allele (DR4) which appears to be associated with a less severe, later onset form of AIH. In Japan, where DR3 is absent from the population, the DRB1*0405 variant of DR4 predisposes to AIH and the clinical course appears to be similar to DR4-associated AIH seen in Caucasians. Analysis of the sequences of the DRB gene products in patients and controls has led to the identification of an amino acid sequence (LLEQKR) at positions 67–72 of the DRβ polypeptide present in more than 90% of AIH patients compared to 61–64% of controls, and to the suggestion that this motif may represent the primary determinant of AIH susceptibility [9]. X-ray crystallographic studies of HLA-DR molecules show position 71 to be located at a crucial site for antigen binding and T cell receptor recognition. They also show that polymorphisms encoding for lysine (a highly charged polar amino acid) or alanine (a neutral non-polar amino acid) at this position may be relevant in the presentation of autoantigenic peptide in the MHC groove to autoreactive T cells.

It is unclear whether null mutations of complement factor 4A or mutations within the tumour necrosis factor-α promoter at position −308 represent additional risk factors (Table 3) because they are in linkage disequilibrium with the DR alleles.

Table 3 Summary of genetic associations with autoimmune hepatitis.

Allele/Antigen	Relative risk
HLA A1	1.89
HLA B8	1.96
TNF*2	1.22
C4A deleted	1.91
HLA DRB3*0101	2.08
HLA DRB1*0301	2.11
CTLA-4	2.12

C4 = complement 4; CTLA = cytotoxic T lymphocyte-associated antigen; HLA = human leukocyte antigen; TNF = tumour necrosis factor.

Non-major histocompatibility complex associations

The immune response is regulated by the interaction of a series of complex networks of different polypeptides. Many of the genes encoding these proteins are polymorphic and each one represents a potential candidate gene. One example is the cytotoxic T lymphocyte-associated antigen-4 (CTLA-4) gene (located on chromosome 2q33). CTLA-4 is a T cell surface molecule which interacts, in competition with the costimulatory molecule CD28, with the ligands B7-1 and B7-2 on antigen presenting cells to influence the induction, maintenance and, in particular, termination of peripheral T cell responses. The demonstration that an exon 1 polymorphism (A/G) of the CTLA-4 gene is associated with susceptibility to other autoimmune diseases (including insulin-dependent diabetes mellitus, autoimmune thyroid disease and primary biliary cirrhosis) led to a study of this polymorphism in European Caucasoid patients with AIH and ethnically matched control subjects. The G allele was more common in patients with AIH type 1 (odds ratio 2.12), and the GG genotype was associated with a significantly higher mean serum aspartate transaminase level ($p = 0.03$) [10].

Autoimmune polyendocrine syndrome

Another possible susceptibility gene outside the MHC is that associated with APS1 (also called autoimmune polyendocrinopathy-candidiasis-ectodermal-dystrophy), in which chronic hepatitis (with similarities to AIH) is a serious disease component in 10–18% of patients. APS1 is a rare autosomal recessive disorder encoded by mutations in a single gene called 'autoimmune regulator', located on the long arm of chromosome 21 (21q22.3). In contrast to other autoimmune diseases, APS1 is characterised by 100% penetrance, Mendelian inheritance, lack of both HLA-DR dependence and female preponderance. Recently, two hepatic autoantigens in chronic hepatitis related to APS1 have been identified as CYP4501A2 (CYP1A2) and CYP2A6 [11]. This is of interest in relation to aetiopathogenesis, as the only other disease in which anti-CYP1A2 autoantibodies have been described is AIH induced by dihydralazine (Table 2).

Pathogenesis of liver damage

The study of the pathogenesis of AIH has been hampered by the lack of a satisfactory animal model. Current insight is somewhat fragmentary. HLA class 1 molecules that present intracellular peptides to CD8+ T cells are known to be expressed on hepatocytes in AIH; furthermore, CD8+ T cells are found in the inflammatory T cell infiltrate in the liver. T cell populations infiltrating the liver in human AIH have recently been shown to be oligoclonal and mainly of the CD8+ subset. This suggests that common antigens presented to CD8+ cells in the context of HLA class 1 molecules are distributed diffusely in the liver in AIH. Thus, cytotoxic activity of CD8+ T cells specific for autoantigen is thought to be one of the mechanisms of tissue damage.

Recent interest has focused on apoptosis induced by Fas/Fas ligand (FasL) interactions. Fas is highly expressed on hepatocytes in the liver, whereas Bcl-2, the anti-apoptotic protein, is expressed at low levels. Studies in two mouse systems of hepatitis suggest that Fas ligand expressed on activated T cells induces apoptosis of hepatocytes in these models [12].

☐ CLINICAL MANIFESTATIONS AND NATURAL HISTORY

The disease mainly affects women (female:male, 4:1), and a young woman with 'lupoid hepatitis' exemplifies the traditional patient with AIH. However, it is now realised that the disease is heterogeneous and may present at any age [13]. The presence or absence of symptoms at presentation often bears little relationship to histological disease severity, and unfortunately many, if not most, patients present with cirrhosis. The syndrome may present as asymptomatic aminotransferase elevation detected on routine screening. Many patients have an insidious, sometimes fluctuating, course with fatigue predominating. Prior icteric episodes may be reported. Others may present with arthralgias, amenorrhoea and jaundice, with a biochemical profile that mimics acute hepatitis. Recognition and appropriate treatment of the patient with an acute presentation are critical and potentially life saving; the previous doctrine that six months of disease duration is required before investigation is erroneous.

It remains controversial whether AIH type 1 carries a natural history different from that of the type 2 variant. The original report of the anti-LKM positive variant, the so-called AIH type 2, describes a more aggressive clinical course than the classic ANA/SMA positive form of the disease. Recent studies, however, show that anti-LKM positive autoimmune hepatitis in children has a disease severity and long-term outcome similar to the type 1 (ANA/SMA positive) variant [13].

☐ TREATMENT

Drug therapy

Current therapeutic regimens, based on prednisolone alone or prednisolone in lower dose combined with azathioprine, were devised three decades ago but their efficacy is remarkable, with the vast majority of patients achieving a clinical, biochemical and histological remission. The presence of cirrhosis does not affect steroid responsiveness, and the 10-year survival (93%) is the same as that of an age- and sex-matched normal population (94%). The incidence of relapse after the cessation of treatment may be as high as 50–70%, indicating that for many patients treatment may indeed be lifelong. Azathioprine monotherapy at a dose of 2 mg/kg is effective for maintaining remission, but many clinicians do not feel that the benefit of a steroid-free regimen outweighs the long-term toxicity of azathioprine.

Despite their success, currently available treatment regimens are flawed. Corticosteroids are not free from complications, and this has led to interest in budesonide, a second-generation steroid with a high first-pass clearance by the liver, low systemic availability, and metabolites without glucocorticoid activity. Preliminary studies suggest that it may be as effective as prednisolone with a reduction in systemic side effects, but confirmation by long-term studies is unavailable.

Other immunosuppressive drugs currently used to prevent rejection in solid-organ transplantation (Fig. 3) may prove of value in future treatment of AIH, but

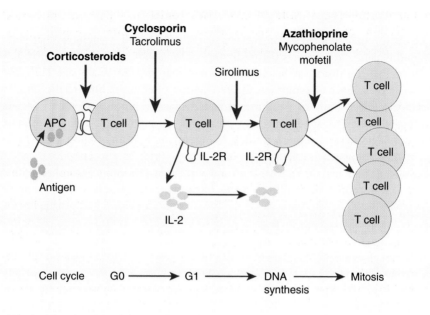

Fig. 3 Sites of action of immunosuppressive agents during immune response (APC = antigen presenting cell; IL = interleukin).

most data are anecdotal. Oral cyclosporin has been used in adults and children refractory to steroid treatment, and as an alternative to prednisolone for inducing remission in children. In a pilot multicentre clinical trial involving 32 children [14], cyclosporin alone was administered for six months to induce remission, followed by combined low doses of prednisone and azathioprine for one month, after which cyclosporin was stopped. Of the 30 patients who remained on treatment, 83% achieved a biochemical remission, and the regimen was well tolerated with few adverse effects. A controlled trial comparing this induction protocol with traditional prednisolone and azathioprine treatment is now underway. Although there are a few case reports of patients with AIH treated with tacrolimus, methotrexate or mycophenolate mofetil, these drugs should be used at present only in patients resistant to, or intolerant of, standard regimens.

Liver transplantation

Liver transplantation should be considered in all patients with decompensated AIH. There are no findings prior to therapy that will predict immediate and long-term prognosis, so the transplantation decision should be deferred, if possible, until after a treatment trial of corticosteroids. Some patients with advanced liver disease, ascites and/or encephalopathy at presentation can be resurrected with immunosuppressive therapy and immediate transplantation avoided.

The five-year survival after transplantation is more than 90%, but recurrence of AIH in the graft is a common event (20–30%), the incidence increasing over time as immunosuppression is reduced [15]. Most units now advocate prolonged continuation of low-dose steroid therapy in patients transplanted for decompensated AIH and maintenance of adequate tacrolimus or cyclosporin blood levels.

REFERENCES

1 Krawitt EL. Autoimmune hepatitis. *N Engl J Med* 1996; **334**: 897–903.

2 Alvarez F, Berg PA, Bianchi FB, *et al.* International Autoimmune Hepatitis Group: review of criteria for diagnosis of autoimmune hepatitis. *J Hepatol* 1999; **31**: 929–38.

3 Czaja AJ, Manns MP. The validity and importance of subtypes in autoimmune hepatitis: a point of view. *Am J Gastroenterol* 1995; **90**: 1206–11.

4 Czaja AJ, Cassani F, Catalata M, *et al.* Frequency and significance of antibodies to actin in type 1 autoimmune hepatitis. *Hepatology* 1996; **24**: 1068–73.

5 Griem P, Wulferink M, Sachs B, *et al.* Allergic and autoimmune reactions to xenobiotics; how do they arise? *Immunol Today* 1998; **19**: 134–41.

6 Wies I, Brunner S, Henninger J, *et al.* Identification of target antigen for SLA/LP autoantibodies in autoimmune hepatitis. *Lancet* 2000; **355**: 1510–5.

7 Kanzler S, Weidemann C, Gerken G, *et al.* Clinical significance of autoantibodies to soluble liver antigen in autoimmune hepatitis. *J Hepatol* 1999; **31**: 635–40.

8. Gough A, Chapman S, Wagstaff K, *et al.* Minocycline induced autoimmune hepatitis and systemic lupus erythematosus-like syndrome. *Br Med J* 1996; **312**: 169–72.

9 Donaldson PT, Albertini RJ, Krawitt EL. Immunogenetic studies of autoimmune hepatitis and primary sclerosing cholangitis. In: Krawitt EL, Wiesner RH, Nishioka M (eds). *Autoimmune liver diseases.* Amsterdam: Elsevier Science, 1998: 141–65.

10 Agarwal K, Czaja AJ, Jones DEJ, Donaldson PD. Cytotoxic T lymphocyte antigen-4 (CTLA-4) gene polymorphisms and susceptibility to type 1 autoimmune hepatitis. *Hepatology* 2000; **31**: 49–53.

11 Clemente MG, Meloni A, Obermayer-Straub P, *et al.* Two cytochromes P450 are major hepatocellular antigens in autoimmune polyglandular syndrome type 1. *Gastroenterology* 1998; **114**: 324–8.

12 Kondo T, Suda T, Fukayama H, *et al.* Essential roles of the Fas ligand in the development of hepatitis. *Nat Med* 1997; **3**: 409–13.

13 Gregorio GV, Portmann B, Reid F, *et al.* Autoimmune hepatitis in childhood: a 20 year experience. *Hepatology* 1997; **25**: 541–7.

14 Alvarez F, Ciocca M, Canero-Valasco C, *et al.* Short-term cyclosporine induces a remission of autoimmune hepatitis in children. *J Hepatol* 1999; **30**: 222–7.

15 Davila R, Keeffe EB. Prednisolone withdrawal advocates: beware of recurrent autoimmune hepatitis. *Hepatology* 1999; **30**: 338–9.

☐ SELF ASSESSMENT QUESTIONS

1 A diagnosis of autoimmune hepatitis can be made:
  (a) Only if smooth muscle antibodies (SMAs) are present
  (b) If antinuclear antibodies, SMAs and liver kidney microsomal antibodies are all negative
  (c) If serum transaminases are normal
  (d) If serum immunoglobulin levels are normal
  (e) When the liver biopsy shows established cirrhosis

2   Autoimmune hepatitis:
     (a) Is an autosomal recessive disease
     (b) Is associated with human leukocyte antigen (HLA) B27
     (c) Is associated with HLA B8, DR3 haplotype
     (d) Can be induced by treatment with minocycline
     (e) Can be triggered by infection with Epstein-Barr virus

3   The prognosis of autoimmune hepatitis:
     (a) Is good, with a five-year untreated survival of >90%
     (b) Is poor, with a five-year untreated survival of <50%
     (c) Can be improved dramatically by a short course (<6 months) of
         corticosteroids
     (d) Is worse if the patient's disease relapses frequently
     (e) Depends almost entirely on the presence of underlying cirrhosis

4   In the treatment of autoimmune hepatitis:
     (a) Corticosteroids should be withheld for six months as the disease may
         resolve spontaneously
     (b) Remission should be induced with azathioprine monotherapy
     (c) Remission can be maintained with azathioprine monotherapy
     (d) Immunosuppressive therapy can be withdrawn in >50% of patients
     (e) Immunosuppressive therapy is required lifelong in >50% of patients

ANSWERS

1a False	2a False	3a False	4a False
b True	b True	b True	b False
c False	c True	c False	c True
d False	d True	d True	d False
e True	e True	e False	e True

Haemochromatosis

Adrian Bomford

☐ HAEMOCHROMATOSIS

Clinical features

Hereditary haemochromatosis is a common inherited disorder of iron metabolism in which iron balance breaks down because increased amounts of iron are absorbed from a normal diet. In the absence of a regulated pathway for iron excretion, long-term positive iron balance leads to progressive accumulation of iron in the parenchymal cells of the liver, pancreas and other organs. Eventually, iron overload leads to widespread organ damage and loss of function, and a characteristic clinical picture emerges. In its most severe form this includes cirrhosis, hepatocellular cancer, diabetes mellitus, a widespread destructive arthritis, sexual dysfunction due to hypogonadotrophic hypogonadism, cardiomyopathy and generalised skin pigmentation.

As with other conditions leading to symptoms and signs in multiple systems, the diagnosis of haemochromatosis requires a high index of clinical suspicion, particularly when the presenting feature is a relatively common clinical problem such as heart failure, diabetes or arthritis. The pathological hallmark of haemochromatosis is excess stainable iron in the parenchymal cells of the liver demonstrated by Perls' stain (Fig. 1). The biochemical features of marked tissue iron overload are increased serum iron and transferrin saturation and elevated serum ferritin levels. A summary of diagnostic criteria that indicate the fully expressed phenotype is given in Table 1.

The clinical expression of haemochromatosis is variable because the rate of iron accumulation, and hence the asymptomatic phase of the illness, varies greatly between individuals. However, most patients become symptomatic and come to

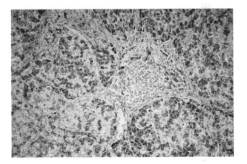

Fig. 1 Liver biopsy stained with Perls' stain showing heavy deposition of iron (grade 4 siderosis). Iron in the form of blue granules is present in every hepatocyte. An expanded portal tract is shown in the centre of the field, and linking fibrous bands are beginning to enclose islands of parenchyma leading to the formation of nodules (cirrhosis).

Table 1 Diagnostic criteria reflecting the iron burden of fully-expressed haemochromatosis [1].

Criteria
1   Stainable iron in hepatic parenchymal cells: grade 3 and 4 (max grade 4)
2   Hepatic iron concentration >80 μmol/g dry weight
3   Hepatic iron index >1.9 (hepatic iron concentration in μmol/g dry weight/age in years)
4   Removal of >5g of iron by initial course of venesection

medical attention by their fourth or fifth decade. Hepatic iron stores vary by as much as ten-fold between patients presenting in middle adult life [2]. The reason for such heterogeneity is not known but it is likely that genetic and environmental factors play a role. Alcohol and dietary factors that augment or reduce iron absorption may also play a part, and iron stores will be limited in women through menstruation and parturition. In addition, there is now growing interest in the possibility that other genetic loci may influence the absorption and distribution of iron, and influence phenotype [3].

The importance of HLA linkage

The observation in 1975 by Simon and colleagues [4] that the frequency of the human leukocyte antigen (HLA) A3 was increased in a group of unrelated haemochromatosis patients proved to be of fundamental importance, changing clinical practice and providing the direction for future research. Their studies provided definitive evidence for the genetic basis of the condition, showed that it was inherited as an autosomal recessive trait, and localised the gene responsible to the region of the major histocompatibility complex (MHC) on the short arm of chromosome 6 (6p). It also became clear that a high proportion of haemo-chromatosis chromosomes carried A3, a finding consistent with the idea that the original haemochromatosis mutation occurred on a founder or ancestral haplotype that became dispersed by population migration. In clinical practice, HLA-linkage has been widely used to assign disease chromosomes during screening of affected pedigrees so that the risk of developing iron overload can be predicted. When combined with clinicopathological studies, gene tracking has allowed the phenotype of homozygous and heterozygous individuals to be defined:

- ☐   homozygotes demonstrate progressive hepatic iron overload

- ☐   heterozygotes may have partial biochemical expression in the form of raised iron indices, but do not progressively accumulate iron [5].

☐ THE HAEMOCHROMATOSIS GENE

Identification, prevalence and penetrance of mutations in *HFE*

The gene for haemochromatosis was identified in 1996 by Feder and colleagues [6]. They used a positional cloning strategy to identify a 250 kb chromosomal subregion on 6p that was conserved on chromosomes carrying the ancestral haplotype. All the genes within this region were identified, and the only mutation that consistently segregated with haemochromatosis was found in the open reading frame of a novel, class I-like gene termed *HFE*. This mutation resulted in the substitution of a cysteine for a tyrosine at position 282 (C282Y), and was predicted to disrupt the structure and function of the gene product. In the USA [6] and in Northern European countries (Table 2), 83% and 90%, respectively, of haemochromatosis patients are homozygous for the C282Y mutation, while in Australia all haemochromatosis is caused by this mutation. In European series, the frequency of homozygosity for C282Y demonstrates a decreasing frequency from north to south, being highest in populations from north-western Europe and lowest in southern Europe (Table 2). Importantly, in southern Italy, 36% of patients who appear to meet diagnostic criteria for haemochromatosis (Table 1) do not have mutations in *HFE*. Some of this genetic heterogeneity can now be explained by mutation at a new haemochromatosis locus, *HFE3* on 7q22 which was described in two families from this region. The finding that the gene mapping to this locus, *Tfr2*, encodes a transferrin receptor [8] has important implications for understanding the pathogenesis of haemochromatosis.

A second mutation, in which aspartic acid replaces histidine at position 63 (H63D), was also described by Feder *et al* [6]. In most series, 2–7% of patients are compound heterozygotes with one chromosome 6 carrying H63D and the other, C282Y (Table 2). This genotype is associated with a modest increase in iron stores, and tissue damage is rare. H63D is definitely a haemochromatosis allele, with both heterozygotes and homozygotes occasionally demonstrating modest iron excess. Other mutations in HFE, such as S65C are very rare but may be associated with iron overload, especially in association with C282Y as a compound heterozygote.

Estimation of population frequencies of the haemochromatosis mutations by random screening indicates that C282Y is confined to European populations or their descendants (USA, Australia and New Zealand). This has led to the suggestion that the gene originated in Celtic or Nordic people. Population studies suggest that the mutation is more common in northern than southern Europe, mirroring the

Table 2 Frequency of C282Y homozygotes and compound heterozygotes (C282Y/H63D) in hereditary haemochromatosis patients from European populations and their descendants [7].

Country/Region	C282Y +/+ (%)	C282Y +/– H63D +/– (%)
Australia	100	0
Northern France	92	2.3
UK	91	2.6
Germany	90	3.5
USA	83	4.5
Austria	77	7.5
Italy	64	6.7

distribution of C282Y in patients from different regions of Europe (Table 2). H63D is common in many populations throughout the world, and probably arose at approximately the same time on widespread chromosomes rather than being introduced through Caucasian admixture.

Before HFE was identified, estimates of the prevalence of haemochromatosis were based on phenotype screening studies of randomly selected individuals or blood donors. The most commonly used measure was elevated serum transferrin saturation (threshold 45–62%). These studies suggested that 3–5 cases per 1,000 of the population of northern European countries or their descendants were homozygous for the haemochromatosis gene and that the carrier frequency was between one in 10 and one in 15. When screening by phenotype (transferrin saturation) was combined with genotyping, the prevalence of C282Y appeared to be similar (Table 3). In two series from the UK the homozygote frequency was as high as one in 145 of the population.

Although these figures suggest that haemochromatosis is a common disease and the most prevalent genetic condition of European populations, many clinicians still regard iron overload as a rare problem with minimal impact on health. This disparity could be due either to the failure to recognise patients with iron overload or to the absence of iron overload and clinical disease in a proportion of homozygous individuals (incomplete penetrance). It was initially thought that penetrance of the homozygous C282Y genotype was high, probably because genotyping was first performed on well characterised groups of iron-loaded patients. As more large-scale population screening data have become available it is becoming clear that only about 50% of homozygous patients develop iron overload [12]. In blood donors, in whom iron stores are reduced by regular donation, the figure may be even lower (Table 3).

Table 3 Prevalence of homozygosity for the C282Y mutation in screening studies using transferrin saturation and genotyping [9].

Country/Region	Prevalence of C282Y homozygotes	Raised ferritin (%)
New Zealand	1 in 213	60
USA	1 in 276	50
Canada	1 in 327	19
Australia	1 in 188	75
UK [10]	1 in 145	–
UK [11]	1 in 145	–

☐ THE HAEMOCHROMATOSIS GENE PRODUCT

The haemochromatosis gene encodes a 348-residue protein, HFE, that shares structural features with the family of MHC class I molecules (Fig. 2). All these proteins are transmembrane glycoproteins that associate with the class I light chain β2-microglobulin and function in the immune system by presenting peptide antigens to T cells. Unlike classical class I molecules, HFE cannot bind peptides because the binding groove is too narrow and the molecule does not appear to have any immune function. Structural and biochemical studies of the wild-type protein however, reveal other unique properties consistent with a role in iron metabolism.

The case for HFE playing a role in iron metabolism also receives strong support from the observation that inactivation of the mouse *Hfe* gene by targeted disruption leads to iron overload in a pattern similar to the human condition. Experiments using cultured cells indicate that at physiological pH HFE forms a complex with the transferrin receptor on the cell surface and becomes internalised, sharing the same intracellular pathway as the receptor. The two proteins dissociate within intracellular endocytic compartments in which the pH is acidic. At the cell surface, HFE appears to compete for binding between the transferrin receptor and its ligand, iron-loaded transferrin, in this way modulating the uptake of iron by the cell. In haemochromatosis, the C282Y mutation disrupts the disulphide bond in the α3 domain of HFE (Fig. 2) and abrogates the binding of β2-microglobulin. In the absence of binding to the class I light chain molecule, cell surface expression and correct orientation of HFE in the cell membrane is disrupted; as a result, the mutant protein remains within the cell and cannot bind to the transferrin receptor. In contrast, the H63D mutation is located in the α1 domain and does not interfere with the binding of β2-microglobulin. Cell surface expression of HFE and association with the transferrin receptor is therefore not impaired.

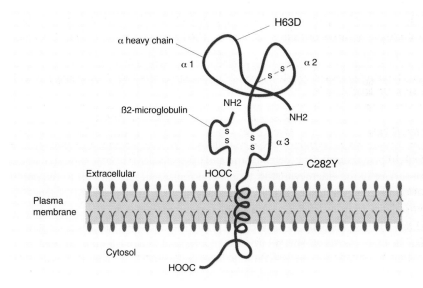

Fig. 2 Model of the HFE protein based on its homology with MHC class I molecules. The single polypeptide chain consists of three extracellular immunoglobulin-like domains, α1, α2 and α3, a membrane-spanning region and short cytoplasmic tail. Between the α1 and α2 domains is a shallow groove that does not bind peptide, while the α3 domain binds β2-microglobulin non-covalently. The approximate locations of the C282Y and H63D mutations are indicated. C282Y eliminates a disulphide bond in the α3 domain, preventing binding of β2-microglobulin and cell surface expression of HFE (from [6] with permission).

☐ REGULATION OF DUODENAL IRON TRANSPORT IN HAEMOCHROMATOSIS

The proximal duodenum demonstrates the highest rates of iron absorption in the different regions of the small intestine because it is here that specific iron transport proteins are expressed by the villus epithelium [13,14]. Villus enterocytes are constantly renewed from a population of stem cells in the duodenal crypts, where they are programmed with information about body iron requirements and modulate their capacity to transport iron accordingly. Normally, a reciprocal relationship exists between the amount of iron transported and body iron stores. This breaks down in haemochromatosis and enterocyte iron transport fails to respond to, or becomes uncoupled from, information about increased iron stores. It is not known with certainty how enterocyte programming occurs, but there is circumstantial evidence to implicate transferrin because the iron saturation of this transport protein varies with iron stores and it binds to transferrin receptors on the basolateral membrane of crypt cells [15]. Wild-type HFE is also expressed predominantly in duodenal crypt cells where, in agreement with results of experiments using cultured cells, it physically associates with the transferrin receptor expressed on the basolateral membrane. HFE may therefore modulate uptake of transferrin iron by crypt cells and participate in the mechanism by which these cells sense body iron stores. In haemochromatosis, in which the expression of mutant HFE is markedly reduced, recycling of the transferrin receptor could be disrupted resulting in reduced delivery of transferrin iron to crypt cells. Relative iron deficiency of the crypt cells could lead to inappropriate upregulation of the enterocyte iron transport pathway and increased absorption of dietary iron [15].

Functional studies indicate that iron transport occurs in three steps:

1   Uptake of iron from the gut lumen by the brush border (apical) membrane.

2   Intracellular processing and transport to the basal region of the cell.

3   Transfer of a proportion of the iron through the basolateral membrane into the portal circulation.

Transporters at both apical and basolateral membranes have now been characterised. DMT1 (divalent metal transporter 1), also known as Nramp2, is a proton-coupled transporter of ferrous iron and other divalent cations, expressed at the apical surface of the enterocyte [13]. Basolateral transfer of ferrous iron to the portal circulation is accomplished by IREG1, the product of *Ireg1* (iron-regulated), a gene that is upregulated in iron deficiency and highly expressed in the duodenum [14]. Both DMT1 and IREG1 are coupled to accessory proteins that change the oxidation state of iron to facilitate transport. Dietary iron in the intestinal lumen is in the oxidised form and requires solubilisation by reduction before transport. The protein responsible for this is a haem-containing, membrane-bound ferric reductase, DcytB (duodenal cytochrome b), that provides ferrous iron directly to DMT1 at the brush border membrane [16]. Hephaestin, a membrane-bound homologue of caeruloplasmin and highly expressed in the small intestine, acts as a multicopper oxidase [17]. It is likely that hephaestin oxidises ferrous ions as they are transported across the basolateral membrane by IREG1 and facilitates the binding of iron to transferrin in the portal circulation. The intracellular processing step remains poorly defined.

Identification of *DMT1* and *Ireg1* provides a means of testing the hypothesis that increased iron absorption in haemochromatosis is caused by increased expression or activity of the two carriers. Increased levels of DMT1 [18] and IREG1 mRNA [14] have been demonstrated in haemochromatosis patients homozygous for the C282Y mutation. DMT1 mRNA is also increased in the mouse model of haemochromatosis [19]. Both mRNA transcripts are regulated at a post-transcriptional level by intracellular iron levels. The link between mutations in HFE and increased expression of the carriers could therefore be the iron status of duodenal crypt cells that appear to be iron deficient because of defective transferrin iron delivery [15]. Further work is required to determine whether net iron absorption is determined by the co-ordinate action of the two carriers or whether independent control can be exerted at apical and basal locations.

☐ TREATMENT AND LONG-TERM MANAGEMENT

The burden in fully expressed haemochromatosis will be at least 5 g (Table 1) but may be as high as 25 g. The iron is removed by regular venesection; this is conveniently performed by taking a unit of blood (ca 600 ml) at weekly intervals. Most patients are able to tolerate this frequency of phlebotomy which should be continued if the haemoglobin level is above 11 g/dl. It is not necessary to monitor serum ferritin levels frequently because this information is not used to decide whether phlebotomy should be performed. Each unit of blood contains about 250 mg of iron, so heavily iron-loaded patients may need to donate 100 units to deplete iron stores fully. Venesection should be continued until the patient has been rendered iron-deficient.

Once iron depletion has been achieved, maintenance phlebotomy should be carried out three or four times a year to prevent re-accumulation and to maintain normal iron balance. The frequency of maintenance phlebotomy should be varied to ensure that:

☐   serum ferritin levels remain below 50 µg/l, and

☐   serum transferrin saturation is less than 35%.

If a patient is diagnosed in the pre-cirrhotic stage of the condition, iron depletion will prevent the progression to cirrhosis and restore normal life expectancy. Once cirrhosis has supervened, venesection prolongs survival and leads to symptomatic improvement but does not appear to reduce the risk of developing hepatocellular cancer. Although the effectiveness of regular screening by ultrasound and α-fetoprotein is under debate, this is widely practised by hepatologists managing patients with haemochromatosis and is certainly effective in detecting tumours at an early stage.

REFERENCES

1   Powell LW. Hereditary hemochromatosis. *Pathology* 2000; **32**: 24–36.
2   Summers KM, Halliday JW, Powell LW. Identification of homozygous hemochromatosis subjects by measurement of hepatic iron index. *Hepatology* 1990; **12**: 20–5.

3   Levy JE, Montross LK, Andrews NC. Genes that modify the hemochromatosis phenotype. *J Clin Invest* 2000; **105**: 1209–16.

4   Simon M, Pawlotsky Y, Bourel M, *et al*. Hemochromatose idiopathique: maladie associée à l'antigene tissulaire HLA-A3? *Nouv Press Med* 1975; **4**: 1432.

5   Bulaj ZJ, Griffen LM, Jorde LB, *et al*. Clinical and biochemical abnormalities in people heterozygous for hemochromatosis. *N Engl J Med* 1996; **335**: 1799–805.

6   Feder JN, Gnirke A, Thomas W, *et al*. A novel MHC class I-like gene is mutated in patients with hereditary haemochromatosis. *Nat Genet* 1996; **13**: 399–408.

7   Bacon BR, Powell LW, Adams PC, *et al*. Molecular medicine and hemochromatosis: at the crossroads. *Gastroenterology* 1999; **116**: 193–207.

8   Camaschella C, Roetto A, Cali A, *et al*. The gene *TFR2* is mutated in a new type of haemochromatosis mapping to 7q22. *Nat Genet* 2000; **25**: 14–5.

9   Adams PC. Population screening for haemochromatosis. *Gut* 2000; **46**: 301–3.

10   Merry-Weather Clark AT, Worwood M, Parkinson L, *et al*. The effect of HFE mutations on serum ferritin saturation in the Jersey population. *J Haematol* 1998; **101**: 369–73.

11   Jackson HA, Carter K, Guttridge MG, *et al*. Haemochromatosis – prevalence and penetrance in blood donors resident in Wales (abstract). *Blood* 1999; **94**: 407a.

12   Olynyk JE, Cullen DJ, Aquilia S, *et al*. A population-based study of the clinical expression of the hemochromatosis gene. *N Engl J Med* 1999; **341**: 718–24.

13   Gunshin H, Mackenzie B, Berger UV, *et al*. Cloning and characterisation of a mammalian proton-coupled metal-ion transporter. *Nature* 1997; **388**: 482–8.

14   McKie AT, Marciani P, Rolfs A, *et al*. A novel duodenal iron-regulated transporter, IREG1, implicated in the basolateral transfer of iron to the circulation. *Mol Cell* 2000; **5**: 299–309.

15   Waheed A, Pakkila S, Saarnio J, *et al*. Association of HFE protein with transferrin receptor in crypt enterocytes of human duodenum. *Proc Natl Acad Sci USA* 1999; **96**: 1579–84.

16   McKie AT, Barrow D, Pountney D, *et al*. Molecular cloning of a B-type cytochrome reductase implicated in iron absorption from mouse duodenal mucosa. *Bioiron'99* 1999; abstract pp 95.

17   Vulpe CD, Kuo YM, Murphy TL, *et al*. Hephaestin, a ceruloplasmin homologue implicated in intestinal iron transport, is defective in the *sla* mouse. *Nat Genet* 1999; **21**: 195–9.

18   Zoller H, Pietrangelo A, Vogel W, Weiss G. Duodenal metal-transporter (DMT1, NRAMP2) expression in patients with hereditary haemochromatosis. *Lancet* 1999; **353**: 2120–3.

19   Fleming RE, Migas MC, Zhou X, *et al*. Mechanism of increased iron absorption in murine model of hereditary hemochromatosis: increased duodenal expression of the iron transporter DMT1. *Proc Natl Acad Sci USA* 1999; **96**: 3143–8.

☐ SELF ASSESSMENT QUESTIONS

1   In hereditary haemochromatosis:
  (a) Sexual dysfunction is due to primary testicular failure
  (b) The diet contains excess iron
  (c) The metabolic fault is the reduced excretion of iron
  (d) Liver biopsy is the only way to quantify body iron stores
  (e) Dietary advice forms an important part of the management

2   People heterozygous for hereditary haemochromatosis:
  (a) Rarely demonstrate increased body iron stores
  (b) May have partial biochemical expression with abnormal iron biochemistry
  (c) Should be offered genetic counselling
  (d) Are at increased risk of developing hepatocellular cancer
  (e) Comprise approximately 10% of northern European people

3   HLA typing:
(a) Provided essential data in the search for the haemochromatosis gene
(b) Can be used to confirm the diagnosis of haemochromatosis in family studies
(c) Has been superceded by genotyping
(d) Can be used to identify the ancestral haemochromatosis haplotype
(e) Is of value in predicting if haemochromatosis patients will develop diabetes

4   The C282Y mutation in the haemochromatosis gene:
(a) Is confined to people of northern European extraction
(b) Shows complete penetrance
(c) Leads to the production of a mutant protein
(d) Can be detected only by sequencing the gene
(e) Is the only known mutation in the gene

5   The HFE protein:
(a) Has features in common with MHC class I molecules
(b) Plays a role in maintaining iron balance
(c) Binds to the transferrin receptor on the cell surface
(d) Is expressed in crypt cells in the duodenal mucosa
(e) Presents peptide antigens to T lymphocytes

ANSWERS

1a False	2a True	3a True	4a True	5a True
b False	b True	b True	b False	b True
c False	c True	c True	c True	c True
d False	d False	d True	d False	d True
e False	e True	e False	e False	e False

Endoscopic ultrasound

Paul Swain

□ INTRODUCTION

Endoscopic ultrasound (EUS) allows close contact or close proximity imaging of the gastrointestinal (GI) tract and retroperitoneal and mediastinal structures which cannot be obtained by more conventional imaging methods. This chapter provides a brief overview of recent developments in GI endosonography, and surveys recent applications for EUS in clinical practice.

□ PRINCIPLES OF ULTRASOUND ENDOSCOPY

Ultrasound transducers convert electrical energy into ultrasonic energy which is transmitted into soft tissue, reflected back to the transducer, and reconverted into electronic signals for display [1]. They are made of an array of piezoelectric crystals which vibrate in response to an applied electrical voltage and in this way generate sound waves. Sound waves generated at a frequency greater than that detectable by the human ear (20–20,000 cycles per second) are termed ultrasound. The ultrasound wave energy reflected from target tissue and tissue boundaries is called the echo. This is deformed when it returns to the transducer array, producing voltage changes which can be amplified and displayed on a monitor. These voltages can be presented as a two-dimensional display, or B-mode (brightness mode) image, which yields information regarding the size and nature of soft tissue structures and is usually viewed in real time.

Transmission of sound waves in tissue depends on the specific tissue density. Air is the enemy of ultrasound. Ultrasound waves are not readily transmitted through air due to its very low density. Bones and other calcified or hard structures such as gallstones also transmit sound waves poorly due to their low compressibility resulting in a high degree of reflectivity. EUS has the advantage that it places the piezoelectric transducer directly on or closely adjacent to the target tissue, in this way avoiding the need to transmit sound waves across air in the form of lung air or bowel gas or across calcified structures such as the sternum, ribs or pelvis, as is often the case using conventional transcutaneous ultrasound. The advantage of combining ultrasound with endoscopy is that high-resolution images of internal organs can be obtained which are unmatched by current alternative imaging techniques such as computed tomography (CT) or magnetic resonance imaging (MRI).

The frequency of the ultrasound wave is an important determinant of imaging depth. The higher the ultrasound frequency used, the greater the degree of image resolution but the more limited the depth of tissue penetration. Transducers working at frequencies of 5.0 MHz and 7.5 MHz are capable of imaging well beyond the gut wall, but allow relatively limited resolution of the mural morphology of the GI tract; 12.0 MHz and 20 MHz transducers give high resolution of GI wall layer anatomy, but have limited ability to penetrate into adjacent organs and structures. It is possible to switch frequencies during an endoscopic examination.

EUS can give astonishing images of the gut wall as a five-layered structure of differing echogenicities alternating between hyperechoic and hypoechoic layers [1,2]. These layers correlate quite well with the histology of the five layers of the gut wall: mucosa, muscularis mucosa, submucosa, muscularis propria and serosa (Fig. 1). There is some distinction between histological thickness and ultrasound 'thickness': the latter is proportional to the time an ultrasonic pulse takes to travel to and return from a reflective interface, and the sound velocity varies with the acoustic impedance of each layer of the gut wall. High-resolution transducers sometimes identify extra layers which have been shown to correlate with the thin layer of connective tissue separating the inner circular and outer longitudinal components of the muscularis propria. Figure 2(a) shows an example of a patient with a lower oesophageal narrowing, seen on a barium swallow, due to a myopathy in which the hyperechoic layers correspond to the muscularis mucosa and muscularis propria. The oesophageal wall thickness is seen to increase from 3 mm to 10 mm by this pathological process (Fig. 2(b)).

□ SUBMUCOSAL LESIONS AND GUT WALL ANATOMY

A variety of lesions arising submucosally may produce a mass-like effect when viewed endoscopically. Compression of the GI tract by an adjacent organ or vascular

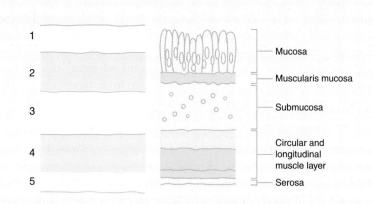

Fig. 1 Endoscopic ultrasound gives astonishing images of the gut wall as a five-layered structure of differing echogenicities, alternating hyperechoic and hypoechoic layers. These layers correlate well with the histology of the five layers of the gut wall.

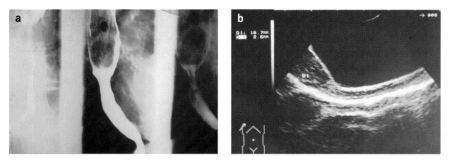

Fig. 2 (a) A barium swallow shows lower oesophaeal narrowing due to myopathy. **(b)** The oesophageal wall thickness is seen to increase from 3 mm to 10 mm by this pathological process. The dark echo-dense muscular layers are particularly thick.

structure, whether abnormal or normal, may produce an appearance of a submucosal mass. Barium X-ray or conventional endoscopy is poor at determining what these submucosal lesions are. Endoscopic forceps biopsies rarely penetrate deeply enough to give a tissue diagnosis of lesions such as a leiomyoma (now called stromal cell tumour) (Fig. 3). EUS is the only currently available technique which has been proven to be useful for evaluating submucosal lesions and determining their underlying structural origin [2–4].

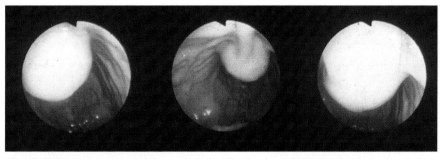

Fig. 3 Endoscopic ultrasound is particularly effective in determining the layer from which submucosal tumours arise such as this gastric leiomyoma (gastric stromal cell tumour).

☐ ENDOSCOPIC ULTRASOUND EVALUATION OF DEPTH OF TUMOUR PENETRATION IN OESOPHAGEAL AND GASTRIC CANCER

EUS is highly accurate and superior to CT scanning for the pre-operative staging of oesophageal and gastric carcinoma [2–5]. It is important to stress that EUS is not a substitute for a CT scan for this situation but, rather, a useful adjunct. It is particularly useful in assessing the depth of wall penetration of cancers (ie T staging) (Table 1). EUS is accurate in confirming the early stages of the disease and in detecting advanced, unresectable oesophageal carcinoma. If the ultrasound endoscope cannot pass through an obstructing oesophageal tumour, the stage is usually T3; this can be confirmed by the use of mini-ultrasound probes. EUS provides a more sensitive and

Table 1 T, N, M classification for staging cancer.

Stage	0	1	2	3	4
Primary tumour confined to T stage		Mucosa only	Mucosa and submucosa	Mucosa, submucosa and muscularis propria	All layers to serosa
Lymph node Infiltration N stage	No nodes	Adjacent to primary	Within field of excision	Distant from primary	
Metastases M stage	No metastases	Metastases			

reliable determination of local vascular involvement compared with a CT scan. Figure 4 shows a T3 oesophageal tumour involving the mucosa, submucosa and deep muscle. Thin alternating hypoechoic and hyperechoic lines separate the serosal surface from the pericardium suggesting that this tumour may still be operable.

Although EUS is better than CT at assessing the presence of lymph nodes, it is not equivalent to histological assessment of sampled tissue. There are sonographic features which make it statistically more likely that such lymph nodes are malignant rather than benign. Lymph nodes, which are larger than 1 cm, round and hypoechoic with distinct borders (Table 2), are more likely to be malignant (Fig. 5).

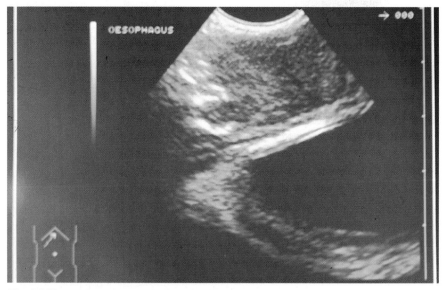

Fig. 4 A T3 oesophageal tumour is shown involving the mucosa, submucosa and deep muscle. Thin alternating hypoechoic and hyperechoic lines separate the serosal surface from the pericardium suggesting that this tumour may still be operable.

Table 2 Features suggestive of malignancy in lymph nodes seen with endoscopic ultrasound.

	Malignant	**Non-malignant**
Size	>1 cm	<1 cm
Echogenicity	Hypoechoic	Hyperechoic
Margins	Distinct	Indistinct
Shape	Round	Ovoid

If all four features favouring malignancy were identified the chance of an individual lymh node being malignant would be 80%. All four features were identifiable in only 25% of malignant lymph nodes [7].

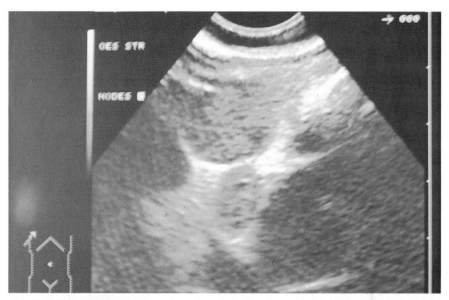

Fig. 5 Multiple enlarged lymph nodes adjacent to the stomach show features, suggestive of malignant involvement. Some are larger than 1 cm, hypoechoic, round with distinct borders.

EUS without biopsy, like CT, cannot predict the presence of malignancy in an individual lymph node with an accuracy higher than 80% [6–8]. EUS is not good at identifying distant metastases in the lung, bone and even in the liver. Whereas it provides outstanding views of the parts of the liver that are closer to the endoscope, it may miss peripheral metastases.

In order to improve the accuracy of EUS regional lymph node evaluation, EUS-guided fine-needle aspiration of suspected malignant nodes has become possible using a linear array ultrasound endoscope [7–10]. This is designed to permit ultrasound scanning parallel to the long axis of the endoscope, and therefore permits ultrasound-guided needle biopsy. The needle moves in this axis and can be viewed not only by the endoscope but also by the EUS transducer as it penetrates the GI tissue. The needle can be seen in real time on the ultrasound screen in the centre of the field moving through tissue to penetrate the lymph node (Figs. 6 and 7). Fine-needle aspiration appears safe even in mediastinal biopsy.

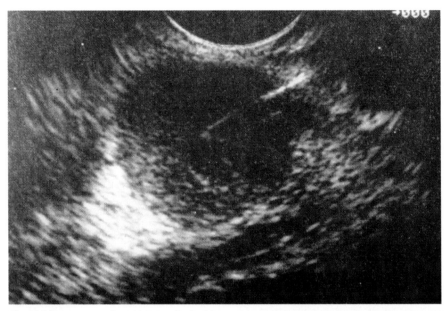

Fig. 6 A linear array echo-endoscope is used to pass a needle into a large mediastinal lymph node adjacent to the wall of the oesophagus to aspirate tissue for cytological analysis.

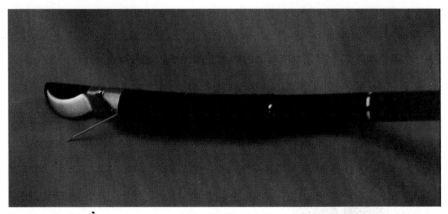

Fig. 7 A view of a linear array echo-endoscope with a needle protruding from its biopsy channel.

Ideally, a CT scan should be performed first to detect distant metastases (M stage). If no distant metastases are detected, EUS should be performed to determine the depth of tumour penetration and the presence of regional lymphadenopathy (T, N stage).

☐ VALUE OF ENDOSCOPIC ULTRASOUND EXAMINATION IN PATIENTS WITH OESOPHAGEAL AND GASTRIC CANCER

Diagnostic EUS can alter the clinical management of patients with oesophageal and gastric cancer by providing accurate pre-therapeutic staging information which is helpful in giving a prognosis for patients presenting with these diseases. Accurate staging of cancer is useful only if the results of such staging have an impact on treatment. At present, where surgery is considered the main therapeutic modality, patients benefit from diagnostic EUS evaluation only when the results of such evaluations demonstrate advanced disease and surgery is in consequence avoided.

☐ VALUE OF ENDOSCOPIC ULTRASOUND IN PATIENTS WITH PANCREATO-BILIARY DISEASE

EUS has allowed high-resolution imaging of the pancreas and biliary tree (Fig. 8), and can distinguish structures as small as 1–2 mm diameter with excellent accuracy [2,6,9,11].

EUS is currently the most sensitive imaging modality for detecting chronic pancreatitis, with a sensitivity (in a series of 81 patients) of 88%, (CT 75%, endoscopic retrograde cholangiopancreatography (ERCP) 74%, abdominal ultrasound 58%), and specificity of 100% (CT 95%, ERCP 88%, abdominal ultrasound 75%) [9]. Patients with chronic pancreatitis who are suspected of having cancer or have focal hypoechoic areas that look like tumours on abdominal ultrasound are challenging to diagnose. The specificity of EUS for distinguishing focal chronic pancreatitis from cancer is at best 75%. However, if fine-needle aspiration is performed at the time of EUS the diagnosis may be clarified [2,10]. EUS is also more sensitive than magnetic resonance cholangiopancreatography at imaging small bile-duct stones [11].

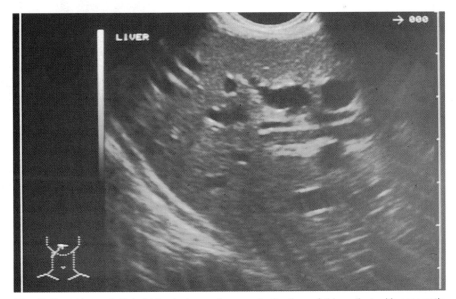

Fig. 8 Clear views of dilated bile ducts can be seen in the liver of this patient with pancreatic malignancy. Structures of less than 2 mm in diameter can be easily identified.

Pseudocysts can be assessed and drained with EUS [2], and the presence or absence of varices over the proposed puncture site can be determined and visualised with colour doppler. New large-channel therapeutic linear array EUS instruments allow the passage of 10 French stents into the pseudocysts.

A clinical dilemma with patients found to have pancreatic cysts is whether to recommend surgical resection or 'watchful waiting'. If the carcino-embryonic antigen (CEA) in the cystic fluid aspirated at EUS is less than 5 ng/ml the cysts are usually benign [12]. EUS is currently the most sensitive method for localising pancreatic endocrine tumours [2].

EUS staging of pancreatic cancer seems accurate [13]. In a series of 99 patients with pancreatic resection, 59 underwent surgical resection. EUS had an accuracy of 87% for T stage, 80% for N stage and 95% for determining vascular invasion [14].

☐ LIMITATIONS OF ENDOSCOPIC ULTRASOUND

EUS equipment was first available commercially in 1985 in Europe. It is widely used in Japan, the USA and parts of Europe including France, Germany and Italy, but has gained slow acceptance in the UK. There are several reasons for this. It is expensive, costing at least £55,000 for the most basic equipment and £120,000 for a standard radial instrument and ultrasound processor. There is also a long training process: at least 100 cases are required to achieve reasonable competence in assessing oesophageal cases, and 300 cases to become reasonably competent with pancreato-biliary cases.

The equipment has evolved slowly. Video-echo-endoscopes have only recently been introduced by Olympus. Fibre-optic echo-endoscopes are still being made by Pentax, whose linear array device is standard equipment for endoscopists performing therapeutic procedures. The endoscopes are still bulky, stiff, clumsy and have the feel of endoscopes made 20 years ago; they could easily be improved. There is, of course, continued competition from ongoing improvements in spiral CT and MRI. The many well-conducted studies which have demonstrated the diagnostic superiority of EUS over CT and MRI may lose their validity as the external scanners improve.

In the UK, there is a sense of therapeutic nihilism about the treatment of oesophageal and pancreatic cancer. In few patients is there any attempt at staging and only a minority are referred for consideration of surgery or oncological treatment once stented. This nihilism is reflected in the limited availability of EUS in the UK.

There has been a slow but steady increase in the use of EUS worldwide. More US trainees are learning EUS than ERCP. The advent of an increasing variety of therapeutic indications for the use of EUS is likely to ensure its viability as a technology at least in the short term.

REFERENCES

1 Kimmey MB, Martin RW. Fundamenals of endosonogaphy. *Gastrointest Endosc Clin North Am* 1992; 2: 557–73.

2 Rosch T (ed). Endoscopic ultrasonography. State of the art 1995. *Gastrointest Endosc Clin North Am* 1995; 5: 475–884.

3 Murata Y, Suzuki S, Hashimoto H. Endoscopic ultrasonography of the upper gastrointestinal tract. *Surg Endosc* 1988; **2**: 180–3.

4 Palazzo L, Landi B, Cellier C, *et al*. Endosonographic features predictive of benign and malignant gastrointestinal stromal cell tumours. *Gut* 2000; **46**: 88–92.

5 Van Dam J. Endosonographic evaluation of the patient with esophageal cancer. *Chest* 1997; **112**: S184–90.

6 Allescher HD, Rosch T, Willkomm G, *et al*. Performance, patient acceptance, appropriateness of indication and potential influence on outcome of EUS: a prospective study in 397 consecutive patients. *Gastrointest Endosc* 1999; **50**: 737–45.

6 Tio TL, Kallimanis G. Endoscopic ultrasonography of perigastrointestinal lymph nodes. *Endoscopy* 1994; **26**: 776–9.

7 Bhutani MS, Hawes RH, Hoffman BJ. A comparison of the accuracy of echo features during endoscopic ultrasound (EUS) and EUS-guided fine-needle aspiration for diagnosis of malignant lymph node invasion. *Gastrointest Endosc* 1997; **45**: 474–9.

8 Mallery S, DeCamp M, Bueno R, *et al*. Pretreatment staging by endosonography does not predict complete response to neoadjuvant chemoradiation in patients with esophageal cancer. *Cancer* 1999; **86**: 764–9.

9 Buscail L, Escourrou J, Moreau J, *et al*. Endoscopic ultrasonography in chronic pancreatitis: a comparative prospective study with conventional ultrasonography, computed tomography, and ERCP. *Pancreas* 1995; **10**: 251–7.

10 Vilmann P, Jacobsen GK, Henricksen FW, Hancke S. Endoscopic ultrasonography with guided fine needle aspiration biopsy in pancreatic disease. *Gastrointest Endosc* 1992; **11**: 762–5.

11 De Ledinghen V, Lecesne R, Raymond JM, *et al*. Diagnosis of cholelithiasis: EUS or magnetic resonance cholangiography? A prospective controlled study. *Gastrointest Endosc* 1999; **49**: 26–31.

12 Hammel P, Levy P, Viotot H, *et al*. Preoperative cyst fluid analysis is useful for the differential diagnosis of cystic lesions of the pancreas. *Gastroenterology* 1995; **108**: 1230–5.

13 Tio TL, Sie LH, Tytgat GNJ. Endosonography and cytology in diagnosing and staging pancreatic body and tail carcinomas. *Dig Dis Sci* 1993; **38**: 59–63.

14 Gress F, Savides T, Zaidi S, Sherman S, *et al*. Endoscopic ultrasound (EUS) staging correlates with survival in patients with pancreatic cancer. *Gastrointest Endosc* 1995; **41**: 423–6.

☐ SELF ASSESSMENT QUESTIONS

1 Ultrasound:
  (a) Ultrasound waves are readily transmitted through air due to its very low density
  (b) Ultrasound frequencies are higher than 18,000 cycles per second
  (c) B-mode is a method of representing three-dimensional images
  (d) The higher the frequency the greater the degree of image resolution but the more limited the depth of tissue penetration
  (e) Transducers are made of an array of pixels which vibrate in response to an applied electrical voltage, and in this way generate sound waves

2 The gut wall and endoscopic ultrasound (EUS):
  (a) EUS shows the gut wall as a four-layered structure
  (b) Stromal cell tumours of the gastrointestinal tract were formerly called leiomyomas
  (c) Endoscopic forceps biopsy is usually helpful in the diagnosis of submucosal tumours

(d) Vascular abnormalities can look like submucosal tumours at endoscopy
(e) Spiral computed tomography (CT) scan is as good as EUS at determining the structural origin of submucosal tumours

3   In patients with oesophageal and gastric cancer:
(a) If the EUS scope will not pass through the tumour the stage is usually T3
(b) CT scan is not necessary if an EUS examination is complete
(c) A radial rather than a linear array EUS allows the needle path to be seen during biopsy
(d) EUS provides excellent views of much of the liver but can miss peripheral metastases
(e) CT scan is best performed after EUS

4   In patients with pancreatic tumours:
(a) Insulinomas and gastrinomas are readily identifiable with CT and selective angiography
(b) Carcino-embryonic antigen of 17 ng/ml aspirated from a 1 cm pancreatic cyst at EUS is suggestive of malignancy
(c) EUS is less good than angiography in determining vascular invasion by pancreatic malignancy
(d) EUS can distinguish chronic pancreatitis from pancreatic cancer with an accuracy better than 90%
(e) EUS can stage pancreatic cancer more accurately than CT

5   Using EUS:
(a) EUS can be used to treat intractable pain from chronic pancreatitis
(b) Stenting of pseudocysts can be accomplished via an EUS endoscope
(c) Bile duct stones can be more safely and accurately identified at EUS than at endoscopic retrograde cholangiopancreatography (ERCP)
(d) EUS is not more sensitive and specific for the diagnosis of early chronic pancreatitis than CT and ERCP
(e) Identifying the layer from which submucosal tumours arise allows for safer endoscopic submucosal resection

ANSWERS

1a False	2a False	3a True	4a False	5a True
b True	b True	b False	b True	b True
c False	c False	c False	c False	c True
d True	d True	d True	d False	d False
e False	e False	e False	e True	e True

Screening for colorectal cancer – time to start?

Richard F A Logan

Colorectal cancer is estimated to be the fourth most common cancer in the world at present, with approximately 677,000 new cases diagnosed each year. Only cancers of the lung (886,000), stomach (785,000) and breast (719,000) are more common. The lifetime risk of developing colorectal cancer in the UK is about one in 20 (Table 1). This figure conceals the fact that most of these cancers are found in people over the age of 65, in contrast to breast cancer which is currently being detected in one in 20 women below age 65.

Less than 40% of all patients with colorectal cancer in the UK survive five years from diagnosis. This is mainly accounted for by the large proportion of patients with advanced cancer (Duke's C and D) at diagnosis. Early cancer has a much better survival: around 90% at five years for Duke's A (tumours confined to the bowel wall) and about 60% for Duke's B (tumours penetrating the bowel wall but without lymph node spread). Colorectal cancer fulfils two of the three prerequisites for possible consideration for screening, namely:

☐ it is of public health importance, and

☐ there is evidence of better survival when diagnosed early.

A third prerequisite is the availability of suitable screening tests. Only faecal occult blood (FOB) tests and flexible sigmoidoscopy are currently being seriously considered for population screening.

Table 1 Lifetime risk of colorectal cancer (based on cancer incidence in England and Wales, 1995).

		% Developing cancer		
		0–64 years	**0–84 years**	**Lifetime risk**
Men	Lung	1.9	8.4	1 in 12
	Colorectum	1.3	5.3	1 in 19
Women	Breast	5.0	9.5	1 in 11
	Colorectum	0.9	4.7	1 in 21

☐ SCREENING TESTS

Faecal occult blood

The most commonly used FOB tests rely on the peroxidase activity of haemoglobin to change the colour of a chromogen, guaiac, when applied to faeces on a test card. Unfortunately, peroxidase-like activity can also be present in some dietary constituents of faeces as well as in blood originating from the small intestine and upper gastrointestinal tract. Normally, 3–6 tests are performed. The sensitivity of a series of tests for detecting cancer has been estimated to be 50–80%. If the test cards are rehydrated before applying the chromogen indicator, the sensitivity increases and specificity decreases. Although the tests themselves are cheap, investigation of positive results requires either a colonoscopy or sigmoidoscopy and barium enema, all of which are relatively expensive. Thus, the specificity of the test is a key factor in the cost of screening.

Flexible sigmoidoscopy

Flexible sigmoidoscopy with a 60-cm scope has the attraction of direct visualisation of most of the left side of the colon in which 60% of colorectal cancers arise. Sigmoidoscopy can also detect colonic polyps, of which the adenomatous variety are believed to be the precursors of most, if not all, colorectal cancers. In skilled hands, flexible sigmoidoscopy takes 6–10 minutes, but the preceding laxative enema is perhaps the most trying aspect of the procedure. Depending on the findings, there is debate as to when a full colonoscopy should then be performed. About 25% of the remaining proximal colon cancers (40% of cancers) are also associated with left-sided adenomas, thus increasing to 70% the potential detection arising from the initial sigmoidoscopy.

Improved screening tests

The demonstration that screening for colorectal cancer using FOB tests is effective has spurred efforts to devise better screening tests, including:

- ☐ adaptations of guaiac-based tests
- ☐ tests based on an immunochemical approach, testing for the presence of human haemoglobin, and
- ☐ attempts to assess the amount of haemoglobin in stools.

None of these alternatives to the Hemoccult FOB test has been assessed in large studies for its cancer yield, specificity and compliance.

Colonoscopy has also been proposed as a mass screening tool on the grounds that it is the most sensitive and specific test available and also offers the possibility of carrying out polypectomy at the initial examination. However, it is not without serious complications such as perforation, and compliance is likely to be considerably less than with flexible sigmoidoscopy.

☐ EVIDENCE OF EFFECTIVENESS OF SCREENING

Screening for colorectal cancer using FOB tests results in a good yield of colorectal cancers, often at an early stage. Unfortunately, this sort of evidence can be regarded as only preliminary evidence that screening for a cancer is effective. Three factors influence and contribute to the invariably remarkably good figures obtained from uncontrolled, non-randomised assessments of screening:

☐ lead time bias: living longer with the diagnosis of cancer

☐ duration or length time bias: the tendency of screening to detect less aggressive cancer, and

☐ selection bias: preferential uptake of screening programmes by health conscious, low-risk individuals.

Because of these three potential sources of bias, it is crucial that, first, the effectiveness of cancer screening is demonstrated in randomised controlled trials (RCTs) and, secondly, in countries in which healthcare is predominantly state-funded, and in which the decision to set up screening is made centrally in competition with other demands for healthcare, two other criteria need to be satisfied, namely, the acceptability and cost-benefit of screening. Investing in a national screening programme which is either unacceptable (ie people will not use it) or much more costly than other healthcare programmes producing similar benefits is a poor investment of a nation's limited healthcare resources.

Screening by faecal occult blood tests

Four large RCTs of FOB screening involving about 330,000 people in four countries (Table 2) have used the Hemoccult test (SmithKline Diagnostics). In two of the trials (Minnesota and Gothenburg) the test area was rehydrated before testing, increasing the sensitivity of the test but inevitably also reducing its specificity (Table 3). The changes in sensitivity and specificity might not appear large, but the consequence is a much higher colonoscopy rate in those two trials. Indeed, it has been suggested that much of the mortality reduction in the group undergoing annual screening in the Minnesota trial can be accounted for by its high colonoscopy rate. Nevertheless, even in this group screening detected only 50% of the colorectal cancers that subsequently occurred in the screened group.

A recent meta-analysis of these four trials found that those offered screening had a 16% reduction (relative risk (RR) 0.84; 95% confidence interval (CI) 0.77–0.93) in the risk of dying from colorectal cancer. When this figure was adjusted for attendance, the benefit increased to 23% (RR 0.77; 95% CI 0.57–0.89) for people who had actually attended for screening. On the basis of these results, it was estimated that between eight and nine deaths from colorectal cancer would subsequently be prevented over a 10-year period in countries with similar risks of colorectal cancer for every 10,000 people aged 45–75 offered screening, assuming two-thirds of people attended for at least one test.

Table 2 Results of randomised controlled trials of faecal occult blood (FOB) screening using Hemoccult (adapted from [1]).

	Minnesota		Nottingham	Funen (Denmark)	Gothenburg
FOB test frequency	Annual	Biennial	Biennial	Biennial	Twice
Follow-up (years)	18	18	8	10	8
FOB test	Rehydrated (83%)		Unhydrated	Unhydrated	Rehydrated
Tests +ve (%)	10	10	2	1	6
Sensitivity (%)	92	92	64	46	81
Colonoscopy rate (%)	38	28	3	3	6
% of all cancers detected	50	39	27	25	28
CRC mortality (per 10,000):					
screened	95	112	47	66	35
controls	141	141	55	80	80
CRC mortality reduction (%)	33	21	15	18	12
(95% CI)	(17–49)	(3–38)	(1–26)	(1–32)	(+12–31)

CI = confidence interval; CRC = colorectal cancer.

Table 3 Impact of rehydration on faecal occult blood tests (from [2]).

	Unhydrated	Rehydrated
Rate of positive tests (%)	2.4	9.8
Sensitivity (%)	81	92
Specificity (%)	98	90
Positive predictive value (%)	5.6	2.2

Screening by sigmoidoscopy

In some parts of the world, particularly in the US, a sigmoidoscopy has been a long established part of the routine periodic health check. Initially, this was performed with the 25-cm rigid sigmoidoscope but the flexible sigmoidoscope has been increasingly used since the 1980s. Sigmoidoscopy can detect adenomatous polyps as well as cancers, so the screening strategy differs from that for FOB tests. Those screened and found to have adenomatous polyps, depending on the size and histology, are then offered a colonoscopy in order to check the rest of the colon and have other polyps (or proximal cancers) removed. These subjects then join an adenoma surveillance programme in which colonoscopy is performed every five years. Subjects with a normal screening sigmoidoscopy are regarded as being at low risk of developing colorectal cancer and would possibly need no further screening procedures in their lifetime.

Observational studies

Several observational (ie non-randomised) studies have shown impressive reductions in the risk of rectal and sigmoid cancers following rigid sigmoidoscopy when used in routine health checks. The best of these is a case-control study [3] which used the comprehensive medical records of the Kaiser Permanente Health Maintenance Organisation in California to compare the screening sigmoidoscopy histories of people who died from colorectal cancer with those of matched controls (Table 4). Most case-control studies of screening cannot assess the effect of the selection bias mentioned earlier. In this study, however, the relative protection offered by sigmoidoscopy was found only for cancers occurring within 20 cm of the anus, and not when deaths from more proximal cancers were considered. Thus, selection bias appears to have been negligible in this study since, if present, an apparent benefit from having a sigmoidoscopy would have been seen with the more proximal cancers. Two other case-control studies have also shown a reduced risk of dying from distal cancers after sigmoidoscopy, although both were less able to allow for the biases inherent in this type of evaluation.

Table 4 Case-control evaluation of screening by rigid sigmoidoscopy (from [3]).

Distance of cancer from anus	Records indicate previous sigmoidoscopy			
	Cases: deaths from colorectal cancer (%)	Controls (%)	RR	95% CI
<20 cm (n = 261)	9	24	0.41	0.3–0.7
>20 cm (n = 268)	23	25	0.96	0.6–1.5

CI = confidence interval; RR = relative risk of colorectal cancer death, adjusted for history of colorectal cancer, family history and number of health checks.

Randomised controlled trials

No RCTs of screening by flexible sigmoidoscopy have yet been completed, but some are now in progress in several countries. In the UK, 65,000 people aged 55–64 have been randomised to receive an invitation for a once-only flexible sigmoidoscopy. People with high-risk adenomatous polyps (>3 polyps, >1 cm in size, severe dysplasia, tubulo-villous or villous histology) are invited to have a colonoscopy followed by regular colonoscopic surveillance. People found to have cancer are treated in the usual way. In the pilot study, 9% of the first 1,000 screened were found to have adenomatous polyps, of which half were in the high-risk group, and five had cancers (4 Duke's A) detected. The controls are 130,000 people of the same age randomised not to have an invitation for screening. The results of this Medical Research Council (MRC) trial are likely to be available in 8–10 years' time. A similar study is in progress in Italy.

□ EVIDENCE OF ACCEPTABILITY

Table 5 shows the overall acceptability of FOB testing in the four RCTs. Even in Minnesota, where the trial recruited volunteers, compliance declined markedly with

Table 5 Acceptability of faecal occult blood screening.

	Population	Age group (years)	≥1 screen	All screens
			Screen accepted	
Minnesota:				
Annual	Volunteers	50–80	90	46
Biennial			90	60
Nottingham	General	45–74	60	38
Funen	General	45–75	67	46
Gothenburg	General	60–64	68	60*

* only two screens performed.

repeated tests. Unlike some screening tests, FOB testing requires the active participation of the subject and many find the test embarrassing or unpleasant.

The acceptability of flexible sigmoidoscopy in the UK pilot studies has been around 30% for the general population. However, in the pilot study of the MRC trial which first identified people interested in screening (60% of those approached), 72% of those randomised attended for the sigmoidoscopy.

As with other screening procedures, compliance increases with greater education and when there is a history of colorectal cancer in relatives or friends. Compliance with regular screening colonoscopy reached 80% in the US National Polyp Study, which involved surveillance of subjects who had previously had an adenomatous polyp removed. Nevertheless, current figures indicate that in the UK no more than two-thirds of the general population find FOB testing acceptable, and less than half are prepared to undergo repeated tests. These figures would be expected to improve considerably if a national programme were introduced with appropriate widespread health education, as has been seen with the breast cancer screening programme.

□ EVIDENCE OF FAVOURABLE COST-BENEFIT BALANCE

The benefits and costs of screening can be considered under the headings listed in Table 6. Screening offers a substantial benefit to those who would have otherwise died of colorectal cancer. However, even for a common cancer such as colorectal cancer, the size of this group is small: no more than nine people in 10,000 over a 10-year period, according to the meta-analysis discussed above. In addition, some cases of colorectal cancer detected by screening may avoid having the more radical curative treatment that would have been necessary if their cancer had been detected later. It has been suggested that screening also provides benefit by reassuring those with negative screening results. This benefit presupposes that there is already a degree of widespread anxiety about colorectal cancer. Unlike breast cancer, this does not appear currently to be the case in the UK, but might well change if a national screening programme were introduced.

For several groups, the results of screening are not beneficial and may even be harmful (Table 6). Fortunately, the degree of harm is usually not great, and the level

Table 6 Benefits and costs of screening.

Benefits:
- Improved prognosis for *some* cases detected by screening
- Less radical treatment for some early cases
- Reassurance for those with negative test results

Costs:
- Longer morbidity in cases whose prognosis is unaltered
- Over-treatment of non- or slowly progressing disease
- False reassurance for those with false negative results
- Anxiety and morbidity for those with false positive results
- Unnecessary medical intervention for false positives
- Hazards of screening test
- Resource costs: diversion of scarce resources to screening

---

of anxiety and inconvenience involved in attending for investigation of false positive tests has been regarded as acceptable.

Attention has focused on the risk of perforation and bleeding from colonoscopy, estimated to occur in 0.4% and 1.2%, respectively, of colonoscopies involving polypectomy. In the Nottingham trial involving almost 1,500 colonoscopies, there were seven serious complications, of which five were perforations and none was fatal.

Resource costs

Many of the costs considered in Table 6 are intangible, and difficult to value in monetary terms. Tangible costs are the health service resource costs of screening. Assessment of these costs in the Nottingham trial showed that the cost of the test cards was only £1.13 (1990 prices), but the total cost per person screened, taking into account the staff time, administration and subsequent investigations, was estimated at £5.33 and the cost per cancer detected at £2,705. Rehydration of the test doubled the cost per person screened, resulting in a 50% increase in the cancer detected cost.

In a cost utility analysis, the Nottingham group calculated on the basis of their trial results that the cost per quality-adjusted life year (QALY) gained (1995 prices) was £5,685 for men and £4,951 for women after a median of eight years of trial follow-up. The lower cost in women reflects their longer life expectancy (ie a woman who does not die of colorectal cancer can expect to live longer than a man). Computer modelling indicates that these costs more than halve when lifetime costs and outcomes are considered rather than only those accruing within the trial follow-up period. These figures can be compared with a similar analysis for breast cancer screening of £3,500 in 1984 (about £6,000 per QALY gained at 1995 prices).

It has been estimated that biennial screening using FOB testing for the entire UK population aged 45–74 (around 18 million) would cost £40 million per year. This figure ignores any extra costs of treatment, and also the substantial and immediate investment necessary to establish the infrastructure for a national programme.

How does colorectal cancer screening compare with other screening programmes?

Calculating the number needed to screen to prevent one death has been suggested as a suitable way of comparing different screening programmes. Using this approach, Table 7 compares colorectal cancer screening with breast cancer and cardiovascular disease screening. The negative values for some of the 95% CIs show that screening for some of these conditions has not significantly reduced mortality. In general, the numbers needed to screen to prevent death are much lower for cardiovascular conditions than for cancer, but such an analysis ignores any of the subsequent treatment costs involved. Costs for treatment with a statin can vary from £250–600 per year, making the cost per life year gained by screening over £25,000. Even hypotensive therapy with a low-cost regimen (£45 per year), for which 1,307 people would need to be screened to prevent one death, would incur drug costs of over £10,000 per year for treating the 235 hypertensives detected by screening. Thus, although the yield of colorectal cancer screening is low, the costs per life year gained are comparable to those for established programmes in cardiovascular disease.

☐ FUTURE DEVELOPMENTS

The randomised trials have proved that colorectal cancer screening works, and that biennial FOB testing has the potential to reduce mortality from colorectal cancer by about 20%. With a compliance rate of around 60%, screening people aged 50–69 years of age would prevent about 1,200 such deaths per year in the UK. Two

Table 7 Comparison of number needed to screen to prevent one death in five years (adapted from [4]).

Disease	Prevalence of untreated disease	Screen (treatment)	No. needed to screen	95% CI
All-cause mortality				
Dyslipidaemia	0.26*	Lipid profile:		
		pravastatin	418	235 to 79,720
		diet	590	292 to –610
Hypertension	0.18	Sphygmomanometer:		
		diuretics, diastolic ↓ 10	274	165 to 1,546
		diuretics, diastolic ↓ 6	1,307	834 to 3,386
Coronary artery disease		Aspirin**	354	155 to –795
Colorectal cancer		Hemoccult (standard)	3,034	157 to –145
Breast cancer		Mammography (standard)	–11,029	1,369 to –967
Cancer-specific mortality				
Colon cancer		Hemoccult (standard)	1,374	955 to 2,802
Breast cancer:				
60–69 years		Mammography (standard)	1,251	853 to 3,058
50–59 years		Mammography (standard)	2,451	1,576 to 7,651

*low-density lipoprotein >4.14 mmol.
**if not contraindicated.
CI = confidence interval.

pilot studies to examine the feasibility of a national programme have just started, with the aim of resolving issues about the FOB test, and defining the best method of investigating those who test positive. The trials so far have relied on colonoscopy and conventional barium enema, but computed tomographic colography offers the possibility in the future of a rapid and painless examination, although colonoscopy would still be required for those found to have polyps.

Other possibilities are the development of interventions to prevent recurrent adenomas. Calcium supplements have recently been shown to reduce adenoma recurrence rates by 19%, and several randomised trials of various agents including aspirin and folic acid are in progress.

REFERENCES

1   Towler B, Irwig L, Glasziou P, *et al.* A systematic review of the effects of screening for colorectal cancer using the faecal occult blood test, Hemoccult. *Br Med J* 1998; **317**: 559–65.
2   Mandel JS, Bond JH, Church TR, *et al.* Reducing mortality from colorectal cancer by screening for fecal occult blood. *N Engl J Med* 1993; **328**: 1365–71.
3   Selby JV, Friedman GD, Queensberry CP, *et al.* A case-control study of screening sigmoidoscopy and mortality from colorectal cancer. *N Engl J Med* 1992; **327**: 653–7.
4   Rembold CM. Number needed to screen: development of a statistic for disease screening. *Br Med J* 1998; **317**: 307–12.

FURTHER READING

1   Northover J (ed). Review in depth: screening for bowel cancer. *Eur J Gastroenterol Hepatol* 1998; **10**: 195–233.
2   Robinson MHE, Hardcastle JD, Moss SM, *et al.* The risks of screening: data from the Nottingham randomised controlled trial of faecal occult blood screening for colorectal cancer. *Gut* 1999; **45**: 588–92.
3   Winawer SJ, Fletcher RH, Miller L, *et al.* Colorectal cancer screening: clinical guidelines and rationale. *Gastroenterology* 1997; **112**: 594–642.
4   Young GP, Rozen P, Levin B (eds). *Prevention and early detection of colorectal cancer.* London: WB Saunders, 1996.
5   Atkin WS. Implementing screening for colorectal cancer. *Br Med J* 1999; **319**: 1212–3.
6   Atkin WS. Screening for colorectal cancer: the heart of the matter. *Gut* 1999; **45**: 480–1.

☐ KEY POINTS

▶ Faecal occult blood (FOB) screening (two-yearly) will reduce mortality by 16–23%

▶ Currently, 50-60% will accept FOB screening in the UK

▶ Cost utility (cost per quality-adjusted life year gained) is similar to breast cancer

▶ Optimal investigation of FOB positives unclear

▶ Pilot studies have now started in the UK

▶ Results of flexible sigmoidoscopy trial should be available in 5–10 years

☐ SELF ASSESSMENT QUESTIONS

1   Colorectal cancer:
    (a) Is more common than breast cancer worldwide
    (b) By age 85 the cumulative incidence is about 5% in the UK
    (c) Most cases occur after age 65
    (d) In the UK, overall five-year survival after diagnosis is about 50%
    (e) Only adenomatous polyps are precursors of cancer

2   Faecal occult blood (FOB) screening using Hemoccult:
    (a) Relies on the presence of peroxidase activity found only in haemoglobin
    (b) Is best done using a rehydrated test
    (c) Rehydration increases the specificity of the test
    (d) Is taken up by only 50–60% of people approached
    (e) Can be expected to reduce mortality from colorectal cancer by over 30% when performed every two years

3   Screening using flexible sigmoidoscopy:
    (a) Is mainly aimed at adenoma detection
    (b) Has been shown to be effective only in observational studies
    (c) Observational studies of cancer screening are prone to selection bias
    (d) Can result in the detection of 80% of all colorectal cancers
    (e) Is more acceptable than FOB screening

4   The following are true when the costs and benefits of colorectal cancer screening are being considered:
    (a) In the UK, when 10 years' biennial FOB screening is offered to 10,000 people aged 45–75, it can be expected to prevent more than 25 deaths from colorectal cancer
    (b) FOB screening has not been shown to reduce mortality from all causes
    (c) A major benefit of FOB screening is the colonoscopic examination of people with positive FOB tests
    (d) The cost per quality-adjusted life year obtained is greater than that for breast cancer screening
    (e) Screening for cardiovascular risk factors is generally no more cost-effective than colorectal cancer screening

ANSWERS

1a False	2a False	3a True	4a False
b True	b False	b True	b True
c True	c False	c True	c False
d False	d True	d False	d False
e True	e False	e False	e True

Impact of coxibs

Christopher J Hawkey

□ INTRODUCTION

Coxibs are selective inhibitors of the inducible cyclooxygenase (COX)-2, newly designated by the World Health Organization as a subclass of non-steroidal anti-inflammatory drugs (NSAIDs). Members of the subclass currently available for clinical use are rofecoxib (Vioxx) and celecoxib (Celebrex)[1].

□ BACKGROUND

NSAIDs reduce pain and the symptomatic manifestations of inflammation by inhibiting prostaglandin (PG) synthesis. The same pharmacological property is central to ulcerogenic actions which result in an estimated 1,200 deaths each year in the UK. For many years it was thought that there was only one COX enzyme, and that there could be no therapeutic gain without the adverse effects of COX inhibition. Much pragmatic drug development reinforced the notion that effective COX inhibition at sites of pain or joint inflammation was inevitably accompanied by COX inhibition in the stomach and duodenum, with consequent ulceration.

□ EARLY CLUES

A number of observations suggested that COX activity could rise in inflammation and be inhibited by steroids. Investigations arising from these observations, together with a programme to identify early inducible genes, led to the discovery of a second COX enzyme, (COX-2), on chromosome 1. COX-1 is on chromosome 9, but they are remarkably similar:

- □ They both have a molecular weight of 72 kDa.

- □ There are 599 amino acids in COX-2 and 604 in COX-2.

- □ Both enzymes are highly conserved between species.

- □ The two proteins are approximately 60% identical at an amino acid level, although homology is much greater for the amino acids lining the COX enzyme.

- □ Both COX-1 and COX-2 have a polar arginine molecule halfway down the channel at position 120, to which non-selective enzymes bind (Fig. 1).

COX-1   **COX-2**

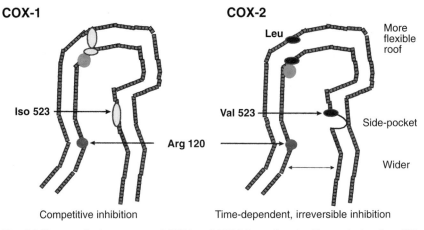

Fig. 1 Differences in the structure of COX-1 and COX-2 (reproduced, with permission, from [1]).

☐ DIFFERENCES BETWEEN COX-1 AND COX-2

There are major differences between COX-1 and COX-2 which relate to their activation:

☐   COX-2 has a more extensive promoter region than COX-1, with receptor binding sites for many signalling molecules involved in gene activation by inflammatory compounds or growth factors, including a TATA box. By contrast, COX-1 is characterised by multiple start sites and an absence of such transcription factor receptor binding elements, characteristic of a constitutive enzyme.

☐   COX-2, but not COX-1, has multiple AAUUUA instability sequences consistent with a short half-life and rapid degradation.

From these and other observations, the notion has arisen that COX-1 is widely expressed and serves protective housekeeping functions, including maintenance of gastroduodenal mucosal integrity, whilst COX-2 is a pathological enzyme induced by cytokines and growth factors at sites of inflammation and in malignancy. This has made COX-2 an attractive target for drug development.

There are also major differences between COX-1 and COX-2 relevant to drug development.

☐   The COX-2 channel is wider than the COX-1 channel. Simple steric hindrance may be insufficient to block enzyme activity.

☐   There is an important difference at position 523 where the amino acid in COX-1 is isoleucine, whilst in COX-2 it is valine. Because valine is smaller than leucine by a methyl group, this leucine/valine substitution in COX-2 leads to a defect in its inner lining shell of amino acids, exposing a side-pocket (the COX-2 pocket) that selective drugs can access and which is important for drug selectivity [2]. Many, but not all, selective COX-2 inhibitors have a tricyclic structure capable of binding within the COX-2 pocket.

☐ Other structural differences in the roof of COX-2 make this more flexible ˜than the roof of COX-1, again giving rise to the possibility of selective drug activation. Accessing the flexible roof may be important for non-coxib compounds such as meloxicam that have some selectivity [1].

☐ In contrast to COX-1 inhibition, selective binding of COX-2 inhibitors appears to be largely irreversible and requires a time-dependent conformational change in the COX-2 enzyme for its activity to be inhibited.

☐ ASSESSING SELECTIVITY

No consensus has emerged on a method to compare the selectivity of individual drugs. Two broad approaches have been taken involving:

☐ recombinant enzymes in expression vectors, or

☐ the activity of COX-1 in platelets and COX-2 induced in monocytes in whole blood.

It is important to be aware that selectivity ratios are generally much higher in recombinant enzyme systems than in whole blood assays [3,4]. The latter can be used to assess the effects of drugs both *in vitro* and *ex vivo*. COX-1 activity is measured in terms of the release of platelet-derived thromboxane (TX) during clotting under controlled conditions, whilst COX-2 is assayed in heparinised blood exposed to lipopolysaccharide to induce COX-2, particularly in monocytes (Fig. 2).

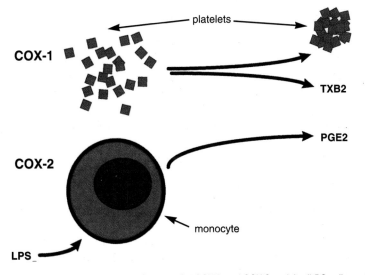

Fig. 2 Schematic representation of assays for COX-1 and COX-2 activity (LPS = lipopolysaccharide; PGE = prostaglandin E; TXB = thromboxane B).

Even here, subtle differences in protocol make comparisons impossible between drugs assessed in different studies. Moreover, COX-2 potency may be underestimated if there is drug degradation during its induction. This has led to the development of a modified whole blood COX-2 assay (the William Harvey modified assay). Monocyte-originated A549 cells are exposed to interleukin-1 for 24 hours before being incubated in heparinised blood and stimulated by calcium ionophore to induce PGE2 synthesis over 30 minutes [4]. This assay has been used to compare a wide range of drugs. Ratios of IC80 values for some drugs of interest are shown in Fig. 3.

□ AVAILABLE COXIBS

Rofecoxib

The sulphone tricyclic drug rofecoxib is probably the most selective COX-2 inhibitor currently available for clinical use [4–6]. In addition to selectivity against COX-2 in recombinant enzyme and whole blood assays, rofecoxib does not affect *ex vivo* gastric mucosal PG synthesis in healthy *Helicobacter pylori*-negative human volunteers, even at high doses. In earlier acute endoscopic studies, 12% of healthy volunteers given rofecoxib at a very high dose (250 mg, 10 times the top daily dose in osteoarthritis) for one week had erosions, compared to 8% on placebo, 94% on aspirin 650 mg four times a day, and 71% on ibuprofen 800 mg three times a day.

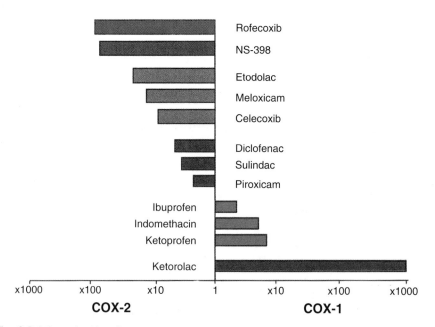

Fig. 3 Relative selectivity of some non-steroidal anti-inflammatory drugs of interest (derived from data in [4]).

Efficacy studies

Dental pain. Single doses of rofecoxib 50 mg have similar maximum efficacy to ibuprofen 400 mg and a longer duration of action. Rofecoxib 50 mg was superior to celecoxib 200 mg (see below) in a direct comparative study [6] (Fig. 4).

Arthritis. In osteoarthritis studies of 6–52 weeks' duration, rofecoxib 12.5 mg and 25 mg showed efficacy equivalent (according to predefined criteria) to ibuprofen 2.4 g or diclofenac 150 mg daily. At present, only phase II data are available for rheumatoid arthritis.

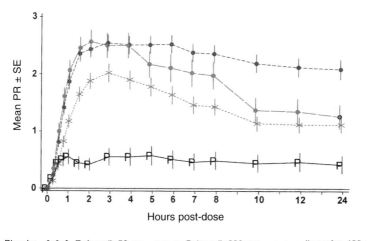

Fig. 4 Dental pain relief with placebo, rofecoxib, celecoxib and ibuprofen (reproduced, with permission, from [6]) (© (1999) National Academy of Sciences USA) (PR = pain relief; SE = standard error).

Gastrointestinal safety

In two large, 26-week controlled endoscopic studies, the primary aim of which was to investigate gastroduodenal safety in patients with osteoarthritis, rofecoxib 25 mg and 50 mg showed substantial reductions in erosions compared to ibuprofen 800 mg three times a day [7]. Over the period of placebo comparison (12 weeks), rofecoxib 25 mg was equivalent (according to predefined criteria) to placebo, whilst rofecoxib 50 mg did not differ significantly from placebo (Fig. 5).

Short-term studies also suggest that rofecoxib lacks the toxicity of NSAIDs to other parts of the gastrointestinal (GI) tract. In a seven-day study [5], the well-known ability of indomethacin (150 mg daily) to damage the small intestine causing enhanced permeability to probe modules was confirmed, whilst rofecoxib 25 mg and 50 mg did not differ significantly from placebo. Similarly, in a one-month study, ibuprofen 800 mg three times a day increased chronic microscopic blood loss into stools, but rofecoxib 25 mg and 50 mg again did not differ significantly from placebo.

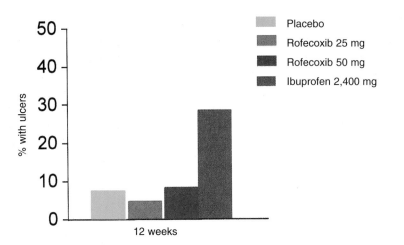

Fig. 5 Rates of ulceration over 12 weeks with placebo, rofecoxib and ibuprofen (reproduced, with permission, from [7]).

Perforations, ulcers and bleeds. A total of 5,435 patients have received rofecoxib during phase IIb and III studies. A meta-analysis of these studies, which also involved placebo, ibuprofen, diclofenac and nabumetone as comparators, identified 38 patients who developed confirmed clinically significant ulcers, GI bleeding or perforation [8]. Event rates on rofecoxib were reduced compared to the NSAID comparators (Fig. 6) and appeared similar to those on placebo, although numbers were small. A prospective randomised study to confirm these data is underway.

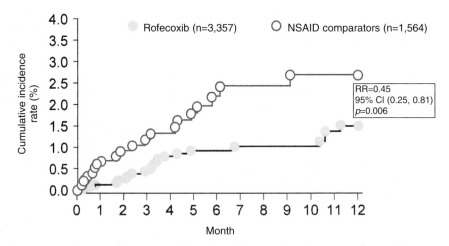

Fig. 6 Cumulative incidence of upper gastrointestinal perforations, ulcers or bleeds in patients taking rofecoxib or comparator non-steroidal anti-inflammatory drugs (NSAIDs) (ibuprofen, diclofenac or nabumetone) (reproduced, with permission, from [8]) (CI = confidence interval; RR = relative risk).

Celecoxib

Celecoxib is a diaryl substituted pyrrazole derivative containing a sulphonamide substituent [8]. It is a selective inhibitor of COX-2, with a selectivity ratio of 375 for recombinant enzyme. However, in the William Harvey modified COX-2 assay it was only approximately ninefold selective for COX-2, less than rofecoxib and similar to the non-coxib inhibitor meloxicam [4]. It is currently unclear why celecoxib has relatively low selectivity in the whole blood assay, and whether this is intrinsic to the drug or reflects the kinetics of the assay. Despite apparently lower biochemical selectivity than rofecoxib, it shows a similar profile of high efficacy and low toxicity in clinical studies.

Efficacy studies

Dental pain. In dental pain studies celecoxib 200 mg was more effective than placebo, and not significantly different from aspirin. However, single doses of celecoxib 100 mg or 200 mg have been reported to be less effective than rofecoxib 50 mg, ibuprofen 400 mg or naproxen sodium 550 mg. Because celecoxib has not been evaluated in a second acute pain model, it has so far failed to obtain a licence from the Food and Drug Administration for this indication.

Arthritis. In contrast to rofecoxib, available phase III data show that celecoxib is an effective treatment for rheumatoid arthritis as well as for osteoarthritis [9,10]. Celecoxib 100 mg or 200 mg twice daily has been shown to be as effective as diclofenac 150 mg or naproxen 1 g daily for symptom relief in both diseases.

Gastrointestinal safety

Many patients in arthritis efficacy trials with celecoxib have undergone endoscopy. Those studies in which endoscopy was performed only at the start and end of the study inevitably reported lower ulcer rates than those involving sequential endoscopy. As with rofecoxib, celecoxib caused significantly fewer ulcers than comparators (Fig. 7), with the exception of one study in which there was no difference from an unexpectedly low rate on diclofenac [9,10]. Ulcer rates on celecoxib 50–400 mg daily were similar to those on placebo, although formal equivalence analyses were not conducted.

Unlike rofecoxib, there are no data about the effect of celecoxib on human gastric mucosal PG synthesis, so this benefit is presumed – rather than proven – to be due to sparing of gastric PGs. Evaluation of celecoxib doses in a short-term volunteer study showed an amount of injury close to that seen with placebo. There have been no reported studies of the effect of celecoxib on intestinal permeability or whole gut microscopic blood loss.

Perforations, ulcers and bleeds. During the phase IIb/III programme evaluating celecoxib only two patients had ulcer complications (perforations, obstructions or bleeds) compared to nine on comparator NSAIDs [11]. A prospective randomised

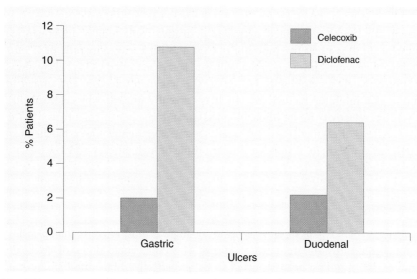

Fig. 7 Percentage of patients with ulcers after six months' treatment with celecoxib 200 mg twice daily or diclofenac SR 75 mg twice daily (redrawn, with permission, from [10]).

study to confirm a reduction in clinically significant ulcer presentations with celecoxib is underway.

☐ RENAL EFFECTS

One interesting consequence of the development of COX-2 inhibitors has been to remind prescribers how much more common is cardiovascular disease than ulcer disease and the renovascular consequences of NSAIDs than their GI consequences.

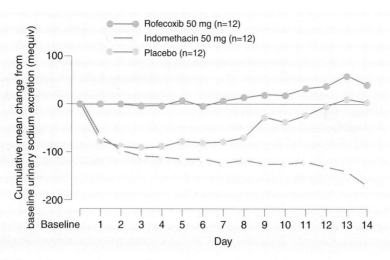

Fig. 8 Cumulative mean change in urinary sodium excretion in elderly subjects taking rofecoxib, indomethacin or placebo daily (reproduced, with permission, from [12]).

It seems clear that COX-2 inhibitors share the ability of non-selective NSAIDs to cause salt and water retention (Fig. 8) and to increase blood pressure [9,12]. This is probably a class effect, although there is no consensus on this. This effect of COX-2 inhibitors is not surprising, given the constitutive expression of COX-2 in the macula densa and its importance in the renin-angiotensin system. These observations have, in turn, led to what may be an overstatement, namely that COX-2 inhibitors share all the renal effects of NSAIDs. It is in fact far from clear that COX-2 inhibitors would share the ability of non-selective NSAIDs to enhance pre-existing renal failure, since renal blood flow may be predominantly COX-1 dependent. Sufficient direct data on patients with pre-existing renal insufficiency taking COX-2 inhibitors are lacking, but should be sought as this may be a significant advantage over non-selective NSAIDs.

□ CARDIOVASCULAR DISEASE

Cardiovascular disease is currently of more interest than GI disease. There are good data establishing that aspirin can prevent cardiovascular disease, low doses being more potent than high doses and selective inhibition of TX the likely mechanism. It is not known whether non-selective NSAIDs, which also inhibit platelet TX synthesis but lack selectivity (they also inhibit endothelial prostacyclin), promote or prevent cardiovascular disease. Concerns have been expressed that switching patients from non-selective NSAIDs, with which there may be inadvertent – albeit partial – protection against cardiovascular disease via inhibition of platelet COX-1 derived TX, to COX-2 inhibitors which lack this property might result in increased levels of cardiovascular disease. These anxieties have been heightened by the recent demonstration that in healthy individuals COX-2 contributes substantially to vascular prostacyclin [13]. However, large numbers of patients have now taken COX-2 inhibitors and the feared epidemic of cardiovascular disease has failed to materialise. It is too soon to be certain that COX-2 inhibitors will not promote

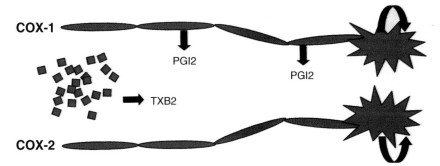

Fig. 9 Schematic representation of COX-1 (blue) and COX-2 (pink) as sources of pro-aggregatory thromboxane (TX) B2 and anti-aggregatory prostaglandin (PG) I2. COX-1 was previously thought to be the dominant source of PGI2 during hypoxia, but COX-2 inhibitors have been shown substantially to reduce excretion of PGI2 metabolites [12]. However, COX-2 is also expressed in plaques where COX-2 derived products could contribute to vascular disease. Further empirical data will be needed to define the net effect of COX-2 inhibitors on vascular disease.

vascular disease. The observations have, however, prompted further reassessment of their possible role, and a realisation that COX-2-derived prostacyclin synthesis may conceivably be accompanied by synthesis of other harmful COX-2 products at sites of inflammation in vascular plaques. This raises the interesting possibility that COX-2 inhibitors might even protect against vascular disease (Fig. 9).

□ CONCLUSIONS

COX-2 inhibitors are unquestionably a major advance over non-selective NSAIDs in preserving (but not enhancing) efficacy, whilst substantially reducing or even eliminating GI toxicity. They probably cause some dyspepsia (though less than non-selective NSAIDs), and appear to have the same potential to cause salt and water retention, predisposing patients to increases in blood pressure and heart failure. It is unclear whether they also exacerbate pre-existing renal failure. Their impact on the cardiovascular system is currently of the greatest interest and may ultimately influence their final evaluation. The interim verdict is, however, highly favourable.

REFERENCES

1 Hawkey CJ. COX-2 inhibitors. *Lancet* 1999; **353**: 307–14.
2 Luong C, Miller A, Barnett J, *et al.* Flexibility of the NSAID binding site in the structure of cyclooxygenase-2. *Nat Struct Biol* 1996; **3**: 927–33.
3 Patrignani P, Panara MR, Sciulli MG, *et al.* Differential inhibition of human prostaglandin endoperoxide synthase-1 and -2 by non-steroidal anti-inflammatory drugs. *J Physiol Pharmacol* 1997; **48**: 623–31.
4 Warner TD, Giuliano F, Vojnovic I, *et al.* Non-steroidal anti-inflammatory drug selectivities for cyclooxygenase-1 rather than cyclooxygenase-2 are associated with human gastrointestinal toxicity: a full *in vitro* analysis. *Proc Natl Acad Sci USA* 1999; **96**: 7563–8.
5 Scott LJ, Lamb HM. Rofecoxib. *Drugs* 1999; **58**: 499–505.
6 Malmstrom K, Daniels S, Kotey P, *et al.* Comparison of rofecoxib and celecoxib, two cyclooxygenase-2 inhibitors, in postoperative dental pain: a randomized, placebo- and active-comparator-controlled clinical trial. *Clin Ther* 1999; **21**: 1653–63.
7 Hawkey CJ, Laine L, Simon T, for the Rofecoxib Osteoarthritis Endoscopy Multinational Study Group. Comparison of the effect of rofecoxib (a cyclooxygenase-2 inhibitor), ibuprofen and placebo on the gastroduodenal mucosa of patients with osteoarthritis. *Arthritis Rheum* 2000; **43**: 370–7.
8 Langman MJ, Jensen DM, Watson DJ, *et al.* Adverse upper gastrointestinal effects of rofecoxib compared with NSAIDs. *JAMA* 1999; **282**: 1929–33.
9 Boyce EG, Breen GA. Celecoxib: a COX-2 inhibitor for the treatment of osteoarthritis and rheumatoid arthritis. *Hosp Formulary* 1999; **34**: 405–17.
10 Emery P, Zeiler H, Kvien TK, *et al.* Celecoxib versus diclofenac in long-term management of rheumatoid arthritis: randomised double-blind comparison. *Lancet* 1999; **354**: 2106–11.
11 Goldstein JL, Agarwal NM, Silverstein E, *et al.* Celecoxib is associated with a significantly lower incidence of clinically significant upper gastrointestinal (UGI) events in osteoarthritis (OS) and rheumatoid arthritis (RA) patients as compared to NSAIDs. *Gastroenterology* 1999; **11**: G0758; A17.
12 Catella-Lawson F, McAdam B, Morrison BW, *et al.* Effects of specific inhibition of cyclooxygenase-2 on sodium balance, hemodynamics, and vasoactive eicosanoids. *J Pharmacol Exper Ther* 1999; **289**: 735–41.
13 McAdam BF, Catella-Lawson F, Mardini IA, *et al.* Systemic biosynthesis of prostacyclin by cyclooxygenase (COX)-2: the human pharmacology of a selective inhibitor of COX-2. *Proc Natl Acad Sci USA* 1999; **96**: 272–7.

Medical management of obesity

Nick Finer

☐ INTRODUCTION: THE OBESITY PANDEMIC

Obesity is the largest and fastest growing public health problem worldwide. Figure 1 shows the increase in prevalence of obesity in the UK. In 1997, 20% of adult women and 17% of men were obese (a body mass index (BMI) >30) and more than 50% overweight (BMI >25). Obesity impairs quality of life, increases morbidity and leads to premature mortality (Fig. 2). Economic surveys in the USA, Australia and France have estimated that obesity accounts for 6–8% of health service costs; in the UK this cost is about £350 million each year [1]. There is now an urgent need for governments to focus on prevention, but there is also a need for effective treatment for those who are already obese and who will become so in the future.

Obesity develops from a chronic net excess of energy intake over energy expenditure. The rising prevalence in most developed or developing countries relates to the interaction of societal changes with individuals who have a susceptible genotype. Societal changes that have led to low levels of energy expenditure (and increasing sedentariness), together with the ready availability of high fat, high energy dense foods, seem to be important causes, and the term 'toxic environment' has been

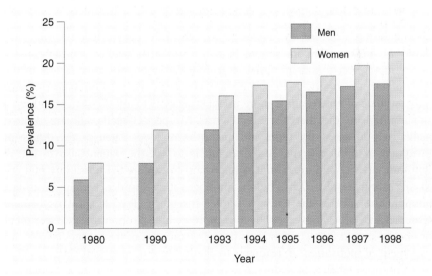

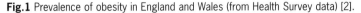

Fig.1 Prevalence of obesity in England and Wales (from Health Survey data) [2].

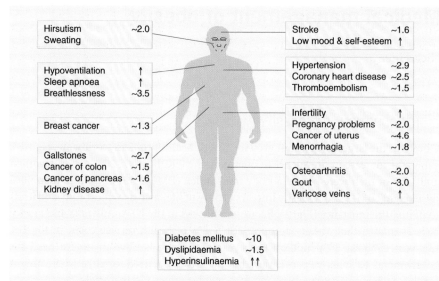

Hirsutism ~2.0	Stroke ~1.6
Sweating	Low mood & self-esteem ↑
Hypoventilation ↑	Hypertension ~2.9
Sleep apnoea ↑	Coronary heart disease ~2.5
Breathlessness ~3.5	Thromboembolism ~1.5
Breast cancer ~1.3	Infertility ↑
	Pregnancy problems ~2.0
	Cancer of uterus ~4.6
	Menorrhagia ~1.8
Gallstones ~2.7	Osteoarthritis ~2.0
Cancer of colon ~1.5	Gout ~3.0
Cancer of pancreas ~1.6	Varicose veins ↑
Kidney disease ↑	

Diabetes mellitus ~10
Dyslipidaemia   ~1.5
Hyperinsulinaemia ↑↑

Fig. 2 Schematic representation of some of the major complications of overweight and obesity and their approximate relative risks for body mass index greater than 27–30.

coined to describe our modern lifestyle. While effective prevention strategies are desperately needed, there is an equally pressing need for effective obesity treatment.

☐ HOW SHOULD WE TREAT THE OBESE PATIENT?

Since obesity is a disease, the doctor's approach to the patient who presents with obesity or its complications should be as in any other medical consultation. A history may give clues about social, psychological or physiological factors in the development of obesity. A formal dietary history is likely to be a considerable underestimate of intake, and a more useful strategy is to ask the patient to keep a contemporaneous diet diary for several weeks. No special dietetic skills are required qualitatively to assess the types and quantities of foods eaten or the degree of disruption of meal patterns. A refinement is to ask the patient also to list all significant activity and exercise. It is important to explore the possibility of a co-existing eating disorder such as bulimia or binge eating disorder (perhaps by using a questionnaire such as the Eating Disorder Inventory (Psychological Assessment Resources Inc, USA) and, especially in men, to exclude alcoholism, since treatment for obesity should follow rather than precede treatment of the eating disorder. An assessment of motivation or 'readiness to change' is also important since, whether intervention with behavioural therapies or drugs is instituted, only those patients at an appropriate stage will succeed in lifestyle modifications. While they rarely present with obesity, patients with a history suggestive of hypothyroidism and Cushing's syndrome will need further evaluation. It is important to elicit a history of the symptoms associated with obesity, since these may be the end-points of greater importance to the patient than reduction of risk factors. Sleep apnoea is common in those with a BMI above 35 [3], especially if collar size is over 43 cm in men, and has profound implications; it is important to ask patients or their partner about symptoms (snoring, apnoea, daytime somnolence) so that appropriate respiratory support can be instituted if apnoea is confirmed with a sleep study. Many drugs can cause or exacerbate obesity (including phenothiazines and other antipsychotic drugs, pizotifen for migraine, anticonvulsants, insulin and thiazolinediones for diabetes, and high doses of corticosteroids). Both weight and height have to be recorded so that BMI can be calculated. Waist circumference (a surrogate measure of visceral obesity) in patients with a BMI over 35 should also be measured since it is an important predictor of medical risk. The currently accepted guidelines for optimal BMI and waist circumference are shown in Table 1. Anthropometric standards for non-Caucasians are being established. Examination should include signs of potential primary causes of obesity (hypothyroidism, Cushing's syndrome, chromosomal abnormalities which are often associated with altered gonadal status, hypothalamic-pituitary disease) and its consequences (dyslipidaemia, hypertension assessed with an appropriate-sized cuff, cardiovascular disease, diabetes mellitus, skin changes such as acanthosis and intertrigo). Investigations should include thyroid function tests, fasting lipids and glucose, liver function tests (minor enzyme changes may indicate non-alcoholic steatohepatitis or alcohol abuse).

Table 1 Suggested categories from assessing risk from obesity and waist circumference (from clinical guidelines of US National Heart, Lung and Blood Institute [4]).

| | | Disease risk relative to normal weight and waist circumference | |
| | | Men = 102 cm | Men >102 cm |
Category	BMI	Women = 88 cm	Women >88 cm
Underweight	< 18.5	–	–
Normal*	18.5–25.0	–	–
Overweight	25.0–29.9	Increased	High
Obese	30.0–34.9	High	Very high
	35.0–39.9	Very high	
Extreme obesity	= 40.0	Extremely high	Extremely high

These data apply to Caucasians: the ranges for optimal health of both body mass index (BMI) and waist circumference are lower in Asian populations.
*Even at normal weight, disease risk increases with increasing waist circumference.

Specialist investigations are rarely needed for management. Resting metabolic rate can be measured by indirect calorimetry, or estimated from measures of lean body mass using electrical bio-impedance or dual-energy X-ray absorptiometry (DEXA). While this can reassure the clinician when faced with patients who persist in the belief that they can maintain weight on a low-energy diet, it rarely convinces such patients. Measures of lean body mass may be useful to feed back progress to patients who incorporate exercise in their regimen. While visceral fat can be measured using computed tomography or magnetic resonance imaging, it adds nothing to routine clinical management. Fasting insulin or measures of insulin sensitivity can be helpful in the failing type 2 diabetic, to predict whether weight loss might restore glycaemic control or to determine that pancreatic beta-cell 'exhaustion' has occurred and that the patient is truly insulin dependent.

In cases of an unusually early and rapid onset of obesity, especially if associated with pubertal delay, plasma leptin levels should be measured since a handful of cases of leptin deficiency have now been described and characterised [5], and can lead to successful treatment.

□ WHAT SHOULD BE THE GOALS OF OBESITY TREATMENT?

Obesity treatment aims to produce weight loss and weight loss maintenance sufficient to improve health status in its broadest sense. In those who have already developed obesity-related complications, the comorbid diseases should be reversed or ameliorated; for those still at risk, effective treatment will normalise the risk without other penalties. Although few well-designed studies have examined the long-term effects of intentional weight loss, two evidence-based reviews from the National Institutes of Health [4] and the Scottish Intercollegiate Guidelines Network [6] confirm that a 10% weight loss is a worthwhile medical goal. Pharmaceutical regulatory authorities have also adopted 10% weight loss as a satisfactory target for proof of drug efficacy, but will also accept lesser weight loss if it is associated with amelioration of obesity comorbidity such as hypertension or diabetes mellitus. Table 2 lists the size of health gain with a 10% weight loss. Despite this evidence, medical practitioners commonly set obese patients much greater targets for weight loss, and often suggest that these targets can be achieved in weeks (eg before a hip operation). At the same time, obese patients are frequently dissatisfied with whatever loss they achieve, and this seems to be an important factor in causing them to abandon further efforts at weight control. The marked disparity between realistic medical goals and patient expectations was shown in a study by Wadden and

Table 2 Health benefits from a 10 kg weight loss.

Mortality	20–25% fall in total mortality
	30–40% fall in diabetes-related death
	40–50% fall in obesity-related cancer deaths
Blood pressure	Fall of ~10 mmHg systolic and diastolic
Diabetes	Risk of developing diabetes reduced by >50%
	Fall of 30–50% in fasting blood glucose
	Fall of 15% in HbA1c
Lipids	Fall of 10% in total cholesterol
	Fall of 15% in LDL
	Fall of 30% in triglycerides
	Increase of 8% in HDL

HbAlc = glycated haemoglobin; HDL = high-density lipoprotein; LDL = low-density lipoprotein.

colleagues [7]. Patients entering a weight management programme with a mean initial weight of 99.1 kg, wanted to lose, on average, 37.7 kg. They described a 25 kg loss as 'acceptable', but the mean loss described as 'disappointing' was 17.4 kg.

Figure 3 schematically describes various weight loss curves (a–f) that might be achieved with interventions. The natural history of body weight is that it increases with increasing age (b). Ineffective programmes will not alter this course and, even if they produce initial weight loss, will be seen to fail within about six months (a and b). Few patients will normalise their weight (e) but, if judged by the criteria of a 10% loss with maintenance for at least two years (d), it is now possible to achieve success in about 50% of unselected patients. Excessive weight loss (f) to unhealthily low body weight is undesirable, and may result from the development or unmasking of an eating disorder. Similarly, patients who show frequent fluctuations of weight loss and gain are not improving their health and may have a disorder such as bulimia.

Successful treatment can result only from permanent changes in energy intake and/or energy expenditure. Such changes can be brought about by processes that are predominantly under the patient's voluntary control (lifestyle modifications) or by using drugs or surgery that 'enforce' a change in either energy intake or expenditure (Table 3). While the evidence suggests an important aetiology for low levels of energy expenditure in obesity, severely obese patients may find it difficult (or even dangerous) to engage in strenuous activity at first; reducing energy intake is a more successful initial step to produce weight loss, while increasing activity seems to have particular value in weight loss maintenance.

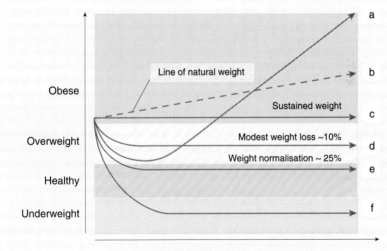

Years of weight management programme

Fig. 3 Schematic representation of the results of weight loss programmes. In most programmes, only a minority of patients achieve even modest weight loss (d), and many patients will show rebound after initial loss (a). When judging outcomes, it is important to remember that the untreated clinical course is shown in (b), and stability (c) represents an improvement. Excessive weight loss (f) is an undesirable outcome and may represent the development of an eating disorder. Few patients with current therapies achieve normalisation (e).

Table 3 Theoretical approaches to weight loss.

Energy intake	Energy expenditure
Voluntary	
Diet	Activity, sport
Energy prescribed	Decreased sedentariness
Macronutrient prescribed	
Very low calorie (liquid) diet	
Involuntary	
Pharmacological	Pharmacological
Satiety	Thermogenic
Anorexia	
Malabsorption	
Surgical	
Restrictive	
Satiety	
Malabsorption	

☐ WHAT CAN DIETARY AND LIFESTYLE TREATMENT ACHIEVE?

The mainstay of obesity treatment hitherto has been 'the diet'. This is most often undertaken as a self-directed process with instruction from a book or slimming club in the community, or often just by self-induced restraint. Since many consumer surveys have found that at any one time about 70% of the population is dieting, it seems (since obesity prevalence is increasing) to be relatively ineffective. The profusion of both medical and non-medical approaches to dieting (low fat, low carbohydrate, high protein) attests to the confusion and fashions that have dictated such advice. Modern dietary treatment should be healthy in terms of preventing cardiovascular disease and be in line with general recommendations for the population. It should provide essential nutrients to minimise loss of lean body mass in the setting of energy deficiency. The diet should be adapted to the patient's social, financial and religious requirements but, above all, be positioned as a long-term change to produce weight loss maintenance, rather than a short-term fix.

Low calorie diets are commonly constructed to restrict daily energy intake to 5.0–6.3 MJ (1,200–1,500 kcal). This can be achieved by calorie counting, scoring by 'fat units', or constructing a diet based on relatively fixed portions of fat and 'protein-foods', and adjusting the number of portions consumed each day from a list of 'carbohydrate-foods'. Such diets aim to achieve the Committee on Medical Aspects of Food Policy (COMA) guidelines [8]. Another approach has focused on tailoring the energy prescription of the diet to an individual's estimated (or measured) energy requirements based on height, weight, age and sex. A modest reduction (eg 2.1 MJ (500 kcal)/day) below energy needs, and/or those that focus on fat reduction may improve compliance and initial success.

Very low calorie or low calorie liquid (milk) diets (VLCDs) aim to maximise weight loss using diets that provide an energy intake of 1.7–3.4 MJ (400–800 kcal) daily in the form of liquid diet. COMA recommendations in 1987 were that such diets should be used only under medical supervision and for not longer than four weeks [8]. Such diets are highly successful at inducing weight loss in previously 'weight loss resistant' patients, presumably because patients tolerate and comply with them surprisingly well. VLCDs induce rapid weight loss, and rapidly improve comorbid diseases such as poorly controlled glycaemic control in diabetes and sleep apnoea, but used alone they are almost universally followed by weight gain. Hopes that combining such diets with behavioural therapy would lead to long-term weight loss maintenance have proved disappointing. An example of one such programme run from the Obesity Clinic at Luton and Dunstable Hospital is shown in Figs. 4 and 5 [9]. Initial weight loss was excellent and follow-up over 18 months suggests good weight loss maintenance. However, few patients (ca 12%) are still attending after 18 months, and the assumption is that those defaulting had regained weight. In practice, the expectations from the success in the first weeks of the VLCD seem to undermine the more complex messages concerning cognitive and behavioural change. These combined programmes are expensive to deliver, and in many countries the specialist dietary and psychology skills may be scarce. An alternative strategy is to use a drug as a second intervention to maintain weight loss after a VLCD (this is discussed later).

Advice and support for patients to increase activity and exercise may produce health benefits independent of weight loss and improve adherence to dietary restraint. Incorporating cognitive and behavioural therapy (often as a group) will

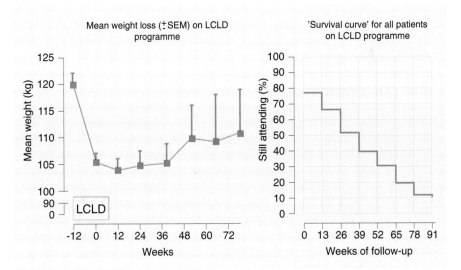

Fig. 4 Mean weight loss in 115 patients treated in a group cognitive-behavioural programme consisting of six weeks of an 800–1,000 kcal/day low calorie liquid diet (LCLD) with six weeks re-feeding, and two-weekly one-hour group meetings. Follow-up was at two weeks, and then at 12-weekly intervals. Note the attrition rate in the number of patients attending, shown as a Kaplan-Meier survival curve (data from [9]).

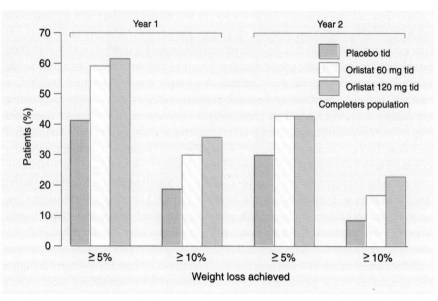

Fig.5 Number of patients achieving weight loss 'targets' after one and two years of orlistat treatment in two doses or placebo, in conjunction with a hypocaloric diet (data from [10]).

enhance weight loss and weight loss maintenance, but still only a minority of patients succeed long term.

Cognitive-behavioural treatment is still evolving, and attempts to define better strategies at weight loss maintenance are continuing. This may involve broadening programmes to include stress management, self-assertiveness, and tailoring programmes to address specific needs of individual patients. Entering patients into programmes only when they are 'ready' for change may also increase efficacy.

☐ WHAT CAN CURRENT DRUG TREATMENT OFFER?

The poor efficacy of programmes that aim to help the patient make 'voluntary' changes to their lifestyle in order to lose weight is not unique to obesity treatment. Reducing salt intake and relaxation techniques will lower blood pressure; weight loss, exercise and dietary change can improve dyslipidaemia; similar lifestyle modification can control blood glucose in non-insulin-dependent diabetes mellitus. However, few patients (or doctors) expect to have to work so hard. Furthermore, the relative efficacy of pharmacotherapy for these conditions is several-fold greater than diet and lifestyle change. Effective pharmacotherapy would be of great value in obesity treatment. Currently (and previously) available drugs act either to enhance satiety or produce anorexia (fenfluramine, dexfenfluramine, phentermine, phenylpropanolamine, sibutramine), or to decrease dietary fat digestion and absorption (orlistat). No safe thermogenic drugs have yet been developed.

A surprisingly consistent finding in well-conducted clinical trials of a number of these drugs has been a plateau in weight loss after six months, with a mean weight loss of about 10–12%. Such a plateau is an inevitable result of any intervention that has a 'fixed' effect on energy intake, expenditure or both. As body weight falls so does energy expenditure (due to a reducing lean body mass), and the re-establishment of energy balance at a lower body weight is inevitable and synonymous with weight loss maintenance. Such a plateau is often misinterpreted as tolerance, but this is incorrect. Weight loss maintenance can be achieved only with continuing efficacy (just as blood pressure, blood glucose or cholesterol are maintained at a more or less constant, but more desirable, level with antihypertensives, hypoglycaemic or lipid-lowering drugs). Proof that an anti-obesity drug is effective comes from observing weight regain when the drug is withdrawn (again analogous to withdrawing treatment for hypertension, diabetes or hypercholesterolaemia). Effective drug treatment does predicate long-term, if not indefinite, treatment. Such considerations impose on anti-obesity drugs a considerable requirement for cost-efficacy, benefit and safety. Patients (and doctors) must also understand that they are pointless if used as short-term measures to produce short-term weight loss.

Pharmacological treatment works synergistically with diet and lifestyle treatments: the better the adjunctive therapies, the better the overall results.

☐ CURRENT DRUGS FOR TREATING OBESITY

A full review of current pharmacotherapy is beyond the scope of this chapter. Two drugs with differing modes of action are now approved and marketed worldwide, although not all countries have approved both drugs.

Orlistat

Orlistat, a derivative of lipstatin, inhibits gastric and pancreatic lipases to produce fat malabsorption. At a dose of 120 mg thrice daily, inhibition is maximal at about 30% [10]. For a subject consuming 10.5 MJ (2,500 kcal) daily, of which 40% of calories come from fat, about 33 g fat daily will not be absorbed. This is equivalent to a faecal energy loss of about 1.4 MJ (350 kcal). A secondary mode of action may be to enforce a low fat diet, since higher fat intakes are commonly accompanied by gastrointestinal side effects. Virtually none of the drug is systemically absorbed, although its two inactive metabolites can be identified in plasma after oral administration of the drug. No important drug interactions have been identified, but prolonged use is associated with statistically significant falls in plasma levels of fat-soluble vitamins and α-carotene, but generally they remain within the normal reference range.

A number of trials lasting up to two years have evaluated orlistat in obesity, both 'simple' or complicated by hypertension or diabetes. The results of a large controlled trial reported by Rössner and colleagues [11] are similar to three other two-year studies [10]. In conjunction with a hypocaloric diet and regular supervision, mean weight loss at one year (intention-to-treat analysis) was 9.7 ± 6.3% in those receiving orlistat 360 mg daily compared to 6.6 ± 6.8% in those on placebo. Some weight regain occurred over the second year (7.6 ± 7.0% vs 4.5 ± 7.6%). Figure 5 shows the results expressed as percentages achieving given target weight losses. While orlistat significantly improves the chances of 'useful weight loss' compared to placebo and inhibits weight regain, only about 25% of such treated patients achieved a greater than 10% loss. Orlistat treatment was associated with greater falls than placebo in total cholesterol, low-density lipoprotein cholesterol, lipoprotein (a), fasting blood glucose and diastolic blood pressure.

Unwanted effects of the drug are mainly gastrointestinal; these are common, occurring in up to 27% of patients, but are usually well tolerated provided the patient follows a reduced fat diet.

Orlistat represents a novel, non-anorectic, peripherally acting anti-obesity drug that certainly has a place in obesity management. The drug needs to be used with careful and ongoing dietary management, and patients and doctors alike must understand that weight loss will be modest, slow but progressive over at least six months.

Sibutramine

Sibutramine is an orally administered drug whose metabolites enhance satiety, and probably thermogenesis, by inhibiting the re-uptake of released serotonin and noradrenaline from hypothalamic neurons. It reduces food intake and in some studies has been shown to increase energy expenditure acutely. It also reduces in part the decline in energy expenditure seen with weight loss and dieting.

Sibutramine is yet to be approved in the UK and is currently awaiting review by the European Regulatory Agency. It has had an extensive clinical development with two-year controlled trials in 'simple' and complicated obesity. In the Sibutramine Trial of Obesity Reduction and Maintenance (STORM) [12], after two years of treatment, sibutramine at a dose of 15–20 mg daily produced a mean weight loss of 10.2 ± 9.3 kg compared to 4.7 ± 7.2 kg on placebo, and 46% of patients receiving sibutramine maintained a 10% weight loss or greater. Another trial used sibutramine for one year in patients who had lost an average of 7.7 kg during four weeks on a VLCD. Sibutramine-treated patients lost a further 6.1 kg compared to a weight regain of 0.2 kg in those on placebo. Diabetics treated with sibutramine show significant improvement in glycated haemoglobin in conjunction with weight loss.

Sibutramine can produce unwanted cardiovascular effects in some individuals. About 3% of treated patients developed hypertension, palpitations or tachycardia. These effects are consistent with sibutramine's mode of action as a serotonin noradrenaline reuptake inhibitor, and implies that it should not be used in patients with a history of coronary artery disease, heart failure or uncontrolled hypertension. Sibutramine does not adversely affect cardiac valve function.

Leptin

Recent advances in the understanding of appetite and body weight regulation are beginning to influence management of obesity, and offer exciting prospects for the future in terms of new drug developments.

The identification of the *ob* gene and its product, the hormone leptin, has been followed by rapid advances in our understanding of its physiology and pathophysiology (Fig. 6). Unlike mutant mice, in which either the *ob* gene or its receptor is associated with obesity (and diabetes), most human obesity is associated with elevated levels of leptin in keeping with the increased fat mass. Based on the concept of overcoming the insulin resistance of type 2 diabetes by administering supra-physiological doses of insulin, clinical trials administering doses of leptin to elevate circulating levels further, and thereby increasing central nervous system concentrations, have been conducted but with disappointing results. However, the proof that leptin controls appetite and body weight has been demonstrated by O'Rahilly's group at Cambridge [13] who have successfully treated two siblings with *ob* gene mutations and leptin deficiency. Such cases are rare.

Other mutations are important in the pathogenesis of obesity. Point mutations in the melanocortin 4 receptor gene (*MC4-R*) have been detected in a number of obese families [5] suggesting that MC4-R agonists may be useful compounds to treat obesity. Neuropeptide Y is a potent stimulus for food intake, and the development of antagonists is a further target for drug development.

☐ FUTURE PROSPECTS FOR PHARMACOTHERAPY

It seems clear from the results of treatment with current drugs that new and more powerful drugs are needed [14]. It remains to be seen whether obesity treatment will develop like other therapeutic areas in which second and third generation

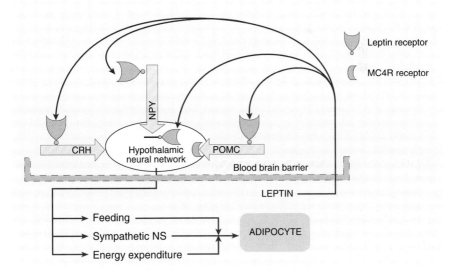

Fig. 6 A schematic design to show the interaction of leptin secreted by adipocytes and its effect on stimulating inhibitory pathways to ingestion (pro-opiomelanocortin (POMC) neurons and corticotrophin-releasing hormone (CRH)) and on inhibiting stimulation by neuropeptide Y (NPY). Mutations of the melanocortin 4 receptor gene (*MC4-R*) are associated with obesity (NS = nervous system).

compounds offer greater efficacy and safety. The redundancy and complexity of neural (and other) pathways to maintain body weight and energy balance may require multiple drugs acting on several control circuits simultaneously. New therapies involving drug combinations may be developed, but the experience with Fen-Phen (the combination of fenfluramine and phentermine that was found to cause cardiac valve lesions [15]) has made many sage physicians wary. Obesity has now reached maturity as a disease, in terms both of its clinical importance and its recognition by public health authorities, but much education is still required to get doctors and patients to treat obesity seriously.

REFERENCES

1   Hughes D, McGuire A. A review of the economic analysis of obesity. *Br Med Bull* 1997; **53**: 253–63.

2   *Health Survey for England* 2000. London: The Stationery Office, 2000.

3   Grunstein RR, Stenlof K, Hedner JA, Sjöstrom L. Sleep apnea is a risk factor for hypertension and hyperinsulinemia in obesity. *Int J Obes* 1993; **17**: 56.

4   National Institutes for Health, National Heart, Lung and Blood Institute. Clinical guidelines on the identification, evaluation, and treatment of overweight and obesity in adults: the evidence report. *Obes Res* 1998; **6** (Suppl 2): 51–290S.

5   Farooqi IS, O'Rahilly S. Recent advances in the genetics of severe childhood obesity. *Arch Dis Child* 2000; **83**: 31–4.

6   Scottish Intercollegiate Guidelines Network. *Obesity in Scotland. Integrating prevention with weight management. A national clinical guideline recommended for use in Scotland.* Edinburgh: Royal College of Physicians of Scotland, 1996.

7   Foster GD, Wadden TA, Vogt RA. Body image in obese women before, during, and after weight loss treatment. *Health Psychol* 1997; **16**: 226–9.

8   Committee on Medical Aspects of Food Policy. *The use of very low calorie diets in obesity.* Report of the working group on very low calorie diets. London: HMSO, 1987.

9   Barrett P, Finer N, Fisher C, Boyle G. Evaluation of a multimodality treatment programme for weight management at the Luton and Dunstable Hospital NHS Trust. *J Hum Nutr Dietetics* 1999; **12** (Suppl 1): S43–52.

10 Hvizdos KM, Markham A. Orlistat: a review of its use in the management of obesity. *Drugs* 1999; **58**: 743–60.

11 Rössner S, Sjöstrom L, Noack R, *et al.* Weight loss, weight maintenance, and improved cardiovascular risk factors after 2 years treatment with orlistat for obesity. European Orlistat Obesity Study Group. *Obes Res* 2000; **8**: 49–61.

12 Hansen DL, Astrup A, Toubro S, *et al.* Predictors of weight loss and maintenance during 2 years treatment by sibutramine in obesity. Results from the European multi-centre 'STORM' trial. *Lancet* (accepted for publication).

13 Farooqi IS, Jebb SA, Langmack G, *et al.* Effects of recombinant leptin therapy in a child with congenital leptin deficiency. *N Engl J Med* 1999; **341**: 879–84.

14 Finer N. Present and future pharmacological approaches. *Br Med Bull* 1997; **53**: 409–32.

15 Kolanowski J. A risk-benefit assessment of anti-obesity drugs. *Drug Saf* 1999; **20**: 119–31.

☐ SELF ASSESSMENT QUESTIONS

1   Body mass index (BMI):
   (a) Can be combined with waist circumference measures to improve risk assessment of obesity

(b) Has a different optimal range for men and women
(c) A BMI greater than 30 is present in about 20% of adults in England
(d) Will continue to fall indefinitely if a patient adheres to a reduced energy diet
(e) Has not increased in the English population over the past 5 years

2   Drug treatment of obesity:
(a) Should be given only for a maximum of 12 weeks
(b) Can be used instead of dietary advice
(c) Is successful at achieving a weight loss of >10% in less than one in two patients
(d) Has been shown to be cost-effective
(e) Has been shown to improve cardiovascular risk factors

3   Dietary advice for the obese patient:
(a) Should reduce energy intake as much as possible
(b) Should be on reducing fat rather than carbohydrate
(c) Rarely leads to weight loss
(d) Should be left to a dietitian
(e) Can be accurately prescribed only if the patient's metabolic rate is measured

4   Obesity:
(a) Is sometimes caused by inherited gene mutations
(b) Is associated with low levels of the hormone leptin
(c) Is harmless if the patient does not have diabetes or heart disease
(d) Substantially increases the risk of uterine cancer
(e) Is commonly caused by thyroid gland disorders

5   Weight loss:
(a) Must be greater than 20% to give medical benefit
(b) Continues for as long as an anti-obesity drug is given
(c) A 10% weight loss reduces systolic blood pressure by 10 mmHg on average
(d) Reduces the risk of developing diabetes by 50%
(e) Reduces all-cause mortality by 30%

ANSWERS

1a True	2a False	3a False	4a True	5a False
b False	b False	b True	b False	b False
c True	c True	c False	c False	c True
d False	d False	d False	d True	d True
e False	e True	e False	e False	e False

New developments in thyroid disease

Anthony P Weetman

Thyroid disease is common: around 2% of women and 0.2% of men will develop hypothyroidism or thyrotoxicosis, while sporadic goiter occurs in 5% of the UK population, again with a female preponderance. These high prevalences mean that even small changes in diagnosis and treatment can have a major effect. They also ensure that the main presenting features are well known, although the diagnosis of thyroid dysfunction is still often overlooked. The development in the 1980s of robust and inexpensive immunoassays for thyroid-stimulating hormone (TSH), free thyroxine (T4) and triiodothyronine (T3) has greatly simplified the determination of thyroid status. As a result, many centres have adopted a staged approach to thyroid function testing, using a normal level of TSH to rule out primary thyroid dysfunction. None the less, there are situations in which reliance on TSH alone can be misleading (Table 1). This chapter provides a brief review of recent developments in the field, especially in the areas of pathogenesis (which may shape future therapy) and treatment. The use of recombinant TSH in follow-up of thyroid cancer is also considered.

Table 1 Causes of abnormal thyroid stimulating hormone (TSH) levels.

Suppressed TSH:
- Thyrotoxicosis (overt or subclinical)
- Recent treatment for thyrotoxicosis
- Thyroid-associated ophthalmopathy
- Sick euthyroid syndrome
- First trimester of pregnancy
- Pituitary or hypothalamic disease
- Drugs (glucocorticoids, dopamine, somatostatin analogues)

Raised TSH:
- Hypothyroidism (overt or subclinical)
- Sick euthyroid syndrome
- TSH secreting pituitary tumour
- Thyroid hormone resistance syndrome
- Adrenal failure

☐ PATHOGENESIS OF THYROID DISEASE

Thyroid-associated ophthalmopathy

Although it is also called Graves' ophthalmopathy, the term thyroid-associated ophthalmopathy (TAO) is preferable because only 90% of patients with TAO have Graves' disease: 5% have autoimmune hypothyroidism and 5% are euthyroid (many develop thyroid dysfunction later). Conversely, around 50% of Graves' disease patients have clinical evidence of ophthalmopathy, while subclinical disease, detectable as enlarged extraocular muscles on imaging, is present in at least 90% of those without clinical signs. These features suggest that the pathogenesis of this enigmatic disorder which, even in mild forms, causes considerable psychological and social problems (Fig. 1) is somehow linked to the autoimmune response in Graves' disease [1]. As all patients with Graves' disease and 10–20% of patients with autoimmune hypothyroidism have autoimmune responses to the TSH-receptor (TSH-R), attention has recently focused on this receptor as a candidate for the long-sought cross-reactive autoantigen present in the thyroid and orbit, which would explain these clinical features. The pre-adipocyte subpopulation of orbital fibroblasts, which can differentiate into fat cells, expresses TSH-R and could therefore be a target for autoimmune processes in Graves' disease and in some patients with autoimmune hypothyroidism.

The extraocular muscles are infiltrated by inflammatory cells, especially activated T cells (Fig. 2). Although antibodies against orbital autoantigens have been found in variable proportions of patients, there is no specific or sensitive test for antibodies which has clinical relevance. Moreover, the absence of orbital involvement in babies with neonatal thyrotoxicosis, in whom there is transplacental transfer of TSH-R stimulating antibodies from a mother who has Graves' disease, argues strongly against a primary pathogenic role for orbital antibodies in TAO. Instead, the proximal pathogenic events in TAO are the release of cytokines, leading to activation of fibroblasts, production of excessive glycosaminoglycans and trapping of water (Fig. 3). It is possibly the site-specific response of fibroblasts in the orbit to cytokines which underlies the striking anatomical localisation of disease (in extreme cases, fibroblasts elsewhere may become involved, as in pretibial myxoedema).

Smoking is the most important risk factor for the development of TAO in patients with Graves' disease. The adverse effects of smoking may be due either to an alteration of the cytokine profile, favouring a more inflammatory response in the orbit, or to an increase in glycosaminoglycan production under conditions of mild

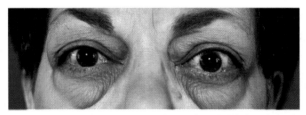

Fig. 1 Moderate thyroid-associated ophthalmopathy, with periorbital oedema, chemosis and lid retraction.

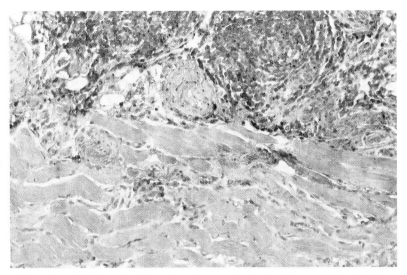

Fig. 2 Lymphocytic infiltrate in the extraocular muscle in thyroid-associated ophthalmopathy. Activated/memory T cells are stained red in this preparation. The muscle fibres are intact but separated by oedema.

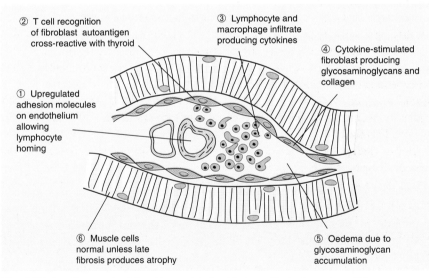

② T cell recognition of fibroblast autoantigen cross-reactive with thyroid

③ Lymphocyte and macrophage infiltrate producing cytokines

④ Cytokine-stimulated fibroblast producing glycosaminoglycans and collagen

① Upregulated adhesion molecules on endothelium allowing lymphocyte homing

⑥ Muscle cells normal unless late fibrosis produces atrophy

⑤ Oedema due to glycosaminoglycan accumulation

Fig. 3 Likely pathogenesis of thyroid-associated ophthalmopathy (redrawn from [3]).

hypoxia. Another risk factor is radioiodine treatment for hyperthyroidism, which worsens ophthalmopathy in up to 15% of patients, particularly in smokers [2]. Activation of T cells occurs 1–3 months after radioiodine; this may explain the deterioration of ophthalmopathy if thyroidal T cells, cross-reactive with an orbital antigen such as TSH-R, are being stimulated through release of thyroid antigens from the damaged gland. Worsening of TAO after radioiodine can be prevented by a short course of prednisolone, starting at the time of I^{131} treatment [2].

Glucocorticoids are also used to treat severe or congestive ophthalmopathy which occurs in 2–5% of patients. Other medical measures have been used to treat TAO (Table 2), but they are at best only partially effective and often have major side effects. Decompression and corrective surgery continue to have important roles in patient management. Our improved understanding of the pathogenesis of TAO should see the introduction early in the new millennium of better treatments, including cytokine antagonists and even antigen-specific immunomodulation.

Table 2 Medical treatment of severe thyroid-associated ophthalmopathy (worsening diplopia, corneal damage with marked soft tissue changes, optic nerve compression).

Glucocorticoids:
prednisolone 60–80 mg daily, tapered over >3 months and/or intravenous pulses of methylprednisolone, 0.5–1 g daily for 3 or more days
locally administered steroids less effective

Orbital radiotherapy:
10 x 2 Gy fractions, sometimes given with glucocorticoids

Cyclosporin A:
less effective than glucocorticoids when used alone, but effective with glucocorticoids when the latter alone have failed

Other immunosuppressive drugs:
azathioprine and cyclophosphamide, but no controlled studies to show benefit

Intravenous immunoglobulins:
similar effectiveness to radiotherapy and glucocorticoids

Somatostatin analogues:
effectiveness probably similar to glucocorticoids

Plasma exchange:
effective only when combined with other immunosuppressive agents

Genetic disorders

Molecular biology has recently unravelled the underlying defects in many genetic disorders of the thyroid (Table 3). They may be broadly classified as arising from mutations in the thyroid hormone receptors (thyroid hormone resistance syndrome), mutations in the TSH-R or its signalling pathway (causing hypothyroidism or hyperthyroidism) and mutations in the genes regulating either hormone synthesis (dyshormonogenesis) or thyroid gland development (congenital hypothyroidism) [4,5]. Autoimmune thyroid disease, non-endemic goitre and differentiated thyroid epithelial cancer also have genetic components, but these are complex, multifactorial disorders and their genetic basis will require much further work for a comprehensive picture to emerge.

Pendred's syndrome

One of the commonest genetic disorders is Pendred's syndrome, an autosomal recessive condition characterised by deafness (it accounts for around 8% of all cases

Table 3 Genetic disorders of the thyroid.

Disorder	Cause
Thyroid hormone resistance syndrome	Mutation in one allele of β thyroid hormone receptor, causing dominant negative inhibition of normal receptor
Hyperthyroidism	Activating mutations of the TSH-receptor or Gsα protein (McCune-Albright syndrome)
Hypothyroidism	Inactivating mutations of the TSH-receptor
Dyshormonogenesis:	
Iodide transport defect	Mutation in sodium/iodide symporter
Iodide organification defect	Mutation in *pendrin* (Pendred's syndrome) or thyroid peroxidase
Loss of iodide reutilisation	Mutation in dehalogenase
Defective thyroid hormone synthesis	Mutation in thyroglobulin
Congenital hypothyroidism	Mutation in *TTF1*, *TTF2*, *PAX8* or TSH-receptor genes

of congenital deafness), goitre and mild hypothyroidism. The mutations responsible occur in the recently cloned *pendrin* gene, which is a chloride and iodide transporter. As yet, it is unclear how this gene relates to thyroid function, and the role of mutations in causing the characteristic Mondini malformation of the cochlea, in which the gene is also expressed, is unknown. There is probably considerable underascertainment of Pendred's syndrome, as only half the affected siblings identified through a known proband display both goitre and deafness [6]. These data support the wider diagnostic use of the perchlorate discharge test (Table 4) in the work-up of congenitally deaf patients, particularly those with radiological abnormalities of the cochlea.

Table 4 Perchlorate discharge test.

- Administer tracer dose of radioiodine (I^{131} or I^{123})
- Measure thyroid uptake 2 hours later
- Administer 1 g potassium perchlorate (adult dose)
- Continue measurement of thyroid radioiodine content over 1 hour
- Decrease in content >10% over 1 hour = positive test

Positive test found in inherited defects of iodide organification (Pendred's syndrome, thyroid peroxidase abnormalities), some patients with Hashimoto's thyroiditis and after radioiodine treatment for hyperthyroidism.

Medullary carcinoma

Familial medullary carcinoma of the thyroid, especially in the context of multiple endocrine neoplasia type 2, is a genetically determined malignancy affecting the calcitonin-secreting C cells rather than thyroid epithelial cells. The discovery that it is usually the result of mutations in the *ret* proto-oncogene [1] has led to a revolution in screening family members once a proband has been identified. Genetic testing avoids the need for annual and unpleasant pentagastrin stimulation testing with calcitonin measurement; it also means that surgery can be planned at an early stage, even before premalignant changes, such as C cell hyperplasia, have occurred.

☐ DIAGNOSIS

Recombinant thyroid-stimulating hormone

The optimum treatment for most well differentiated malignancies of the thyroid epithelium, whether papillary or follicular carcinoma, is total thyroidectomy, radioiodine ablation of any thyroid remnant and lifelong treatment with T4 in doses sufficient to suppress TSH. Up to 30% of patients treated in this way may develop recurrent disease, sometimes many years after the original presentation, so lifelong follow-up is necessary. With optimal treatment, the cause-specific survival rate at 20 years is 95% for papillary carcinoma (which accounts for around 80–90% of thyroid epithelial malignancies) and 80% for follicular carcinoma. Early detection of recurrent or metastatic disease is associated with a better outcome; it can be dealt with by radioiodine ablation in doses which have a lower risk of complications than those given if disease is widespread.

Follow-up of these patients has increasingly relied on the measurement of serum thyroglobulin (Tg), a specific and sensitive tumour marker in patients who have undergone thyroid ablation as initial treatment. This marker is supplemented by whole body I^{131} scanning, which is particularly useful in localising recurrent disease, and also when Tg antibodies (present in up to 25% of patients) interfere with Tg estimation. Practice varies between centres, but many now rely on Tg measurement alone for long-term follow-up, provided that the whole body I^{131} scan is negative 6–12 months after the initial thyroid ablation. The sensitivity of both Tg measurement and whole body I^{131} scanning is increased by withdrawing T4 treatment, allowing TSH levels to rise – indeed, this is mandatory to obtain satisfactory scans (Fig. 4). Patients judged to be at low risk may have Tg measured while on T4, but withdrawal is required to optimise the value of Tg measurement in those at high risk.

Unfortunately, T4 withdrawal for 2–3 weeks to achieve the necessary rise in TSH may be accompanied by marked symptoms of hypothyroidism. The recent introduction of recombinant TSH, which can be given intramuscularly, allows follow-up scans or Tg levels to be obtained under optimum TSH conditions without the need to stop T4, and thus avoids any symptoms of hypothyroidism [8]. However, the preparation is expensive and its exact place in follow-up has still to be determined. Many patients clinically have a low risk of recurrence, while others, who require TSH-stimulated measurements, may tolerate T4 withdrawal. None the less, recombinant TSH will be a valuable tool in the management of thyroid cancer, not only in follow-up but also in allowing uptake of ablative doses of I^{131} in patients who cannot accept T4 withdrawal or cannot produce endogenous TSH because of hypopituitarism.

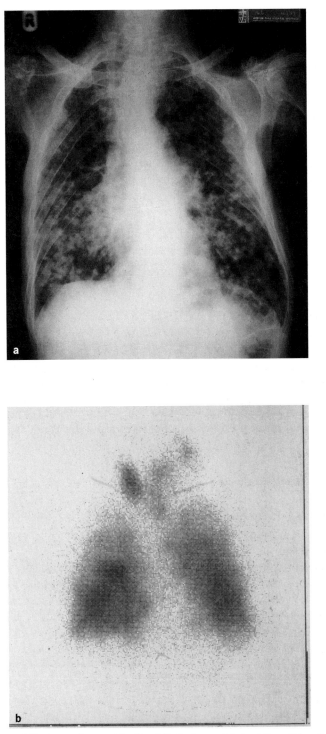

Fig. 4 Metastatic follicular carcinoma of the thyroid in the lungs: **(a)** chest X-ray, **(b)** radioiodine scan showing uptake in the lungs and the neck, including thyroid bed.

☐ TREATMENT

Goitre

The commonest cause of goitre in the absence of altered thyroid function and in iodine-sufficient countries is 'simple' (or 'colloid') goitre (Table 5). The aetiology of simple goitre is unknown and multifactorial. Goitrogens and mild defects in thyroid hormone synthesis probably underlie some cases; in others, disordered regulation of autocrine and paracrine growth factors may be responsible. Long-standing diffuse goitre progresses to multinodularity, and later still may lead to thyrotoxicosis as autonomous hyperfunctioning nodules enlarge. At such a stage, radioiodine is the treatment of choice. However, the treatment of euthyroid diffuse or multinodular goitre has been unsatisfactory – indeed, if the patient is happy to accept the appearance of the goitre and there are no pressure effects, treatment is unnecessary provided that appropriate measures have been undertaken to ensure exclusion of malignancy. Compressive symptoms, including tracheal narrowing, neck discomfort, cosmetic concerns and retrosternal extension are the most important indications for intervention.

T4 treatment has been employed for decades with variable degrees of success [9], at least in part because patients were unselected. The aim of T4 treatment is suppression of TSH, but many patients have varying degrees of thyroid autonomy and suppressed TSH levels at the time of diagnosis. When TSH is suppressed by T4, diffuse goitre may decrease in size by up to 60%, but often treatment is less effective, especially in nodular goitre. Moreover, there is concern about the long-term effects of excessive T4 on the heart (increasing the risk of atrial fibrillation) and the skeleton. Surgery has been the other mainstay of treatment, but goitre may recur in around 20% of cases over the subsequent 10 years and this is not avoidable by T4 replacement.

Table 5 Causes of goitre.

Sporadic goitre:
- •Simple, non-toxic goitre: diffuse or multinodular (colloid goitre)
- Toxic multinodular goitre
- Hashimoto's thyroiditis
- Graves' disease
- Destructive thyroiditis, postpartum thyroiditis, silent thyroiditis, subacute thyroiditis, amiodarone
- Goitrogens and drugs with antithyroid action (eg lithium, iodine)
- Genetic disorders (see Table 3)
- Infiltration (Riedel's thyroiditis, amyloidosis, sarcoidosis)
- Secondary (TSH-secreting pituitary tumour, excessive stimulation from human chorionic gonadotrophin in pregnancy or choriocarcinoma)

Endemic goitre:
- Iodine deficiency
- Goitrogens (eg cassava)

TSH = thyroid-stimulating hormone.

Recently, radioiodine has been used for non-toxic goitre, at doses of 600–3,400 MBq. Size is reduced by over 50% at two years (Fig. 5), although the price to be paid is hypothyroidism in a third of patients after five years. Longer-term data are not yet available. Even very large goitres (>8 times normal size) and those causing tracheal compression can be treated with radioiodine, despite theoretical concerns that radioiodine could cause transient thyroiditis and acute swelling of the thyroid [10].

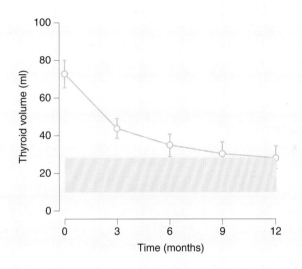

Fig. 5 Mean (±SE) thyroid volume before and after radioiodine therapy for diffuse non-toxic goitre (shaded area represents normal range) (from [7], with kind permission, from © The Lancet Ltd).

Subclinical hypothyroidism

In subclinical hypothyroidism caused by partial thyroid damage, normal levels of free T3 and T4 are maintained by levels of TSH higher than normal. The name implies that these individuals have no symptoms, but this is not always the case, particularly as the progression of even mild disturbances of thyroid function occurs over months or years. The ready availability of TSH testing has meant that many patients are recognised at the subclinical stage of hypothyroidism, and the question arises as to whether treatment is indicated. Follow-up population surveys show that subclinical hypothyroidism progresses over 20 years to overt hypothyroidism (with low free T4 levels) with an odds ratio of 8 in women [11]. However, if accompanied by thyroid antibodies, particularly thyroid peroxidase (previously known as thyroid microsomal) antibodies, the odds ratio increases markedly to 38; thyroid antibody positivity without a raised TSH has the same risk as an isolated elevated TSH level. It is important to note that transient elevation of TSH is not uncommon during recovery from an acute illness; measurements should therefore be repeated after 2–3 months to see whether the raised TSH is sustained. In men, the relative risks of progression from subclinical to overt hypothyroidism are even higher.

T4 treatment therefore seems warranted in any patient with subclinical hypothyroidism and positive thyroid antibodies; follow-up or a therapeutic trial of T4 is indicated in the remainder (Fig. 6). Most of the surprisingly few therapeutic trials of T4 in this condition have shown a benefit in a modest proportion of patients, particularly in psychometric performance and mood [12]. Moreover, subclinical hypothyroidism is 2–3 times more common than expected in

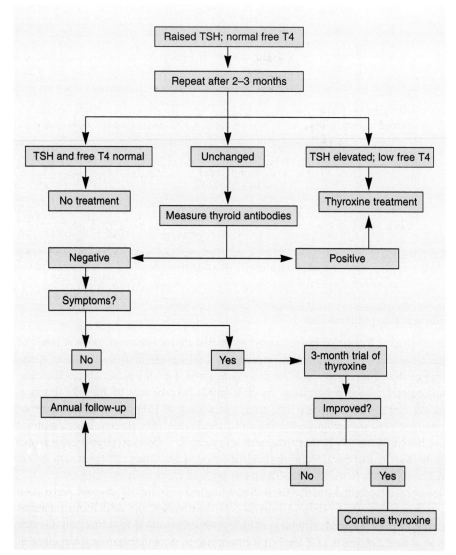

Fig. 6 Management algorithm for subclinical hypothyroidism (T4 = thyroxine; TSH = thyroid-stimulating hormone).

populations with hypercholesterolaemia, and treatment with T4 may lower cholesterol, albeit modestly (around 0.4 mmol/l). Given the large population with subclinical hypothyroidism, its recognition and treatment is probably akin to hypertension in cost-benefit analysis. In pregnant women, subclinical hypothyroidism may adversely affect the neuropsychological development of their babies, raising the question of screening for hypothyroidism antepartum or even preconception [13].

Triiodothyronine for hypothyroidism?

Conventional wisdom holds that T4 replacement is all that is necessary to restore euthyroidism in hypothyroid patients. T3 is undoubtedly the active thyroid hormone, but even physiologically is largely derived from extrathyroidal T4 de-iodination rather than thyroid secretion. However, as the rate of T4 de-iodination varies between tissues, some organs might be hypothyroid if total reliance is placed on the rate of intrapituitary conversion of T4 to T3, as reflected by normal TSH levels to assess the adequacy of T4 replacement. Some hypothyroid patients feel better with a supraoptimal dose of T4, although there are risks, particularly of atrial fibrillation, if TSH levels are suppressed. The goal of conventional treatment is to normalise TSH levels, ideally titrating T4 to achieve TSH levels below 2 mU/l but above the lower limit of the reference range.

In a five-week trial, substituting 50 μg of the usual dose of T4 with 12.5 μg T3 had a small but significant beneficial effect on mood and neuropsychological function [14]. No long-term studies have been performed to show that improvement is sustained and that there are no adverse effects, particularly on cardiac function. The results certainly challenge current dogma and may lead to the development of novel combinations of T4 and slow-release T3 substitution to mirror more closely normal thyroid hormone patterns.

Graves' disease

The main first-line treatment for Graves' disease in the UK is still antithyroid drugs, although endocrinologists are increasingly using radioiodine as primary treatment as the safety of this is now well established. On the other hand, the very small increased risk of death from thyroid cancer after radioiodine [15] suggests a continuing need for caution in children and adolescents whose growing thyroid may be particularly susceptible to this effect. The main advantages and disadvantages of each treatment are shown in Table 6.

Although there have been many attempts to increase remission rates after antithyroid drugs, long-term (>10 years) remission occurs in 40% of patients irrespective of whether the treatment used is the block-replace or titration regimen (Table 7). Administration of T4 after antithyroid drug treatment has stopped, with the aim of 'resting the thyroid', does not improve remission rates in the UK, despite previous encouraging reports from Japan [16].

Table 6 Comparison of treatments for Graves' disease.

Treatment	Advantages	Disadvantages
Antithyroid drugs	Easy to administer Rapid control of hyperthyroidism Can be given in pregnancy	Low remission rate Side effects: rash, arthralgia, gastrointestinal symptoms, agranulocytosis, hepatitis, lupus-like syndrome
Radioiodine	Can be given as outpatient Effective in 90% after one dose Can easily be repeated	Contraindicated in pregnancy and breast feeding Need for radiation protection for children of patients Theoretical concerns in children and adolescents Side effects: hypothyroidism, worsening of ophthalmopathy
Subtotal thyroidectomy	Allows confirmation of diagnosis if coincidental malignancy suspected Rapid reduction in goitre size	Hospital admission Side effects: hypothyroidism, hypoparathyroidism, recurrent laryngeal nerve damage, haemorrhage and laryngeal oedema

Table 7. Comparison of the titration and block-replace regimens for administering antithyroid drugs.

	Titration	Block-replace
Carbimazole	40 mg daily initially, reduced gradually to 5–15 mg daily	40 mg daily
Thyroxine	Not needed	100–150 µg daily when free T4 levels are normal; titrate to maintain free T4 levels in reference range
Duration	18–24 months	6 months
Use in pregnancy	Yes	No

Remission rate:
  1 year
  10 years
	
	50–60%
	40%
		
		50–60%
		40%

T4 = thyroxine.

REFERENCES

1   DeGroot LJ, Hennemann G, Larsen PR (eds). *Thyroid disease manager.*
    http://www.thyroidmanager.org.

2   Bartalena L, Marcocci C, Bogazzi F, *et al.* Relation between therapy for hyperthyroidism and
    the course of Graves' ophthalmopathy. *N Engl J Med* 1998; **338**: 73–8.

3   Weetman AP. Thyroid-associated ophthalmopathy and dermopathy. In: Volpé R (ed).
    Contemporary endocrinology: autoimmune endocrinopathies. Totowa, NJ, USA: Humana Press
    Inc, 1999.

4   Bodenner DL, Lash RW. Thyroid disease mediated by molecular defects in cell surface and
    nuclear receptors. *Am J Med* 1998; **105**: 524–38.

5   Macchia PE. Recent advances in understanding the molecular basis of primary congenital hypothyroidism. *Mol Med Today* 2000; **6**: 36–42.

6   Reardon W, Coffey R, Phelps PD, *et al.* Pendred syndrome – 100 years of underascertainment? *Q J Med* 1997; **90**: 443–7.

7   Hegedüs L, Bennedbaek FN. Radioiodine for non-toxic diffuse goitre. *Lancet* 1997; **350**: 409–10.

8   Haugen BR, Pacini F, Reiners C, *et al.* A comparison of recombinant human thyrotropin and thyroid hormone withdrawal for the detection of thyroid remnant or cancer. *J Clin Endocrinol Metab* 1999; **84**: 3877–85.

9   Hermus AR, Huysmans DA. Treatment of benign nodular thyroid disease. *N Engl J Med* 1998; **338**: 1438–47.

10   Bonnema SJ, Bertelsen H, Mortensen J, *et al.* The feasibility of high dose iodine 131 treatment as an alternative to surgery in patients with a very large goiter: effect on thyroid function and size and pulmonary function. *J Clin Endocrinol Metab* 1999; **84**: 3636–41.

11   Vanderpump MPJ, Tunbridge WM, French JM, *et al.* The incidence of thyroid disorders in the community: a twenty-year follow-up of the Whickham survey. *Clin Endocrinol (Oxford)* 1995; **43**: 55–68.

12   Weetman AP. Hypothyroidism: screening and subclinical disease. *Br Med J* 1997; **314**: 1175–8.

13   Pop VJ, van Baar AL, Volsma T. Should all pregnant women be screened for hypothyroidism? *Lancet* 1999; **354**: 1224–5.

14   Bunevicius R, Kazanavicius G, Zalinkevicius R, Prange AJ Jr. Effects of thyroxine as compared with thyroxine plus triiodothyronine in patients with hypothyroidism. *N Engl J Med* 1999; **340**: 424–9.

15   Franklyn JA, Maisonneuve P, Sheppard M, Boyle P. Cancer incidence and mortality after radioiodine treatment for hyperthyroidism: a population-based cohort study. *Lancet* 1999; **353**: 2111–5.

16   Wiersinga W. Immunosuppression of Graves' hyperthyroidism – still an elusive goal. *N Engl J Med* 1996; **334**: 265–6.

☐ SELF ASSESSMENT QUESTIONS

1   A suppressed thyroid-stimulating hormone (TSH) may be found in:
   a)   Subacute thyroiditis
   b)   A euthyroid patient who had radioiodine 4 weeks ago for thyrotoxicosis
   c)   Sick euthyroid syndrome
   d)   Thyroid hormone resistance syndrome
   e)   Isolated adrenal failure

2   Causes of goitre include:
   a)   Graves' disease
   b)   Lithium
   c)   Iodine
   d)   Amiodarone
   e)   Subacute thyroiditis

3   In the treatment of Graves' disease:
   a)   Radioiodine should be avoided in young women as it may cause infertility
   b)   Radioiodine should be used with caution in patients with severe thyroid-associated ophthalmopathy
   c)   Antithyroid drugs, in a titration regimen, should be given for six months

d) Antithyroid drugs achieve a remission rate of 60% after 10 years
e) Antithyroid drugs may rarely cause a lupus-like syndrome

4   The perchlorate discharge test is positive in:
(a) Mutations of the sodium/iodide symporter
(b) Pendred's syndrome
(c) Thyroid peroxidase mutation
(d) Some cases of Graves' disease
(e) Some cases of Hashimoto's thyroiditis

5   Measurement of serum thyroglobulin:
a) Is useful in the diagnosis of papillary carcinoma of the thyroid
b) May be interfered with by thyroglobulin antibodies
c) Is indicated in follow-up of medullary carcinoma of the thyroid
d) Is best performed after T4 withdrawal or TSH stimulation in patients at high risk of recurrence
e) Is indicated in primary hyperthyroidism

ANSWERS

1a True	2a True	3a False	4a False	5a False
b True	b True	b True	b True	b True
c True	c True	c False	c True	c False
d False	d True	d False	d False	d True
e False	e True	e True	e True	e False

Monoclonal antibodies in the treatment of cancer

Robert Marcus

☐ INTRODUCTION

It is now 100 years since Paul Ehrlich proposed the use of 'magic bullets' to treat human disease; in his case, the postulated targets were micro-organisms, specifically tuberculosis. The notion of directing therapy to the site of disease is therefore not novel. The discovery of non-toxic and effective antimicrobial chemotherapy in treating infectious disorders reduced the impetus to explore this area further.

The discovery of antibodies to bacteria and in response to vaccination led to a greater understanding of the immune response, but the implications for cancer therapy were not apparent for decades. From a historical perspective, this is understandable: in an era in which there was no effective therapy for malignant disease, the notion that a then ill-understood human defence mechanism against infection could be utilised as an approach to the treatment of malignant disease would have seemed far-fetched. None the less, the idea that the immune response might in some way be exploited in the treatment of cancer was examined, albeit unsuccessfully, in clinical trials of vaccination with autologous leukaemic blast cells in conjunction with chemotherapeutic agents. A number of early studies using polyclonal antibodies raised in horses and rabbits against injected tumour cells also had little success. Major problems included severe reactions in the host to the infusion of these crude antisera, lack of specificity and, where responses were observed, these were only short-lived.

The synthesis of monoclonal antibodies in Cambridge by Köhler and Milstein in 1975 [1] (Fig. 1) was a major advance towards effective therapy for a number of reasons.

First, advances in the technology led to the identification by these antibodies of specific antigens on the surface of haemopoietic and other cells. Within five years, multiple epitopes which defined different stages of B and T lymphocyte differentiation had been described. This, in turn, led to the precise definition initially of acute B and T cell malignancy, and subsequently of other myeloid and lymphoid leukaemias and lymphomas. These epitopes, inelegantly known by their 'clusters of differentiation' or CD numbers have now become a *sine qua non* of diagnostic haematopathology.

Secondly, the ability to synthesise large quantities of such antibodies in sterile non-mammalian systems permitted sufficient amounts to be available for therapy.

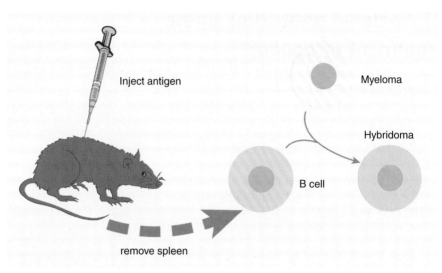

Fig. 1 Production of monoclonal antibodies.

Thirdly, the notion that such antibodies might harness natural effector mechanisms to destroy human tumour cells without the need for toxic chemotherapy was extremely attractive to clinicians used to inducing hair loss, vomiting, sterility and myelosuppression as inevitable consequences of anti-cancer treatments (Fig. 2).

☐ INITIAL CLINICAL STUDIES

Initial clinical studies with murine monoclonal antibodies had limited therapeutic success, for a number of now readily understandable reasons:

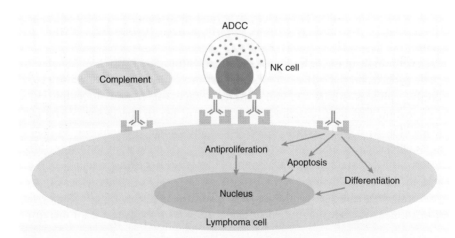

Fig. 2 Mechanisms of recruitment of natural effector mechanisms to antibody coated cells (ADCC = antibody-dependent cell-mediated cytotoxicity; NK = natural killer).

1   These murine antibodies poorly recruited human effector mechanisms.

2   They induced human anti-mouse antibodies (so called HAMA responses).

3   Antigens which act as excellent targets in a diagnostic context may not be useful epitopes.

None the less, the tantalising results of Levy's group at Stanford, who used idiotype as a therapeutic target for their clinical studies utilising murine antibodies in lymphoma [2], stimulated others to adopt this approach.

Campath antibodies

Waldmann's group in Cambridge synthesised a family of antibodies of different immunoglobulin (Ig) subclasses against an antigen present on all B and T cells and some monocyte subclasses [3]. This antibody group, known as campath antibodies, was used in a number of clinical trials in lymphoproliferative disorders. Only the IgG2b subclass seemed to have any useful therapeutic effect, and even this was short-lived and limited by HAMA responses (Fig. 3). This latter problem was solved by grafting the mouse antigen binding region to a humanised form of the antibody to create campath-1H [4]. Unfortunately, the theoretical attractions of this humanised monoclonal antibody were not translated into clinical benefit. Campath is highly immunosuppressive since it binds to and may destroy a significant percentage of all circulating lymphocytes. Although this antibody may have a role in the treatment of chronic lymphocytic leukaemia, its ability to shrink tumour masses of lymphoma cells is limited, for reasons not entirely understood.

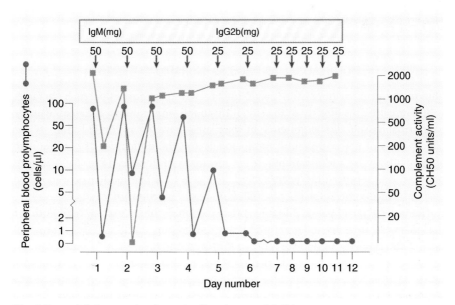

Fig. 3 Campath-1 therapy of malignancies (Ig = immunoglobulin).

The CD20 antigen

The CD20 antigen, present on mature B cells and their malignant counterparts but not on T cells or other haemopoietic cells, has proved to be a more useful target for monoclonal antibody attack. The antigen itself is large, it spans the cell membrane, is present in high antigen density and is not shed or modulated (Fig. 4). Initial clinical results with human/mouse chimeric antibody, initially known as IDEC C2B8 and now licensed as rituximab, showed impressive results in relapsed follicular lymphoma, with up to 50% response rates lasting a median of nearly one year in heavily pretreated patients [5]. Responses in high-grade lymphoma have been less impressive, but the minimal side effects and ease of administration have led to the incorporation of this agent into a number of combined modality approaches to establish its role early in the course of both low- and high-grade lymphoma.

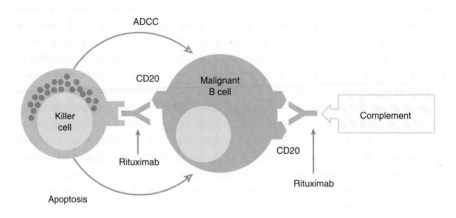

Fig. 4 Potential mechanisms of action of rituximab (ADCC = antibody-dependent cell-mediated cytotoxicity).

☐ BINDING OF MONOCLONAL ANTIBODIES TO RADIO-ISOTOPES

One of the original hopes for 'magic bullets' was the notion that such therapies would target toxins directly to the site of tumours, with minimal collateral damage to normal tissue. Developments in this area have been limited due to the effectiveness of newer unbound monoclonals and the difficulties of binding high activity toxins or radio-isotopes to monoclonal antibodies (Fig. 5). Recently, however, this approach has been revived. The anti-CD20 antibody has been linked by a number of groups to either ^{131}iodine [6–8] or ^{90}yttrium [9].

The advantage of using ^{131}iodine is that the same isotope may be used both for dosimetry and imaging and also for therapy. As a gamma-emitter, ^{131}iodine does not need to enter or be bound to every cell in the tumour mass to effect a useful cytotoxic response. The disadvantage of this approach is that of myelosuppression, with escalating dosages associated with a requirement for reinfusion of previously stored stem cells [10,11]. Other toxicities include hepatotoxicity and high levels of renal excretion. This approach is also being explored in the context of deliberate

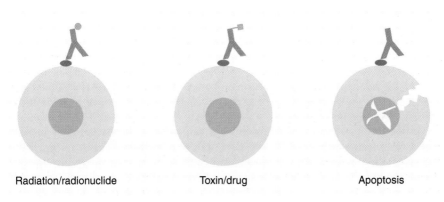

| Radiation/radionuclide | Toxin/drug | Apoptosis |

Fig. 5 Additional killing mechanisms of monoclonal antibodies.

myeloablation for stem cell transplantation in which [131]iodine or [90]yttrium is linked to anti-CD45 specifically to target marrow as a substitute for total body radiotherapy as cytoreductive therapy in acute leukaemia.

The alternative to [131]iodine is [90]yttrium linked to the same anti-CD20 antibody. The advantages of this beta-emitter are that special radiation precautions do not need to be taken, and that handling and administration are simplified.

Non-Hodgkin's lymphoma

Preliminary data suggest that both approaches are effective in relapsed low-grade non-Hodgkin's lymphoma (NHL), but that both are significantly myelosuppressive [8,9]. The role of such antibodies in the overall management of NHL will be determined by the randomised trials now in progress.

Acute myeloid leukaemia

Similar approaches are now being taken in a number of other malignancies. Recently, the CD33 antigen, almost universally present on the surface of the cells of acute myeloid leukaemia (AML), has been used as a target for two different approaches. The first has involved the binding of this antibody to a specific toxin (in this case calcheamicin). The antibody is then infused into patients suffering from AML. This agent (CMA 676 or mylotarg), given every 14 days for 3–4 doses, induces a response in almost 50% of patients with minimal toxicity, and has now been licensed in the USA for the treatment of elderly patients with AML. An unbound anti-CD33 antibody is also being tested in combination with chemotherapy in relapsed AML patients to establish whether such additional therapies may have an impact in these resistant cases.

☐ SOLID TUMOURS

The emphasis in all the earlier studies and initial clinical trials was on haematological malignancy, either leukaemia or lymphoma. This is not due to any intrinsic prejudice on the part of clinicians and scientists against the commoner solid tumours such as breast or colon cancer, but for reasons partly historical and partly scientific. The first monoclonal antibodies were raised against blood-derived cells since these are easier to isolate and disaggregate in large numbers than cells derived from solid tumours. Purified cell lines which maintain all the antigenic characteristics of the original tumour are also easier to grow and maintain when derived from haemopoietic tissue.

Antibodies have been raised not only against surface antigens normally present on the cell surface such as CD20 and CD33 but also against antigens not normally expressed. In theory, such an approach would have the advantage of further specificity, since only aberrant cells would be targeted and not their normal counterparts, but the presence of such characteristics on the cell surface is rare. Recently, however an antibody has been raised against the Her2 surface antigen present on 30% of breast cancer cells [12]. The presence of this surface marker confers a particularly adverse prognosis, with lower response rates to conventional chemotherapy, a higher incidence of metastatic disease, and shorter response times. A humanised monoclonal antibody raised against this antigen (herceptin), in combination with conventional chemotherapy, has been shown in randomised clinical trials [13,14] to prolong remissions by 4–6 months – a statistically significant and clinically meaningful result.

☐ NOVEL APPROACHES

In addition to such approaches, which either utilise natural effector mechanisms such as antibody-dependent cell-mediated cytotoxicity and complement activation or target toxins or radio-isotopes to the tumour site, other novel approaches utilising such antibodies are now entering clinical trials. These include bispecific antibodies which bind to the tumour antigen and simultaneously to a T cell antigen such as CD3 in an effort to recruit such cells to the tumour site, activate them and so enhance tumour cell kill. This is a theoretically attractive approach, but has yet to be proved beneficial [15,16].

Other approaches just beginning to enter clinical trials include:

- ☐ the use of newer technologies specifically to screen for high affinity antibodies

- ☐ utilising multiple antibodies for targeting of tumours, and

- ☐ employing antibodies in novel strategies, such as purging of contaminating tumour cells in stem cell transplantation.

☐ THE FUTURE

It is 50 years since the first cytotoxic drugs were used to treat leukaemia, and 25 years since the first description of monoclonal antibody technology (Fig. 6). In the next decade we can expect to see the further development of antibody technology to

Products/drugs

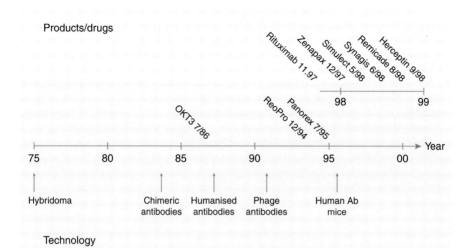

Fig. 6 Twenty-five years of antibody technology (Ab = antibody).

improve the effectiveness and specificity of anti-cancer treatments, with a reduction in the unpleasant and often dangerous toxicities which are currently an inevitable consequence of cancer therapy.

REFERENCES

1   Köhler G, Milstein C. Continuous cultures of fused cells secreting antibody of predefined specificity. *Nature* 1975; **256**: 495–7.

2   Brown SL, Miller RA, Borning SJ, *et al.* Treatment of B-cell lymphomas with anti-idiotype antibodies alone and in combination with alpha-interferon. *Blood* 1989; **73**: 651–61.

3   Riechmann L, Clark MR, Waldmann H, Winter G. Reshaping human antibodies for therapy. *Nature* 1988; **332**: 323–37.

4   Hale G, Dyer MJ, Clark MR, *et al.* Remission induction in non-Hodgkin lymphoma with reshaped monoclonal antibody CAMPATH-1H. *Lancet* 1988; **ii**: 1394–9.

5   Czuczman MS, Grillo-Lûpez AJ, White CA, *et al.* Treatment of patients with low-grade B cell lymphoma with the combination of chimeric anti-CD20 monoclonal antibody and CHOP chemotherapy. *J Clin Oncol* 1999; **17**: 268–76.

6   Vose J, Saleh M, Lister A, *et al.* Iodine-131 anti-B1 antibody for non-Hodgkin's lymphoma (NHL): overall clinical trial experience. *Proc Am Soc Clin Oncol* 1998; **17**: 10.

7   Kaminski MS, Gribbin T, Estes J, *et al.* I-131 anti-B1 antibody for previously untreated follicular lymphoma (FL): clinical and molecular remissions. *Proc Am Soc Clin Oncol* 1998; **17**: 2.

8   Kaminski MS, Zelenetz AD, Press O, *et al.* Multicenter phase III study of iodine-131 tositumomab (anti-B1 antibody) for chemotherapy-refractory low-grade or transformed low-grade non-Hodgkin's lymphoma (NHL). *Blood* 1998; **92**: 1296.

9   Knox SJ, Goris ML, Trisler K, *et al.* Yttrium-90-labeled anti-CD20 monoclonal antibody therapy of recurrent B-cell lymphoma. *Clin Cancer Res* 1996; **2**: 457–70.

10 Press OW, Eary JF, Appelbaum FR, *et al.* Radiolabeled-antibody therapy of B-cell lymphoma with autologous bone marrow support. *N Engl J Med* 1993; **329**: 1219–24.

11 Press OW, Eary JF, Appelbaum FR, *et al.* Phase II trial of 131I-B1 (anti-CD20) antibody therapy with autologous stem cell transplantation for relapsed B cell lymphomas. *Lancet* 1995; **346**: 336–40.

12　Adams GP, Schier R, McCall AM, *et al.* Prolonged *in vivo* tumour retention of a human diabody targeting the extracellular domain of human HER2/neu. *Br J Cancer* 1998; **77**: 1405–12.

13　Stebbing J, Copson E, O'Reilly S. Herceptin (trastuzamab) in advanced breast cancer. Review. *Cancer Treat Rev* 2000; **26**: 287–90.

14　Dilman RO. Perceptions of herceptin, a monoclonal antibody for the treatment of breast cancer. Review. *Cancer Biother Radiopharm* 1999; **14**: 5–10.

15　Kipriyanov SM, Moldenhauer G, Strauss G, Little M. Bispecific CD3 x CD19 diabody for T cell-mediated lysis of malignant human B cells. *Int J Cancer* 1998; **77**: 763–72.

16　Segal DM, Weiner GJ, Weiner LM. Bispecific antibodies in cancer therapy. *Curr Opin Immunol* 1999; **11**: 558–62.

Vaccine strategies for cancer

Mererid Evans, Stephen Man and Leszek K Borysiewicz

Cancer is second only to cardiovascular disease as the most common cause of death in industrialised countries and is a rising cause of mortality in developing countries. Cardiovascular mortality has reduced dramatically over the last 50 years, but cancer mortality rates are more or less stable, stressing the need for novel therapeutic approaches. Immunotherapy, utilising strategies developed for vaccination against infectious diseases, holds considerable promise while also extending the tantalising prospect of active prophylaxis.

Clinical support for the idea that the immune system may restrain the development of cancer emerged in the 1800s when William Coley, a surgeon at Memorial Hospital in New York, noticed regression of tumours in patients with bacterial infections. Since that time, T cell-mediated anti-tumour immunity has been well documented in both human and experimental animal tumour models. In the last few years, great efforts have been made to understand the molecular basis of T cell-mediated anti-tumour immunity and to elucidate the molecular nature of tumour antigens recognised by T cells. The identification of human tumour antigens has made it possible to develop specific immunotherapies based on attacking tumour cells bearing the identified antigens. Several clinical approaches to cancer immunotherapy are now possible and will be discussed in this review.

☐ THE IMMUNE RESPONSE TO TUMOURS

Current approaches to immunotherapy rely mainly on the role of CD8+ cytotoxic T lymphocytes (CTLs), because tumour-specific CD8+ CTLs can lyse tumour cells directly and eradicate tumour masses *in vivo* in animal tumour models. CD8+ cells recognise peptides presented by major histocompatibility (MHC) class I molecules (also known as HLA molecules in humans) on the cell surface. Naïve CD8+ cells are activated by recognition of antigen on the surface of professional antigen presenting cells (APCs) (dendritic cells (DCs), macrophages and B cells) which express high levels of MHC and co-stimulatory molecules (eg B7). Activated CD8+ cells proliferate and differentiate into armed cytotoxic CD8+ T cells that can kill target cells expressing the peptide:MHC complex without the need for co-stimulation. In this way, CTLs monitor the body's cells for microbial infection or malignant transformation. Peptides presented by MHC class I molecules are generated by intracellular processing of proteins by the target cell in a pathway summarised in Fig. 1.

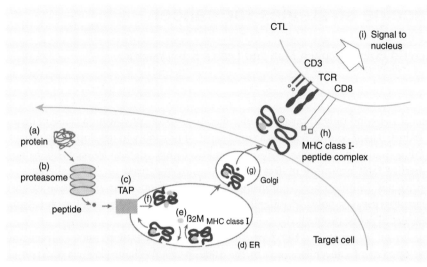

Fig. 1 Generation and presentation of antigenic peptides for cytotoxic T-lymphocytes (CTL). Intracellular proteins (a) are degraded by proteasomes (b) into short peptides which are transported via the transporter associated with antigen processing (TAP) (c) into the endoplasmic reticulum (ER) (d). In the ER, calnexin bound to major histocompatibility complex (MHC) class I heavy chain is displaced by β2-microglobulin (β2M) (e). The MHC-β2M complex associates with TAP and collects the peptide (f). Peptide binding stabilises the trimolecular MHC class I structure which is transported through the Golgi (g) to the cell surface (h). T cell receptor (TCR) recognition of peptide/MHC class I, together with CD8 acting as an adhesion and co-stimulatory molecule, results in signalling to the nucleus via CD3 and activation of the CTL (i).

☐ TUMOUR ANTIGENS

Over recent years, many MHC class I-restricted tumour antigens have been identified, mostly from melanoma. Relatively few tumour antigens have been isolated from other types of cancer because of difficulties in generating specific tumour-reactive T cells. The tumour antigens identified thus far can be classified into several categories, as shown in Fig. 2:

- ☐ *Group I* antigens are patient-specific, and arise as a result of somatic mutations in normal gene products which are incidental to the oncogenic process.

- ☐ *Group II* antigens are tumour-specific (antigens expressed in tumour cells but not in normal tissue), and include viral oncogenes.

- ☐ *Group III* antigens correspond to normal gene products which are not expressed in somatic tissues except the testis, but are reactivated in tumours of various histological types including melanoma; they can be regarded in practice as tumour-specific antigens.

- ☐ *Group IV* antigens correspond to normal tissue-specific gene products, also called 'differentiation antigens', and are more widely distributed.

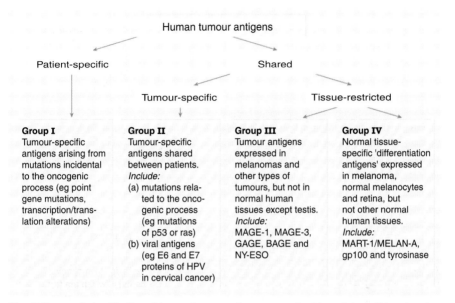

Human tumour antigens

Patient-specific

Shared

Tumour-specific

Tissue-restricted

Group I	Group II	Group III	Group IV
Tumour-specific antigens arising from mutations incidental to the oncogenic process (eg point gene mutations, transcription/translation alterations)	Tumour-specific antigens shared between patients. *Include:* (a) mutations related to the oncogenic process (eg mutations of p53 or ras) (b) viral antigens (eg E6 and E7 proteins of HPV in cervical cancer)	Tumour antigens expressed in melanomas and other types of tumours, but not in normal human tissues except testis. *Include:* MAGE-1, MAGE-3, GAGE, BAGE and NY-ESO	Normal tissue-specific 'differentiation antigens' expressed in melanoma, normal melanocytes and retina, but not other normal human tissues. *Include:* MART-1/MELAN-A, gp100 and tyrosinase

Fig. 2 Proposed classification of human tumour antigens recognised by cytotoxic T lymphocytes from cancer patients [1] (HPV = human papillomavirus).

The aim of specific immunotherapy is to generate an immune response towards a tumour antigen capable of rejecting the tumour *in vivo*. Antigens that can generate a clinically beneficial response are referred to as 'tumour rejection antigens'. The prediction is that tumour-specific antigens (groups I and II) and antigens with highly restricted tissue distribution (group III) should make potent tumour rejection antigens, whereas tissue-specific antigens (group IV) may trigger tolerance to varying degrees and be less effective tumour rejection antigens. Experimental observations to support this view are not conclusive, and group IV antigens have been successful in some clinical trials. In practical terms, patient-specific antigens (group I) are less useful for immunotherapy than shared tumour antigens (groups II-IV) that are applicable to many patients.

Although CD8+ CTL may be the predominant effector arm of the anti-tumour immune response, CD4+ T helper (Th) cells also play a crucial role, primarily in priming and maintaining CD8+ T cell responses. CD4+ Th cells recognise peptides presented by MHC class II molecules, and some MHC class II-restricted melanoma antigens recognised by CD4+ T cells have recently been isolated [2]. It will be essential to include them in effective tumour vaccination protocols.

☐ TUMOUR ESCAPE FROM IMMUNE RECOGNITION

Tumour cells have elaborated strategies to evade an apparently effective immune response, thus allowing them to establish and grow. These strategies may impact on the effectiveness of immunotherapy. Possible mechanisms of tumour escape from CTL are shown in Table 1.

Table 1 Possible mechanisms of tumour escape from immune recognition.

- Downregulation of major histocompatibility complex class I expression
- Tumour antigen or epitope loss variants
- Tumour stroma
- Tolerance to self-antigens
- Secretion of T cell immunosuppressive factors (eg transforming growth factor-β, interleukin-10)
- General immune suppression (eg tumour burden)

Abnormal MHC class I antigen expression, for example, has often been observed in many different tumour types, including melanoma, colon, cervix, breast, lung and laryngeal cancers, and is frequently associated with tumour progression. In a recent study [3], altered MHC class I expression was found in 90% of freshly isolated cervical cancers, ranging from loss of a single MHC class I allele to complete loss of MHC class I expression. The emergence of tumour antigen-loss variants is also a considerable problem: that is, variants lacking that antigen will survive and grow selectively in the face of an effective immune response directed against a specific antigen. This has been shown in a patient with recurrent metastatic melanoma.

An effective vaccination protocol will need to generate an immune response that can overcome the problem of tumour escape. The use of multivalent vaccines containing many tumour antigens will both reduce the probability of selection for antigen-loss variants and increase the likelihood that at least some of the antigens used in the vaccine will be represented in the tumour targeted for elimination. Other factors like the downregulation of the class I presentation pathway are less easily tackled. The true impact of tumour escape on immunotherapy will be revealed only by clinical trials.

□ TRIALS OF IMMUNOTHERAPY

Immunotherapy for cancer may be divided into *active immunotherapy* ('cancer vaccines') and *passive immunotherapy* ('adoptive immunotherapy') as shown in Table 2.

Active immunotherapy by vaccination induces or augments a host immune response and is the focus of this review. Adoptive immunotherapy involves the transfer to a patient of tumour-specific T cells expanded *in vitro*. It has been used successfully for the treatment of Epstein-Barr virus-associated lymphoproliferative disease following bone marrow transplantation [4], and adoptive transfer of tumour-infiltrating lymphocytes (TILs) along with interleukin (IL)-2 in melanoma patients has resulted in objective tumour regression [2].

Most early cancer vaccine trials used non-specific approaches in which patients were immunised with whole cancer cells or subcellular fractions from cancer cells. These approaches have been refined and are still valid. The identification of genes

Table 2 Approaches to cancer immunotherapy based on the identification of the genes encoding tumour rejection antigens.

Active immunotherapy ('cancer vaccines')
Immunisation with:

- immunodominant peptides (native or modified)
- antigen-presenting cells pulsed with protein or peptide
- tumour vaccines
- recombinant viruses encoding the antigen
- 'naked' DNA encoding the antigen

Passive immunotherapy ('adoptive immunotherapy'):

- transfer of cells sensitised *in vitro* to the specific antigen
- transduction of effector cells (or stem cells) with genes encoding T cell receptors that recognise specific antigens

---

encoding tumour antigens, however, has led to the development of specific immunotherapies to attack tumour cells bearing the identified antigens. Several clinical approaches utilising these genes or gene products are currently being tested. Most studies to date are in patients with metastatic melanoma, for several reasons:

☐ melanoma tumour-reactive CTLs are relatively easy to generate

☐ spontaneous remissions suggest that natural immunity occurs

☐ many melanoma tumour-specific antigens have been defined

☐ lesions are easily accessible for study, and

☐ there is no effective treatment for disseminated melanoma.

Examples of human vaccine studies in patients with metastatic melanoma are shown in Table 3.

Peptide vaccines

The identification of the immunodominant peptides in tumour antigens has made it possible to immunise with native synthetic peptides or peptides modified at MHC class I and II anchor sites to increase their immunogenicity.

Many trials of peptide vaccination have been carried out in metastatic melanoma, with varying degrees of success (see Table 3). In one trial [7], 20 melanoma patients were immunised with the MART-1 melanoma antigen in incomplete Freund's adjuvant (IFA). One patient exhibited a complete response. A second patient experienced disappearance of biopsy proven mediastinal and lung metastases and, although an axillary lymph node progressed, resection of the node left him free of disease. Both patients have remained disease-free for the past four years. In a more recent trial [8], melanoma patients were immunised with a gp100 peptide

Table 3. Examples of vaccine studies in patients with melanoma.

Study	Ref.	Vaccine	No.	Outcome
Marchand et al (1995)	5	HLA-A1-restricted MAGE 3 peptide in saline	12	2 partial responses No CTL responses
Jaeger et al (1996)	6	HLA-A2-restricted MART-1, tyrosinase and gp100 peptides	6	No clinical responses T cell responses to MART-1 and gp100 but not to tyrosinase peptides
Cormier et al (1997)	7	HLA-A2 restricted MART-1 peptide in IFA	20	1 complete + 1 partial remission ongoing at 4 years Modest immunity to peptide and tumour
Rosenberg et al (1998)	8	Modified HLA-A2 restricted gp100 peptide with IL-2	31	13 (42%) objective cancer responses
Mukherji et al (1995)	9	'DC-like' cells loaded with MAGE-3 peptide	3	MAGE-specific CTL in blood and TIL of 2 patients
Nestle et al (1998)	10	DCs loaded with melanoma peptides or tumour lysate	16	2 complete responses 3 partial responses
ECOG 1684 (1996)	11	IFN-α2b adjuvant		Increased disease-free survival

CTL = cytotoxic T lymphocyte; DC = dendritic cell; ECOG = Eastern Cooperative Oncology Group; HLA = histocompatibility locus antigen; IFA = incomplete Freund's adjuvant; IFN = interferon; IL = interleukin; MAGE = melanoma antigen gene 1; MART = melanoma antigen recognised by TIL cells; TIL = tumour-infiltrating lymphocyte.

(gp100:209–217) modified at the 210 position to increase MHC binding. The administration of this peptide in IFA in combination with IL-2 to 31 patients with metastatic melanoma resulted in an objective response in 13 patients (42%). There were no clinical responses in 11 patients who received the peptide without IL-2. Interestingly, peripheral blood CTL responses were less frequent when IL-2 was administered with peptide, which may be due to activation of CTL and trafficking to the tumour site. Currently, phase III studies are being planned to treat patients with metastatic melanoma with either IL-2 alone or IL-2 in conjunction with the modified gp100 peptide.

In a phase I–II clinical trial [12], 19 patients with advanced cervical cancer were immunised with a vaccine consisting of two human papillomavirus (HPV) type 16 E7 peptides and one helper peptide. These patients had HPV16-positive cervical carcinomas refractory to conventional treatment. No adverse side effects were observed. In two patients, disease remained stable for one year after vaccination, but the rest developed progressive disease. Following this trial, future studies are planned in patients with less advanced disease.

These trials show that peptide vaccines are safe and warrant further investigation. Some of the problems of peptide vaccination include the emergence of tumour antigen-loss variants and MHC polymorphism. Multivalent vaccines should reduce the outgrowth of antigen-loss variants, and 'generic' vaccines containing multiple epitopes restricted by different MHC molecules could be used in a wider patient population. Vaccines that also include Th epitopes may produce stronger CTL responses by recruiting CD4+ T cells. Another potentially more serious problem is the possibility of inducing tolerance to tumour antigens; this has been seen in animal models. The critical balance between peptides which stimulate or switch off the immune system stresses the need to proceed with caution.

Dendritic cell vaccines

Proteins or peptides can be pulsed on to APCs (primarily DCs) for immunisation. DCs express high levels of MHC and co-stimulatory molecules, and are therefore well equipped to induce antigen-specific CD8+ and CD4+ T cell responses. Techniques to generate large numbers of functionally active DCs by culturing bone marrow or peripheral blood cells in the presence of granulocyte-macrophage colony stimulating factor (GM-CSF) and other cytokines such as IL-4 have been developed over recent years.

In an important trial [10], DCs loaded with a cocktail of melanoma peptides or tumour lysate were used to vaccinate patients with advanced melanoma. Keyhole limpet haemocyanin was added as a CD4 helper antigen. DCs were injected directly into uninvolved inguinal lymph nodes (under ultrasound control) at weekly intervals. Vaccination resulted in objective cancer regression in five of 16 evaluated patients (complete responses 2; partial responses 3). There was dramatic regression of metastases in skin, lung, soft tissue and pancreas in these patients, and both patients exhibiting a complete response remained disease-free 15 months following vaccination. Evidence of antigen-specific immunity induced by DC vaccination was found in 11 patients. Administration of APCs pulsed with idiotypic protein from B cell lymphomas has also resulted in tumour regression of selected patients [13].

These studies show that vaccination with autologous DCs is safe, and promising in terms of clinical effect. Further studies involving more patients are necessary to prove clinical effectiveness.

Tumour vaccines

The use of whole tumour cells or tumour cell extracts is a 'non-specific' immunisation approach that can be applied to cancers where tumour-specific antigens have not yet been identified. The presence of multiple tumour antigens allows the immune system to 'select' the most effective tumour antigens from a mix of antigens presented to it and limits the generation of tumour antigen-loss variants. Induction of autoimmune responses directed against non-tumour-specific self-antigens is a potential problem.

Tumour cells are poor APCs, and attempts have been made to enhance their immunogenicity and generate better anti-tumour responses after vaccination. Genetically modified tumour vaccines (GMTV) have been created by insertion of genes encoding cytokines and growth factors (including IL-2, IL-4, IL-6, IL-12, interferon-γ and GM-CSF). Traditionally, tumour cells have been modified *ex vivo*, but a newer strategy is to modify tumour cells *in situ* by direct intratumoral delivery of genes. Promising results from animal models have been reported, but there have been few clinical studies of GMTV.

Another strategy to increase the immunogenicity of tumour cells is the development of tumour cell-DC hybrids [14]. The hybrids, generated by electrofusion techniques, present antigens expressed by the tumour cell in concert with the co-stimulating capabilities of DCs. Seven of 17 patients (41%) with metastatic renal cell carcinoma immunised by hybrid cell vaccination responded, with a mean follow-up time of 13 months. Four patients completely rejected all metastatic tumour lesions, one presented a 'mixed response', and two had a tumour mass reduction greater than 50%. Induction of specific CTL responses to Muc1 tumour-associated antigen were demonstrated as well as recruitment of CD8+ lymphocytes into tumour challenge sites. The European Group for Hybrid Cell Vaccination is now testing this strategy with different antigenic tumours in a number of European centres.

Fractionation of proteins from tumour cells led to the isolation of heat-shock proteins (HSPs) (or stress-induced proteins) [15]. When injected into animals, HSPs generate a CTL response and cause rejection of the cancers from which they were purified. HSPs are expressed in all living cells in response to heat shock, glucose deprivation, ischaemia and other causes. They are not antigenic *per se* but act as carriers of antigenic tumour proteins. A pilot study of HSPs was conducted in 16 patients to test the logistics of the HSP vaccination approach in humans. No unacceptable vaccine-related toxicities occurred, and six of 12 patients immunised showed a significant increase in the number of MHC class I-restricted tumour-specific CD8+ T cells. As a result of this trial, larger clinical trials are now in progress.

Recombinant viral vaccines

For over a decade, recombinant virus vectors have been used and developed extensively to deliver genes encoding target antigens to host cells. The target antigens are processed and presented via MHC class I to induce antigen-specific CTL responses.

A recombinant vaccinia virus encoding modified forms of HPV16 and 18 E6 and E7 (TA-HPV) was used safely to vaccinate eight patients with recurrent cervical cancer in a phase I–II clinical trial [16]. The use of vaccinia virus, a lytic virus, as well as deletion in the RB-binding site within the E7 gene, reduces the oncogenic potential of TA-HPV. All patients generated anti-vaccinia antibodies, while three of the eight had an anti-HPV antibody response following vaccination. One of the three patients was also shown to have CTL specific for HPV18 post-vaccination and remains disease-free three years later, although the contribution of the vaccine cannot be judged. As a result of this study, a large EORTC trial evaluating the effect of TA-HPV in patients with cervical cancer is currently in progress.

Virus-like particles (VLPs) are non-infectious, DNA-free particles made up of HPV viral capsid proteins (eg HPV L1 or L1/2 proteins) which spontaneously assemble when expressed in yeast or higher eukaryotic cells infected with baculovirus or vaccinia virus vectors. VLPs generate a systemic humoral response sufficient for protection against tumour challenge in animal models and are promising agents for prophylactic vaccination in man. An effective prophylactic vaccine would have major implications in regions such as South America and Africa where mass screening is inadequate, although the most appropriate target population has still not been established. 'Empty' HVP/VLPs may serve as vehicles for the delivery of immunogenic DNA or proteins. A combined prophylactic and therapeutic vaccine for HPV can be envisaged that features tumour-associated viral proteins (eg HPV16 E7) inserted into 'empty' VLPs.

DNA vaccines

Intramuscular or gene gun administration of 'naked' DNA constructs encoding target antigens can generate potent immune responses in experimental animals. Various strategies to improve the immunogenicity of DNA vaccines, for example by co-administration of cytokine encoding DNA, have also been reported in animal models. DNA vaccines, like peptide vaccines, consist of pure antigenic material but, in contrast to peptide vaccination, DNA vaccination results in intracellular processing and endogenous presentation of target antigens, which may be advantageous.

Clinical trials of DNA vaccination in humans have not yet been reported. Potential targets for DNA vaccination are virally-induced cancers; however, DNA vaccination of viral oncogenes such as E6 and E7 of HPV may not be safe, and RNA vaccination may be an alternative useful approach.

☐ FUTURE POTENTIALS

The discovery of new tumour antigens, the increasing number of potential adjuvants, the advances in antigen delivery systems and the development of new vaccination strategies represent a substantial opportunity, as well as a considerable challenge, in selecting and optimising the best approaches for the development of prophylactic and therapeutic cancer vaccines. A combination of vaccination strategies may be the most effective: for example, strong CD8+ T cell responses against malaria have been induced [17] by heterologous prime-boost immunisation, in which the immune response was primed with DNA and boosted with a recombinant vaccinia virus. Alternatively, vaccination combined with antibody-based therapies or adoptive transfer may be most effective. Results from ongoing clinical trials are eagerly awaited and will clarify future directions for cancer immunotherapy.

REFERENCES

1   Gilboa E. The makings of a tumour rejection antigen. *Immunity* 1999; **11**: 263–70.

2   Wang RF, Rosenberg SA. Human tumour antigens for cancer vaccine development. *Immunological Rev* 1999; **170**: 85–100.

3   Koopman LA, Corver WE, Van der Slik AR, *et al.* Multiple genetic alterations cause frequent and heterogeneous human histocompatibility leukocyte antigen class I loss in cervical cancer. *J Exp Med* 2000; **6**: 961–75.

4   Heslop HE, Ng CY, Li C, *et al.* Long-term restoration of immunity against Epstein-Barr virus infection by adoptive transfer of gene-modified virus-specific T lymphocytes. *Nat Med* 1996; **2**: 551–5.

5   Marchand M, Weynants P, Rankin E, *et al.* Tumour regression responses in melanoma patients treated with a peptide encoded by gene MAGE-3. *Int J Cancer* 1995; **63**: 883–5.

6   Jaeger E, Bernhard H, Romero P, *et al.* Generation of cytotoxic T-cell responses with synthetic melanoma-associated peptides in vivo: implications for vaccines with melanoma-associated antigens. *Int J Cancer* 1996; **66**: 162–9.

7   Cormier JN, Salgaller ML, Prevette T, *et al.* Enhancement of cellular immunity in melanoma patients immunized with a peptide from MART-1/MELAN-A. *Cancer J Sci Am* 1997; **3**: 37–44.

8   Rosenberg SA, Yang JC, Schwartzentruber DJ, *et al.* Immunologic and therapeutic evaluation of a synthetic tumour-associated peptide vaccine for the treatment of patients with metastatic melanoma. *Nat Med* 1998; **4**: 321–7.

9   Mukherji B, Chakraborty NG, Yamasaki S, *et al.* Induction of antigen-specific cytolytic T cells in situ in human melanoma by immunization with synthetic peptide-pulsed autologous antigen presenting cells. *Proc Natl Acad Sci USA* 1995; **92**: 8078–82.

10 Nestle FO, Alijagic S, Gilliet M, *et al.* Vaccination of melanoma patients with peptide- or tumour lysate-pulsed dendritic cells. *Nat Med* 1998; **4**: 328–32.

11 Kirkwood JM, Strawderman MH, Ernstoff MS, *et al.* Interferon alfa-2b adjuvant therapy of high-risk resected cutaneous melanoma: the Eastern Cooperative Oncology Group trial EST 1684. *J Clin Oncol* 1996; **14**: 7–17.

12 Van Driel WJ, Ressing ME, Kenter GG, *et al.* Vaccination with HPV 16 peptides of patients with advanced cervical carcinoma: clinical evaluation of a Phase I-II trial. *Eur J Cancer* 1999; **35**: 946–52.

13 Hsu FJ, Caspar CB, Czerwinski D, *et al.* Tumour-specific idiotype vaccines in the treatment of patients with B-cell lymphoma: long-term results of a clinical trial. *Blood* 1997; **89**: 3129–35.

14 Kugler A, Stuhler G, Walden P, *et al.* Regression of human metastatic renal cell carcinoma after vaccination with tumour cell-dendritic cell hybrids. *Nat Med* 2000; **6**: 332–6.

15 Prezepiorka D, Srivastava PK. Heat shock protein-peptide complexes as immunotherapy for human cancer. *Mol Med Today* 1998; **4**: 478–84.

16 Borysiewicz LK, Fiander A, Nimako M, *et al.* A recombinant vaccinia virus encoding human papillomavirus types 16 and 18, E6 and E7 proteins as immunotherapy for cervical cancer. *Lancet* 1996; **347**: 1523–7.

17   Schneider J, Gilbert SC, Hannan CM, *et al.* Induction of CD8+ T cells using heterologous prime-boost immunization strategies. *Immunol Rev* 1999; **170**: 29–38.

☐ SELF ASSESSMENT QUESTIONS

1   Major histocompatibility class I molecules:
   (a) Are present only on antigen presenting cells (APCs) such as dendritic cells
   (b) Present peptides for recognition by CD4+ T helper cells
   (c) May be downregulated on cancer cells

2   Human tumour antigens that represent normal 'differentiation' antigens:
   (a) Are predicted to be the most effective tumour rejection antigens
   (b) Include MART-1/MELAN-A and gp100 melanoma proteins
   (c) Are highly tissue-restricted

3   A problem *not* generally associated with peptide vaccination is:
   (a) Growth of antigen-loss tumour variants
   (b) Induction of tolerance
   (c) Autoimmunity to tumour-associated self-antigens

4   Tumour vaccines may be effective because:
   (a) They may be manipulated *in vitro* to enhance immunogenicity
   (b) Tumour cells are good APCs
   (c) They contain a highly purified mix of tumour rejection antigens

5   The following vaccination strategies do not depend on the identification of tumour-specific antigens:
   (a) Peptide vaccination
   (b) DNA vaccination
   (c) Heat-shock protein vaccination

ANSWERS

1a False	2a False	3a False	4a True	5a False
b False	b True	b False	b False	b False
c True	c False	c True	c False	c True

Diabetic nephropathy: significance, treatment options and future prospects

Aled O Phillips

☐ INTRODUCTION

Diabetic nephropathy (DN) is a common complication of diabetes mellitus which has a major impact on patient morbidity and mortality and therefore a profound impact on the delivery of health care in this country. It affects more than one-third of patients with insulin-dependent diabetes mellitus (type 1 diabetes) and an increasing proportion of patients with non-insulin dependent diabetes mellitus (type 2 diabetes), making it the single most common cause of end-stage renal failure (ESRF) in Western countries. There is a consensus that survival and rehabilitation of diabetic patients on renal replacement programmes continue to be inferior to that of non-diabetic patients. However, survival has greatly improved since the famous report of Ghavamian, *et al*, which concluded:

> there is little prospect of improving the quality of life for patients with diabetic nephropathy and renal failure, and that survival is likely to be short. For some, we only prolong the misery. Dialysis for such patients may be considered as a palliative measure with little likelihood of long term survival [1].

Research in this area over the past 25 years has greatly increased our understanding of the pathophysiology of DN, and there is now clear evidence that numerous therapeutic interventions may delay the progression of renal disease.

☐ DIABETIC NEPHROPATHY: THE CLINICAL PICTURE

One of the earliest renal functional abnormalities in diabetes mellitus is a rise in glomerular filtration rate (GFR), so-called hyperfiltration. Although this is a characteristic finding, there is no evidence that hyperfiltration is in itself detrimental to long-term renal function, and furthermore hyperfiltration does not identify those patients who go on to develop overt renal disease. The first feature of incipient DN is the appearance of microalbuminuria (30–300 mg/24 h); subsequently, persistent albuminuria (>300 mg/24 h) develops. The clinical syndrome of overt DN is therefore characterised by persistent albuminuria, early arterial blood pressure elevation, and a relentless decline in GFR. Although microscopic haematuria may be found in 50% of patients with DN, its presence, particularly in the absence of diabetic retinopathy and non-nephrotic range proteinuria, should alert the clinician to the presence of non-diabetic renal disease.

What accounts for the increasing incidence of DN, referred to as 'a silent epidemic which has been missed by the non-nephrological community'? The increase in the incidence of DN relates to an increase in the rate of ESRF in patients with type 2 diabetes, which has been markedly greater than that for ESRF from other causes. This is all the more poignant considering that until recently type 2 diabetes was considered to have a benign renal prognosis. This concept of a benign renal prognosis in type 2 diabetes is a paradox, given the fact that reports dating back to Cotugno in 1764 [2] and Rayer in 1839 [3] suggested the presence of proteinuria in such patients. Furthermore, the seminal report of Kimmelstiel and Wilson in 1936 [4] concerned seven cases with an average age of 58.6 years and an average duration of diabetes of 3.9 years, almost certainly all with type 2 diabetes. The increased incidence in ESRF from type 2 diabetes is partly explained by an increase in the prevalence of diabetes in the general population, and also by the longer survival of this group of patients.

In addition to being a strain on health care resources (in the USA it is estimated that each patient with diabetes mellitus and ESRF incurs direct medical costs of $53,000 annually), it is clear that the mortality of diabetic patients with ESRF is higher than for any other group of ESRF patients for all treatment modalities [5] (Fig. 1). Although this is also true for renal transplantation, it is worth noting that the gain in survival after transplantation relative to survival for dialysed patients on the waiting list is greater in patients with, than without, diabetes (Table 1) [6]. It is therefore clear that DN will continue to be a major problem in terms of patient morbidity and mortality and also for the provision of health care resources for the medical community for the foreseeable future.

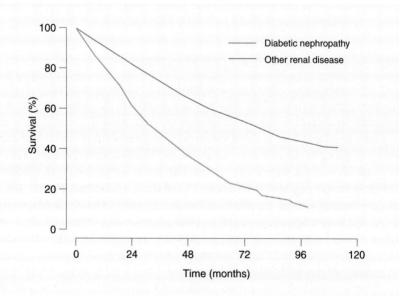

Fig. 1 Survival of dialysed patients with diabetic nephropathy compared to patients with other forms of renal disease (adapted from [5], with permission).

Table 1 Survival of patients with end-stage renal failure according to treatment modality (adapted from [6], with permission).

Treatment modality	Survival (%) 1st year	3rd year	5th year
Patient survival on renal replacement therapy			
non-DM	91	77	65
DM	79	50	30
Patient survival (DM) on dialysis			
haemodialysis	79	52	30
peritoneal dialysis	75	42	25
Patient survival with transplant			
non-DM	96	94	91
DM	87	81	74

DM = patients with diabetes mellitus; non-DM = non-diabetes mellitus patients.

☐ CURRENT TREATMENT OPTIONS

There is a consensus that patients with DN who have developed persistent proteinuria will nearly always progress to ESRF [7,8]. Numerous studies have however demonstrated that it is possible to alter the rate of progression. Studies performed to date have identified three key therapeutic goals which, if implemented rigidly, are known to influence favourably the rate of progression of DN.

Glycaemic control

There is clear epidemiological evidence that the development of nephropathy in both type 1 and type 2 diabetes is related to poor glycaemic control [7,8]. Furthermore, the microvascular complications of diabetes including DN may be influenced by strict glycaemic control. The recently completed Diabetes Control and Complications Trial (DCCT) of 14,000 type 1 patients demonstrates that strict glycaemic control is effective in primary prevention (the development of microalbuminuria), and also secondary prevention (delaying the development of overt nephropathy) (Fig. 2). It is of note that the effect of intensified treatment on the appearance of albuminuria becomes apparent only after a three-year observation period [9]. However, following development of overt nephropathy, strict glycaemic control does not retard progression of renal disease. Recent studies suggest that these findings may also be applied to type 2 diabetes [10,11].

Two years after the end of the DCCT trial, despite the strong evidence supporting the role of strict metabolic control, the difference in diabetic control has not been maintained between the intensive and conventional treatment groups, emphasising the difficulty in implementing evidence-based treatment strategies [12].

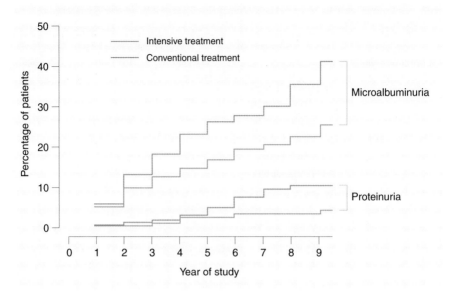

Fig. 2 Cumulative incidence of development of microalbuminuria or overt proteinuria in the intensive or conventional treatment groups (adapted from [9], with permission).

Treatment of hypertension

There is a strong correlation between the degree of hypertension and the rate of progression of overt DN in both type 1 and type 2 diabetes. More direct evidence implicating hypertension in progression of DN comes from the early work of Mogensen *et al* [13] demonstrating a slower rate of progression of nephropathy following aggressive treatment of hypertension. Lowering blood pressure reduces albuminuria and attenuates the rate of loss of GFR in type 1 diabetes (Fig. 3) [7]. The recently published UK Prospective Diabetes Study (UKPDS) also demonstrates that tight blood pressure control reduces the risk of macrovascular and microvascular complications (including nephropathy) in type 2 diabetes [14]. It is now widely accepted that early and aggressive treatment of arterial hypertension is an important goal in the management of DN in both patient groups, with a blood pressure of less than 140/85 mmHg set as an acceptable goal.

Use of angiotensin converting-enzyme inhibitors

The beneficial effects of angiotensin converting-enzyme (ACE) inhibitors in normotensive microalbuminuric type 1 and type 2 patients are now well established, confirming that ACE inhibitors have effects which are divorced from their anti-hypertensive action [15]. They may alter renal haemodynamics and reduce the intra-glomerular hypertension characteristic of diabetes. In addition, recent studies have demonstrated that ACE inhibitors may also affect mesangial cell function as well as intrarenal cytokine generation.

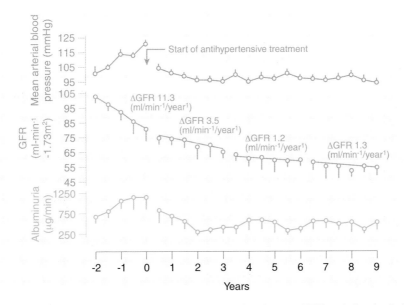

Fig. 3 Relationship between hypertension, glomerular filtration rate (GFR) and albuminuria before and after institution of long-term effective antihypertensive treatment in patients with diabetic nephropathy (adapted from [7], with permission).

These studies suggest that introduction of ACE inhibitors is effective in secondary prevention (ie delaying progression from microalbuminuria to proteinuria). ACE inhibitors also delay the progression of overt nephropathy in type 1 diabetics (Fig. 4), and this effect is above and beyond that conferred by their antihypertensive effects [16]. ACE inhibitors should therefore be considered as the first choice for the treatment of hypertension in patients with incipient and overt DN.

Two recently published studies in both type 1 and type 2 diabetes suggest that ACE inhibitors may also be useful in normotensive normoalbuminuric patients (Fig. 5) [17,18]. These studies raise the question of the use of ACE inhibitors in all diabetic patients, which has major financial implications. Golan *et al* [19] suggested that treating all middle-aged normotensive normoalbuminuric diabetic patients with ACE inhibitors provides additional renal benefit at a modest additional cost (Fig. 6). However, because of the higher incidence of ischaemic nephropathy in type 2 diabetic patients, the use of ACE inhibitors must be carefully monitored. This point is also illustrated by analysis of the recently published and widely cited UKPDS data [20]. This study convincingly demonstrated the beneficial effect of aggressive anti-hypertensive treatment on patient outcome in a population of type 2 diabetic patients. However, it did not differentiate between DN and renal impairment from non-diabetic diseases, such as ischaemic nephropathy, in this population. This probably explains the lack of benefit of ACE inhibition as compared to beta-blockade on renal outcome seen in this study.

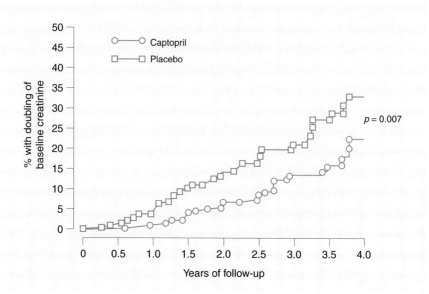

Fig. 4 Progression of nephropathy in insulin-dependent diabetes mellitus treated with captopril or placebo expressed as the cumulative percentage of patients with doubling of the baseline creatinine following treatment (adapted from [16], with permission).

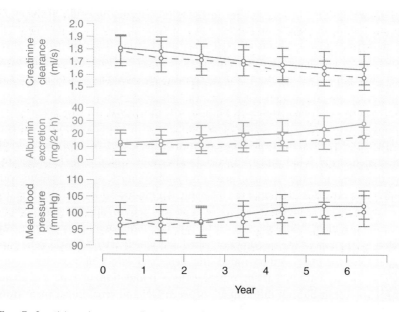

Fig. 5 Creatinine clearance, albumin excretion and mean blood pressure in normotensive, normoalbuminuric patients with type 2 diabetes who received enalapril or placebo (adapted from [18], with permission).

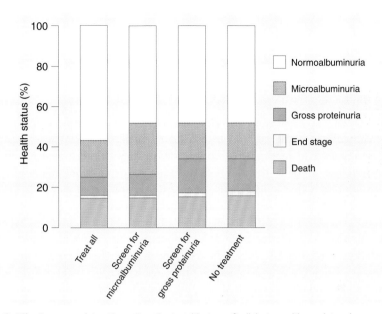

Fig. 6 Effectiveness of treating all patients with type 2 diabetes with angiotensin converting-inhibitors. Distribution of health status after 10 years of each clinical strategy (adapted from [19], with permission).

Other therapeutic options

Dietary protein restriction retards the progression of renal disease in virtually all experimental animal models. Studies in humans, however, are less convincing. All major observational studies of type 1 and type 2 diabetes have failed to show an impact of modification of dietary protein intake on progression of DN. Furthermore, the recommendation of low protein diets in diabetic patients with renal impairment must be tempered by their predisposition to catabolism and malnutrition.

It has also been suggested that hyperlipidaemia accelerates progression of renal disease. Large trials examining the effect of lipid lowering on the progression of DN have not been carried out, and therefore treatment of an abnormal lipid profile in diabetic patients should be considered in the context of other cardiovascular risk factors.

Smoking has also been suggested as a possible risk factor for the development of DN. The prevalence of albuminuria and the rate of progression of renal failure are significantly higher in smoking than non-smoking diabetic patients. This, in addition to 'cardiovascular' considerations, provides a compelling argument to stop smoking.

☐ FUTURE PROSPECTS: LESSONS FROM CELL BIOLOGY

All the treatment options above relate to a decline in the rate of progression of DN, but do not halt its progression or reverse the disease process. The goal of *in vitro* based research is to increase our understanding of the mechanisms involved in the pathogenesis of DN which may lead to the development of targeted therapeutic interventions.

In vitro studies into the mechanisms of diabetic glomerulosclerosis

Diabetic mesangial expansion includes increased cellularity, thickening of the basement membranes and copious extracellular matrix (ECM). When mesangial cells were cultured in high glucose concentration they demonstrated a biphasic growth response; initially there was stimulation of replication, followed by a sustained inhibition after longer incubation periods. Exposure of mesangial cells to high glucose levels also promotes transcriptional activation of type IV collagen and fibronectin genes, and increases the synthesis of their respective proteins. Glucose may also decrease degradation of ECM components which may contribute to this accumulation in the diabetic state. The mechanisms whereby glucose causes these responses are still not fully understood, but they involve specific pathways of glucose transport and metabolism (reviewed in [21]). The effects of glucose on mesangial cell collagen synthesis may be mimicked by the overexpression of the facultative glucose transport protein GLUT 1 [22]. This therefore suggests that it is the increased uptake of glucose into the cell, rather than ambient glucose concentration *per se*, which is the major determinant of exaggerated ECM formation.

Two metabolic consequences of elevated intracellular glucose which are suggested as potential mediators of the effect of high glucose concentrations on cell function are activation of protein kinase C (PKC) and increased polyol pathway activation. Studies in isolated glomeruli and in cultured mesangial cells have demonstrated that high ambient concentrations of glucose activate PKC which has been implicated in increased fibronectin and collagen gene expression in mesangial cells. Polyol pathway activation may also be linked to PKC activation as this may lead to an alteration in the redox state of the cell. Therefore, these postulated mechanisms are not mutually exclusive, which may explain the overlapping effects observed in studies of inhibitors of individual pathways (Fig. 7).

Generation of the ECM is complex and may be modulated by pro-fibrotic cytokines. Of all cytokines studied to date, transforming growth factor (TGF)-β has now emerged as a key mediator of matrix remodelling in health and disease including diabetic nephropathy [23]. Stimulation of collagen gene expression and protein synthesis in mesangial cells by glucose *in vitro* are mediated, at least in part, by autocrine activation of TGF-β. More recent studies by Kolm-Litty *et al* [24] have demonstrated that induction of TGF-β in mesangial cells is mediated by increased glucose metabolism by the hexosamine pathway. In addition to TGF-β, another growth factor implicated in progressive renal injury is platelet-derived growth factor (PDGF). Although the effects of glucose on matrix production by mesangial cells may be mediated by TGF-β, increased TGF-β production following incubation in a high glucose medium is an indirect effect of glucose which occurs via increased production of PDGF. These studies suggest that glucose may influence glomerular ECM turnover by modulating a complex cytokine network.

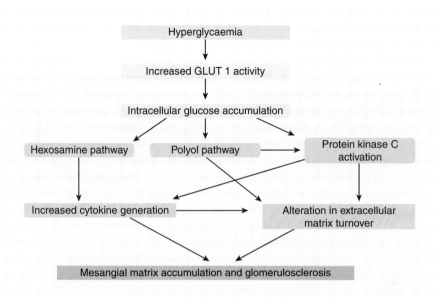

Fig. 7 Consequences of hyperglycaemia on mesangial cell function and its potential contribution to diabetic glomerulosclerosis (GLUT 1 = glucose transport protein).

Insights into renal interstitial fibrosis in diabetic nephropathy

As a result of the increasing awareness of the functional importance of the tubulointerstitium in the progression of diabetic nephropathy, several studies have focused on the mechanisms of induction of these interstitial changes. Proximal tubular epithelial cells are a source of many cytokines as well as expressing receptors for a number of similar molecules (reviewed in [25]).

One aim of our work has been to examine how renal proximal tubular cells may contribute to interstitial fibrosis by alterations in TGF-β generation. Glucose caused an increase in TGF-β mRNA, but TGF-β protein synthesis occurred only after the application of a second stimulus (PDGF or interleukin (IL)-1β) (Fig. 8). Addition of either of these cytokines increased the stability of D-glucose induced TGF-β mRNA. In contrast, incubation of D-glucose primed cells with tumour necrosis factor (TNF)-α did not result in TGF-β production and, unlike IL-1β and PDGF, TNF-α did not influence TGF-β mRNA stability (reviewed in [26]). These observations suggest that post-transcriptional modification of TGF-β mRNA may be limited to specific cytokine stimulation, which may therefore play a crucial role in the control of TGF-β protein synthesis by proximal tubular epithelial cells. More recent data suggest that the mechanisms of this post-translation of TGF-β involves alteration of cytoplasmic protein binding to specific sequences within the 5' untranslated region of its mRNA. The contrasting effects of glucose on the generation of TGF-β by mesangial cells and proximal tubular cells may therefore be an important factor which may explain why only 30% of all diabetic patients develop progressive renal interstitial fibrosis, which ultimately results in renal failure.

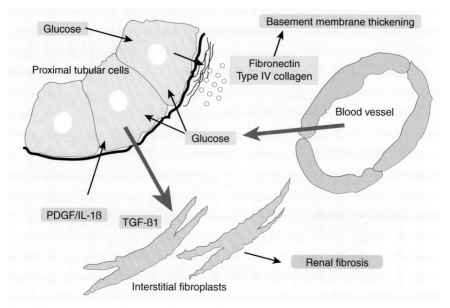

Fig. 8 Postulated mechanisms by which interactions between elevated glucose concentrations and the renal proximal tubular epithelial cell may contribute to the renal interstitial changes associated with diabetic nephropathy (TGF = transforming growth factor; PDGF = platelet-derived growth factor; IL = interleukin).

☐ CONCLUSIONS

Diabetic nephropathy is characterised by glomerular, vascular, tubular and interstitial lesions that initially develop without any measurable renal dysfunction and occur independently of the pathological changes associated with progressive diabetic nephropathy. These early structural changes are consistent with the studies of modulation of proliferation and matrix turnover generated using both cultured mesangial and proximal tubular cells. Furthermore, based on the combined data from *in vitro* and *in vivo* data, new insights into the pathogenesis of progressive DN have identified potentially new therapeutic targets such as TGF-β or PDGF. Presently, at best, short-term intervention studies are available for these new targets, and therefore both the long-term efficacy and safety of such therapeutic interventions remain to be demonstrated. Another important insight provided by experimental work is the demonstration that second stimuli in addition to hyperglycaemia may be necessary to induce pathogenetic mediators and progression of renal disease (Fig. 9). Further identification of such progressive factors in experimental diabetes will have obvious implications for our understanding of the mechanisms that drive the development of nephropathy in only a subset of diabetic patients.

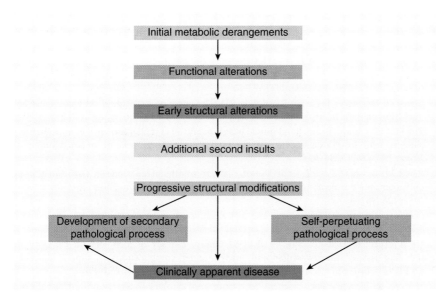

Fig. 9 Schematic outline of potential stages in the development of diabetic nephropathy.

REFERENCES

1 Ghavamian M, Gutch CF, Kopp KF, Kolff WJ. The sad truth about hemodialysis in diabetic nephropathy. *JAMA* 1972; **222**: 1386–9.

2 Cotugno D. De Ischiade Nervosa Commentarius. Bari: Cacucci Editore, 1983.

3 Rayer P. Traite des maladies des reins et des altérations de la sécrétion urinaire étudiées en elles-mêmes et dans leurs rapports avec les maladies des uretères, de la vessie, de la prostate et de l'urètre. Librairie de l'Academie Royal de Médicine, 1839.

4 Kimmelstiel P, Wilson C. Intercapillary lesions in the glomeruli of the kidney. *Am J Pathol* 1936; **12**: 83–98.

5 Marcelli D, Spotti D, Conte F, *et al.* Prognosis of diabetic patients on dialysis: analysis of Lombardy registry data. *Nephrol Dial Transplant* 1995; **10**: 1895–900.

6 Rodriguez JA, Cleries M, Vela E. Diabetic patients on renal replacement therapy: analysis of Catalan registry data. *Nephrol Dial Transplant* 1997; **12**: 2501–9.

7 Parving HH. Renoprotection in diabetes: genetic and non-genetic risk factors and treatment. *Diabetologia* 1998; **41**: 745–59.

8 Ritz E, Stefanski A. Diabetic nephropathy in type II diabetes. *Am J Kidney Dis* 1996; **27**: 167–94.

9 The Diabetes Control and Complications Research Group. Effect of intensive therapy on the development and progression of diabetic nephropathy in the Diabetes Control and Complications Trial. *Kidney Int* 1995; **47**: 1703–20.

10 UK Prospective Diabetes Study (UKPDS) Group. Intensive blood glucose control with sulphonylurease or insulin compared with conventional treatment and risk of complications in patients with type 2 diabetes. *Lancet* 1998; **352**: 837–53.

11 Ohkubo Y, Kishikawa H, Araki E. Intensive insulin therapy prevents progression of diabetic microvascular complications in Japanese patients with NIDDM: a randomised prospective 6-year study. *Diab Res Clin Pract* 1995; **28**: 103–17.

12 Epidemiology of Diabetes Interventions and Complications Research Group. Epidemiology of diabetes interventions and complications. *Diabetes Care* 1999; **22**: 99–111.

13 Mogensen CE. Long-term anti-hypertensive treatment inhibiting progression of diabetic nephropathy. *Br Med J* 1982; **285**: 685–8.

14 UK Prospective Diabetes Study (UKPDS) Group. Tight blood pressure control and risk of macrovascular and microvascular complications in type 2 diabetes: UKPDS 38. *Br Med J* 1998; **327**: 703–13.

15 Ravid M, Savin H, Jutrin I, *et al.* Long-term stabilisation effect of angiotensin converting enzyme inhibition on plasma creatinine and on proteinuria in normotensive type II diabetic patients. *Ann Intern Med* 1993; **118**: 577–81.

16 Lewis EJ, Hunsicker LG, Bain RP, Rohde RD. The effect of angiotensin-converting enzyme inhibition on diabetic nephropathy. *N Engl J Med* 1993; **329**: 1456–62.

17 The EUCLID Study Group. Randomised placebo-controlled trial of lisinopril in normotensive patients with insulin-dependent diabetes and normoalbuminuria or microalbuminuria. *Lancet* 1997; **349**: 1787–92.

18 Ravid M, Brosh D, Levi Z, *et al.* Use of enalapril to attenuate decline in renal function in normotensive, normoalbuminuric patients with type 2 diabetes mellitus. *Ann Intern Med* 1998; **128**: 982–8.

19 Golan L, Birkmeyer JD, Welch G. The cost effectiveness of treating all patients with type 2 diabetes with angiotensin-converting enzyme inhibitors. *Ann Intern Med* 1999; **131**: 660–7.

20 UK Prospective Diabetes Study (UKPDS) Group. Efficacy of atenolol and captopril in reducing risk of macrovascular and microvascular complications in type 2 diabetes: UKPDS 39. *Br Med J* 1998; **317**: 713–20.

21 Sharma K, Ziyadeh FN. Biochemical events and cytokine interactions linking glucose metabolism to the development of diabetic nephroapthy. *Semin Nephrol* 1997; **17**: 80–92.

22 Heilig CW, Concepcion LA, Riser BL, *et al.* Overexpression of glucose transporters in rat mesangial cells cultured in a normal glucose milieu mimics the diabetic phenotype. *J Clin Invest* 1995; **96**: 1802–14.

23 Sharma K, Ziyadeh FN. Hyperglycaemia and diabetic kidney disease. *Diabetes* 1995; **44**: 1139–46.

24 Kolm-Litty V, Sauer U, Nerlich A, *et al.* High glucose induced transforming growth factor β1 production is mediated by the hexosamine pathway in porcine glomerular mesangial cells. *J Clin Invest* 1998; **101**: 160–9.

25 Phillips AO, Janssen U, Floege J. Progression of diabetic nephropathy. Insights from cell culture studies and animal models. *Kidney Blood Press Res* 1999; **22**: 81–97.

26 Phillips AO. Diabetic nephropathy: the modulating influence of glucose on transforming factor β production. *Histo Histopathol* 1998; **13**: 565–74.

□ SELF ASSESSMENT QUESTIONS

1 Development of diabetic nephropathy is usually associated with:
(a) Microscopic haematuria
(b) Nephrotic range proteinuria
(c) Late onset of hypertension
(d) High patient mortality
(e) Poor glycaemic control

2 Tertiary prevention of diabetic nephropathy (prevention of progression of renal impairment) can be achieved by:
(a) Strict glycaemic control
(b) Introduction of angiotensin converting-enzyme (ACE) inhibitors
(c) Aggressive treatment of hypertension
(d) Treatment of hyperlipidaemia
(e) Protein restriction

3   Diabetic nephropathy is generally:
    (a) Only associated with type 1 (IDDM) diabetes
    (b) A contraindication to renal transplantation
    (c) Not amenable to therapeutic intervention
    (d) The commonest cause of end-stage renal failure
    (e) Only seen in poorly controlled diabetic patients

4   Use of ACE inhibitors in diabetic nephropathy:
    (a) Confers no additional benefit to other antihypertensive treatment
    (b) Should be used in all normoalbuminuric normotensive patients
    (c) Should be used only in type 1 diabetes with renal impairment
    (d) Is effective in patients with significant renal impairment
    (e) Is the treatment of choice for all diabetic patients with renal impairment

5   In diabetic nephropathy:
    (a) Renal function correlates to the degree of mesangial expansion
    (b) Patient prognosis has not changed in the last 20 years
    (c) Glomerulosclerosis is the result of protein kinase C activation
    (d) Pathological changes are the result of alterations in transforming growth
         factor-β generation
    (e) Renal function correlates to the degree of interstitial fibrosis

ANSWERS

1a False	2a False	3a False	4a False	5a True
b True	b True	b False	b False	b False
c False	c True	c False	c False	c False
d True	d False	d True	d True	d False
e True	e False	e False	e False	b True

Acute renal failure

John D Firth

Renal function is acutely disturbed in about 5% of hospital admissions, and a conservative estimate suggests that 70 per million population per year develop acute renal failure of sufficient severity to require renal replacement therapy. There are no specific symptoms or signs, hence the need for routine and urgent measurement of 'urea (or creatinine) and electrolytes' on all emergency admissions to hospital.

Acute renal failure, defined as a failure of renal function usually manifest as a rise in serum urea or creatinine which occurs over hours or days, is most commonly seen in the context of circulatory disturbance. Why the kidney seems more vulnerable than other organs in this situation remains unknown, as do the precise mechanisms of damage and recovery. Application of cell biology techniques is throwing increasing light on some aspects of the problem and producing the hope, not yet fulfilled, of new and better treatments. This chapter cannot attempt to cover or do justice to the whole range of issues that might be dealt with under the title of 'acute renal failure'. Mention will be made of 'timeless' clinical priorities [1], and of two areas of particular recent interest and controversy regarding pathophysiology and treatment: the use of growth factors to speed recovery, and the effects of using different types of dialysis membrane.

☐ CLINICAL APPROACH TO THE PATIENT WITH ACUTE RENAL FAILURE

Immediate priorities

If initial assessment suggests problems with the airways, breathing or circulation, the immediate priority must be to resuscitate and ensure adequate ventilation. If these are satisfactory, the most pressing hazard is hyperkalaemia which can cause cardiac arrest without warning. In any particular patient, the risk of this correlates better with the ECG appearance than with the level of serum potassium. Any change more severe than tenting of the T waves – that is, reduction in size of the P waves, increase in PR interval, widening of QRS complex (culminating in sinusoidal wave form) – demands immediate treatment with intravenous calcium chloride. This 'stabilises' the cardiac membranes (mechanism unknown) but does not affect the level of serum potassium. The treatment most commonly employed thereafter is intravenous glucose and insulin, which reduces serum potassium concentration by 1–2 mmol/l over 30 minutes. An alternative to this is intravenous or nebulised salbutamol, which is similarly effective. It is used as routine first-line treatment for dangerous hyperkalaemia in at least two renal units in the UK (Figs. 1 and 2) [2,3].

Both glucose/insulin and salbutamol work by stimulation of sodium/potassium ATPase, causing a shift of potassium from the extracellular to intracellular compartment. Cation exchange resins, administered orally or rectally, can be used to increase gastrointestinal elimination of potassium, but take many hours to have any effect and remove relatively little potassium; most cases of severe hyperkalaemia will require urgent dialysis.

Other life-threatening complications of acute renal failure include pulmonary oedema and (less commonly) profound acidosis. Aside from standard supportive care, these remain indications for emergency dialysis or haemofiltration.

Management of fluids

Many patients with acute renal failure have intravascular volume depletion. There are only two reliable physical signs: a low jugular venous pressure, and a postural drop in blood pressure, which should be estimated with the patient lying and sitting if standing is not prudent. Intravascular volume depletion should be corrected rapidly (using blood, colloid or 0.9% saline, as appropriate) with infusion stopped as soon as the signs of depletion have been corrected. Thereafter, fluid input should equal output, plus an additional 0.5–1 l/day for insensible losses, adjusted in the light of twice daily repeated clinical assessment of the patient's volume status.

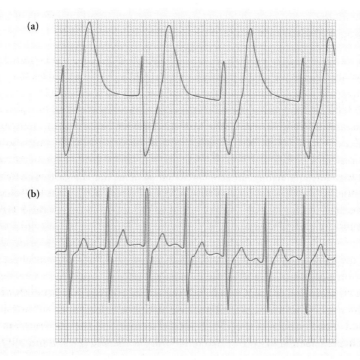

Fig. 1 ECG of a patient with hyperkalaemia **(a)** before (serum potassium 8.7 mmol/l) and **(b)** after (serum potassium 5.9 mmol/l) intravenous administration of salbutamol 0.5 mg (reproduced, with permission, from [3]).

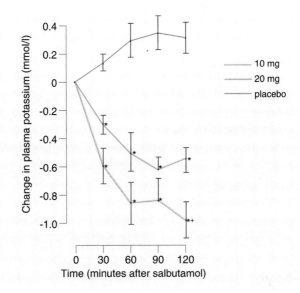

Fig. 2 Effect of nebulised salbutamol, 10 mg or 20 mg, or placebo on plasma potassium concentration in a study of 10 hyperkalaemic chronic dialysis patients, each studied on three occasions. The falls in plasma concentration were significant. Values are means ± standard errors (reproduced, with permission, from [2]).

Diagnosis of the cause

Pre-renal failure will be found in 80–90% of patients with acute renal failure where, by definition, renal function recovers immediately with fluid resuscitation, or acute tubular necrosis, where structural damage to the kidney has occurred and recovery, anticipated in most cases, is delayed. It is vitally important, however, that physicians are alert to the possibility of other diagnoses, particularly in cases where there is no good evidence of circulatory disturbance as a prelude to renal failure. A lazy attitude (eg 'another case of acute tubular necrosis, scarcely worth thinking about') is responsible for some patients being denied curative treatment and condemned to a lifetime on dialysis. The alternative diagnoses to consider are listed in Table 1, and two critical findings illustrated: a cellular cast in the urine (Fig. 3) and an ultrasound showing an obstructed kidney (Fig. 4).

☐ PATHOPHYSIOLOGY OF ACUTE TUBULAR NECROSIS

The basic anatomy of the renal tubule is well known: the proximal tubule leads into the descending limb of the loop of Henle, whose ascending limb leads into the distal convoluted tubule. The flow of tubular fluid in the two limbs runs in a countercurrent manner, allowing the formation of a standing gradient of interstitial osmolality from the renal cortex (300 mosm/l, the same as plasma) to the renal papilla (ca 1,000 mosm/l). The high osmolality of the papillary interstitium allows passive abstraction of water from tubular fluid in the distal nephron in the presence

Table 1 Clinical approach to acute renal failure

Diagnosis	Key clinical features	Key investigation	Immediate treatment
Pre-renal failure & acute tubular necrosis	Common Circulatory disturbance Evidence of volume depletion Sepsis Predisposing drugs	Clinical diagnosis	Volume resuscitation Treatment of precipitating condition Withdrawal of toxic drugs
Urinary obstruction	'Prostatic symptoms' Urinary stones Back pain Palpable bladder Rectal examination	**Ultrasound examination** – but note that up to 5% may have non-dilated obstruction	Urethral catheter Suprapubic catheter Antegrade nephrostomy
Renal inflammation	Multisystem disease Predisposing drugs*	**Stick testing showing proteinuria and haematuria** **Urinary microscopy showing cellular casts**	Depending on precise diagnosis (beyond the scope of this chapter**)
Bilateral renal artery occlusion†	Generalised atheromatous vascular disease	Urinary sodium concentration equal to that in plasma	? Conservative ? Thrombolytic ? Revascularisation

*The commonest predisposing drugs are penicillins, sulphonamides, non-steroidal anti-inflammatory agents and thiazides, but many others have been reported and any drug should be regarded as a potential culprit if the renal biopsy shows acute interstitial nephritis.

**In any case of acute renal failure with haematuria and proteinuria, blood tests should be sent to look for evidence of autoimmune rheumatic disorder or systemic vasculitis. Renal biopsy will almost certainly be justified to determine diagnosis and prognosis and to guide treatment.

† This is rare. Acute complete occlusion of the renal artery usually leads to infarction of the kidney, but a collateral renal blood supply can develop in patients with long-standing atheromatous renovascular disease, and this is sometimes able to maintain viability in the face of complete occlusion of the main renal artery. In one paper it was reported that such patients pass urine containing sodium in equal concentration to that in plasma, but it is not known what the clinical response to this finding should be.

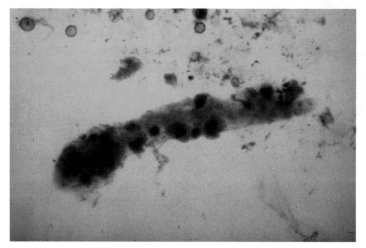

Fig. 3 A red cell cast in the urine of a patient with acute renal failure due to nephritis (red cells are stained blue).

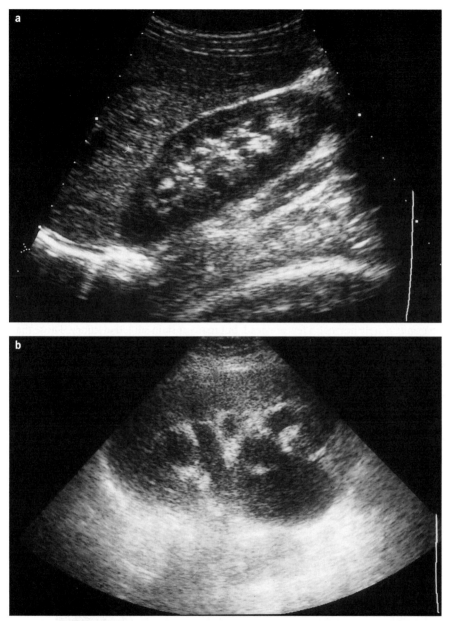

Fig. 4 Renal ultrasound examination of **(a)** a normal native kidney, and **(b)** an obstructed transplant kidney showing dilatation of the renal pelvis and calyces. The appearance of an obstructed and dilated native kidney is similar.

of antidiuretic hormone, which renders the collecting tubules permeable to water. Hence urinary osmolality can approach that of the papillary interstitium when water needs to be conserved.

Less well recognised is the fact that the vasa rectae, which supply blood to the renal medulla, of necessity also run in a countercurrent manner, leading to the development of a standing gradient of oxygen tension within the kidney. The superficial cortex operates at normal tissue levels of oxygen tension, but islands within the deeper cortex and the whole of the renal medulla operate all the time at greatly reduced oxygen tension, as low as 1–3 kPa. This is an inevitable consequence of the anatomy, and is probably correctly regarded as a price paid for the mechanism by which the mammalian kidney performs the critical homeostatic function of modulating water excretion.

The fact that much of the renal tubule, which is metabolically very active, sits in an environment of low oxygen tension appears to render it susceptible to ischaemic or hypoxic damage when the circulation is compromised, a feature further exacerbated by the propensity of the renal vessels to be particularly sensitive to some vasoconstrictor agents. Classic studies published in the 1950s and 1970s demonstrated histologically that patients with persistent acute renal failure following ischaemic or toxic insult often had acute necrosis of some renal tubular cells. Whilst attention focused for some time on the medullary thick ascending limb of Henle's loop as the site most susceptible to damage, it is now clear that the most severe injury occurs in the S3 segment of the proximal tubule.

Work in the past 10 years has emphasised something that always was likely: that, following injury to the kidney, cells are not simply left 'alive or dead'. Many cells are alive and entirely normal, a few are dead, but many sustain sublethal injury. Those that are dead may have died from necrosis or apoptosis – very different processes. In cells that are damaged, dysfunction that has been demonstrated includes loss of polarity, tight junction function and cell-substrate adhesion, exfoliation of viable cells from the tubular basement membrane, and abnormal renal tubular cell-cell adhesion. Alterations in gene expression and cellular dedifferentiation have also been described [4]. The situation is immensely complex, but it is inevitable that improved understanding of the processes involved will lead to the suggestion of novel treatment mechanisms, to be tested first in animal models and then (if promising) in man.

Clinical recovery following acute tubular necrosis typically takes a few weeks. This depends upon restoration of normal function in cells that have sustained sublethal injury. Cells that have died could be replaced by regeneration or their functions could be assumed by others. However, there is much evidence to indicate that cellular regeneration is important. This is a particularly exciting area of research where cell biology and clinical medicine may meet to the benefit of patients.

□ GROWTH FACTORS

There are an increasing number of clinical situations where the use of growth factors is well established. Nephrologists are familiar with the use of erythropoietin. Colony-stimulating factors are given routinely to hasten the regeneration of blood cells in a variety of conditions. As regards acute renal failure, in several animal models there is compelling evidence that administration of exogenous growth factors can accelerate the process of recovery. In the rat with renal ischaemia induced by temporary clamping of the renal artery, both epidermal growth factor and recombinant human insulin-like growth factor-1 (rhIGF-1) increase the rate of cellular regeneration and speed the return of normal function (Fig. 5) [5]. Epidermal growth factor has also been shown to be effective in promoting renal recovery in the rat with mercuric chloride nephrotoxicity, and hepatocyte growth factor is efficacious in a mouse model of acute renal failure.

The first paper describing the use of a growth factor in patients with acute renal failure was published in 1999 [6]. Seventy-two patients with acute renal failure following trauma, surgery or sepsis, with no response to correction of volume depletion, a fractional sodium excretion of more than 1% (a conventional indicator of tubular damage) and no diagnosis other than 'acute tubular necrosis', were randomised to receive placebo or rhIGF-1 100 μg/kg desirable body weight, by subcutaneous injection twice daily for 14 days. The groups appeared to be well matched. The results were very disappointing. Urinary volume and glomerular filtration rate measured by creatinine or iothalamate clearance did not differ significantly at any time in the treated and control groups (Fig. 6). Requirement for, and days spent on, renal replacement therapy were similar in both.

(a)	Cortex		Corticomedullary junction		Glomeruli		Tubules	
	Mean	SE	Mean	SE	Mean	SE	Mean	SE
ARF + vehicle	6,375	±1,992	6,870	±2,133	692	±180	7,565	±2,269
ARF + rhIGF-1	26,354	±3,396	51,115	±9,466	3,203	±679	50,015	±10,898
p	<0.001		<0.002		<0.01		<0.01	

Data expressed as cpm of [³H]thymidine/mg DNA; p values calculated with unpaired t-test (SE = standard error).

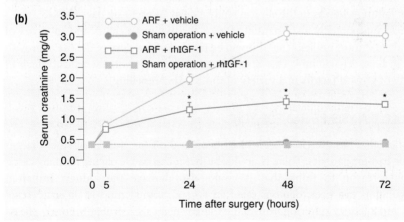

Fig. 5 Effect of administration of recombinant human insulin-like growth factor (rhIGF-1) to a rat with acute renal failure (ARF) induced by clamping both renal pedicles for 60 minutes: **(a)** increased rate of cellular regeneration, as determined by estimation of thymidine incorporation into DNA extracted from several renal tissues 72 hours after the induction of renal failure; **(b)** increased rate of functional improvement, as shown by reduced area under the curve of serum creatinine vs time. Treatment with rhIGF-1 or vehicle was started after the measurement at 5 hours was obtained (p <0.05 vs ARF + vehicle) (with permission, from [5]).

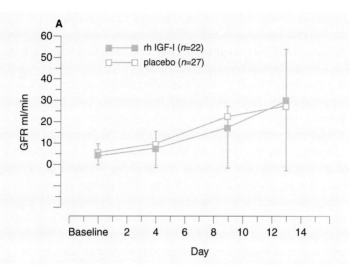

Fig. 6 Glomerular filtration rate (GFR) measured as clearance of iothalamate in all study participants with sufficient urine flow rates. Data are mean ± standard deviations. There is clearly no significant difference between the groups (rhIGF-1 = recombinant human insulin-like growth factor) (with permission, from [6]).

There could be many reasons for this negative result. It is known that rhIGF-1 can act on the human kidney, but there is no doubt that acute tubular necrosis seen in clinical practice – usually the result of severe illness and with multiple insults to the kidney – is different from acute renal failure in the relatively 'clean' rat models that have been used to test the efficacy of growth factor treatments. Furthermore, in the rat models, growth factors have been administered within 24 hours of the onset of renal failure, whereas in the clinical study a delay of up to six days elapsed.

Whilst undoubtedly a substantial setback for the investigators and sponsors of this study, it is most unlikely that this will be the end of the story of the use of growth factors in acute renal failure. The experimental evidence showing beneficial effects of a variety of growth factors in a variety of models is compelling.

□ COULD DIALYSIS BE BAD FOR YOU?

A question that has exercised nephrologists on and off for years is whether dialysis could be bad for patients. There is no doubt that it can be life-saving in many cases, but some reason to think that it could also damage the kidney. Impaired autoregulation has been demonstrated in several animal models of acute renal failure, and a kidney suffering from acute tubular necrosis is probably poorly placed to withstand further episodes of ischaemia. Renal biopsy specimens showing cell necrosis of apparently differing ages support the contention that damage does not happen once and for all, but that serial episodes occur. There is obviously no shortage of possible explanations: patients with acute tubular necrosis often have intermittent hypotension and episodes of apparent sepsis. Since dialysis is an episodic event, sometimes associated with hypotension, it is not at all unreasonable to ask the question 'could dialysis be bad for you?'. However, since patients with severe acute renal failure die without treatment, it is clearly not practical to attempt an answer to the question in its barest form, but the question 'could some types of dialysis be worse for you than others?' has been asked, and there was considerable interest in this in 1999.

Not all dialysis membranes are the same, and for the purposes of this debate they can be divided into bioincompatible and biocompatible (strictly, less incompatible) types (Table 2) [7]. Bioincompatible membranes activate complement and lead to neutrophil activation and infiltration into the kidney. These neutrophils might possibly cause or prolong renal damage by releasing vasoconstrictors and damaging oxygen radicals, suggesting that bioincompatible membranes might delay recovery from acute renal failure.

Table 2 Types of dialysis membrane.

Membrane classification	Type of membrane	Clinical features
'Bioincompatible'	Generally cellulose-based, eg cuprophan, cellulose acetate, hemophan	Activate complement Activate leukocytes Induce free radical release
'Biocompatible'	Generally synthetic, eg polysulfone, polyacrylonitrile	Less of the above

Notes: (i) The terms 'bioincompatible' and 'biocompatible' are relative, not absolute.
(ii) See [7] for further discussion.

In 1994 two randomised controlled studies in 52 and 72 patients, respectively, reported that the use of cuprophan (bioincompatible) membranes adversely affected the duration of oliguria, the rate of renal recovery, the occurrence of sepsis, and the survival rate. The effects reported were substantial and could not be ignored, but they were surprising to many nephrologists. They stimulated much debate, some rather acrimonious, regarding methodology, statistical techniques and possible bias.

An international multicentre group reported the findings of a larger trial in October 1999 of 180 patients with acute renal failure randomly assigned to bioincompatible cuprophan or biocompatible polymethylmethacrylate membranes: 58% of those assigned to cuprophan survived, compared with 60% treated with polymethylmethacrylate membranes. There was no difference in a number of secondary outcomes, including the number of dialysis sessions required or incidence of sepsis [8].

An accompanying editorial in the *Lancet* reviewed this study and 12 others assessing the role of membrane bioincompatibility on outcome of acute renal failure [9]. The conclusion was that complement-activating membranes do not 'confer extraordinary risks'.

REFERENCES

1   Firth JD. The clinical approach to the patient with acute renal failure. In: Davison AM, Cameron JS, Grunfeld J-P, *et al* (eds). *Oxford Textbook of Clinical Nephrology*. 2nd edn. Oxford: Oxford University Press, 1998: 1557–82.

2   Allon M, Dunlay R, Copkney C. Nebulised albuterol for acute hyperkalemia in patients on hemodialysis. *Ann Intern Med* 1989; **110**: 426–9.

3   Lens XM, Montoliu J, Cases A, *et al.* Treatment of hyperkalaemia in renal failure: salbutamol v. insulin. *Nephrol Dial Transplant* 1989; **4**: 228–32.

4   Lieberthal W. Biology of acute renal failure: therapeutic implications. *Kidney Int* 1997; **52**: 1102–5.

5   Ding H, Kopple JD, Cohen A, Hirschberg R. Recombinant human insulin-like growth factor-1 accelerates recovery and reduces catabolism in rats with ischemic acute renal failure. *J Clin Invest* 1993; **91**: 2281–7.

6   Hirschberg R, Kopple J, Lipsett P, *et al.* Multicenter clinical trial of recombinant human insulin-like growth factor I in patients with acute renal failure. *Kidney Int* 1999; **55**: 2423–32.

7   Vanholder R, De Vriese A, Lameire N. The role of dialyzer biocompatibility in acute renal failure. *Blood Purif* 2000; **18**: 1–12.

8   Jorres A, Gahl GM, Dobis C, *et al.* Haemodialysis-membrane biocompatibility and mortality of patients with dialysis-dependent acute renal failure: a prospective randomised multicentre trial. *Lancet* 1999; **354**: 1337–41.

9   Vanholder R, Lameire N. Does biocompatibility of dialysis membranes affect recovery of renal function and survival? Review. *Lancet* 1999; **354**: 1316–8.

☐ SELF ASSESSMENT QUESTIONS

1   In the normal kidney:
  (a) Renal blood flow, expressed in ml/min/g tissue, is higher than that of any other large organ
  (b) Oxygen tension in the renal vein is much higher than that in the veins draining most organs
  (c) Parts of the deep cortex and the whole of the medulla operate at very low oxygen tension
  (d) Renal blood vessels are particularly susceptible to some vasoconstrictors
  (e) Countercurrent flow of blood in the vasa rectae allows the formation of a standing oxygen gradient

2   Reliable signs of intravascular volume depletion are:
  (a) Postural hypotension
  (b) Dry mouth
  (c) Low jugular venous pulse
  (d) Reduced urine output
  (e) Reduced skin turgor

3   In acute renal failure:
  (a) Intravenous calcium chloride reduces the serum potassium concentration
  (b) Nebulised salbutamol can be used to reduce the serum potassium concentration
  (c) Most patients with severe hyperkalaemia will require renal replacement therapy
  (d) Normal renal ultrasound excludes obstruction
  (e) Hyperkalaemia is particularly likely in patients with rhabdomyolysis

4   In acute tubular necrosis:
   (a) Recovery requires cellular regeneration
   (b) Growth factors have been shown to speed recovery in animal models but not in man
   (c) It is rare for patients not to recover renal function
   (d) The damaged kidney is particularly vulnerable to further insult
   (e) Non-steroidal anti-inflammatory agents, converting enzyme inhibitors and aminoglycosides should be avoided

ANSWERS

1a True	2a True	3a False	4a True
b True	b False	b True	b True
c True	c True	c True	c False
d True	d False	d False	d True
e True	e False	e True	e True

Psoriasis

Christopher E M Griffiths

☐ INTRODUCTION

Psoriasis is a common, chronic disease which affects at least 2% of the UK population, although few, if any, epidemiological surveys of prevalence have been performed in this country. Skin diseases are poorly represented in the pantheon of NHS and research priorities. It is true that few people die as a consequence of diseases such as psoriasis, but this statement bears closer scrutiny. Psoriasis affects more people than diabetes or rheumatoid arthritis and, like those diseases, is currently incurable. The burden on the affected individual is immense: it is estimated that the quality of life for patients with psoriasis is the same as – or worse than – that for people with diabetes or ischaemic heart disease, and close to that of patients with cardiac failure [1]. Although psoriasis may not contribute to mortality figures, it destroys people's lives. The major cause of psychosocial stress in our patients comes from avoidance coping: in other words, their lives are significantly constrained in that they actively avoid situations in which others may comment adversely about their skin disease (a process known as automatic vigilance). For instance, patients will not use local swimming pools or go on a public beach – even though they know sunlight alleviates psoriasis – and are embarrassed to stay overnight at the homes of friends and relatives.

The socio-economic burden of psoriasis is difficult to quantify, particularly in the UK. In the US, where figures are more readily available, it is calculated that $1.5 billion is spent per year on psoriasis care. Drug costs are uncertain as few medicines are used solely for the treatment of psoriasis, but are approximately $1.5 billion per year worldwide. Inpatient bed use is still a major healthcare cost; for instance, a recent audit in our 19-bed dermatology unit in Manchester revealed that 50% of bed occupancy was for psoriasis treatment.

Thus, there is a compelling and compassionate need to study pathomechanisms in psoriasis and ultimately to develop effective and perhaps even curative therapies. This review discusses recent progress in our understanding of psoriasis and its management.

☐ CLINICAL PRESENTATION OF PSORIASIS

The characteristic, textbook lesion of psoriasis is a red, heavily-scaled but well-demarcated plaque (Fig. 1) [2]. Such plaques most commonly occur on the extensor aspects of elbows and knees, scalp and lumbo-sacral area (Fig. 2) but may involve any skin surface. Psoriasis may take the following forms (Table 1):

☐ The *chronic plaque form* is the commonest subtype of psoriasis, accounting for 90% of cases.

☐ Confluence of plaques may lead to total skin involvement, known as *erythroderma* (Fig. 3).

☐ *Guttate psoriasis* describes the sudden onset of showers of small, 4–5 mm diameter plaques predominantly on the trunk 2–3 weeks post-streptococcal pharyngitis or tonsillitis (Fig. 4). This form usually clears spontaneously.

☐ *Generalised pustular psoriasis*, like guttate psoriasis, is precipitous in onset and consists of painful red plaques studded with small sterile pustules. Nowadays, this form is seen most often after withdrawal of systemic

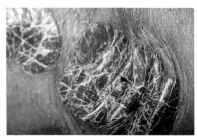

Fig. 1 Plaque of psoriasis.

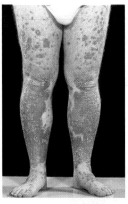

Fig. 2 Chronic plaque psoriasis on legs.

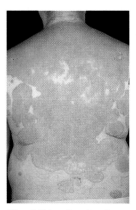

Fig. 3 Extensive chronic plaque psoriasis on the trunk.

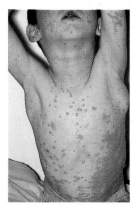

Fig. 4 Guttate psoriasis.

Table 1 Clinical subtypes of psoriasis.

- Chronic plaque
- Erythrodermic
- Guttate
- Generalised pustular
- Palmo-plantar pustular

glucocorticosteroids which, for this reason, should not be used in the management of psoriasis.

☐ *Palmoplantar pustular psoriasis*, a chronic, localised form of pustular psoriasis, which may occur on the palms and soles.

In approximately 50% of patients there are characteristic psoriatic changes on one or more nails, including pitting, onycholysis and dystrophy (Fig. 5). There is a seronegative arthritis in 5–10% of patients (Fig. 6). This so-called 'psoriatic arthritis' is variable in presentation, ranging from arthritis mutilans and sacroiliitis to involvement of distal interphalangeal joints.

There are two distinct ages of onset:

☐ *Type I*, presenting before 40 years of age, with a peak onset at 20 years (75% of cases), and

☐ *Type II*, presenting over the age of 40, and peaking at 55–60 years.

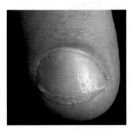

Fig. 5 Nail involvement in psoriasis, showing pitting.

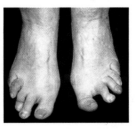

Fig. 6 Psoriatic arthritis.

Type I psoriasis is more severe, usually familial and strongly associated with human leukocyte antigen (HLA) Cw6, whereas type II psoriasis is less aggressive, sporadic and only weakly associated with HLA Cw6.

☐ GENETICS OF PSORIASIS

The strong familial incidence indicates that genetic predisposition is key for development of psoriasis. To date, four genetic loci have been identified on chromosomes 6p, 17q, 4q and 1q, known as psoriasis genes 1, 2, 3 and 4, respectively. At least six other loci are known, and it is clear that psoriasis will be revealed as several subtypes identified by genotype. One possible early spin-off of the molecular genetic work is the development of a good animal model for the disease. Currently, none exists as humans are the only species to develop psoriasis.

In addition to research into the genetics of psoriasis, there is a considerable weight of evidence that it is a T cell-mediated, possibly autoimmune, condition [3], the putative autoantigen being a component of keratin. Psoriatic plaques are characterised by epidermal keratinocyte proliferation and a T cell infiltrate, predominantly CD8+ cells in the epidermis and CD4+ cells in the dermis (Fig. 7). The efficacy of T cell-targeted drugs such as cyclosporin, anti-CD4 monoclonal antibodies and an interleukin (IL)-2 fusion toxin bear out this observation. The intraplaque cytokine milieu in psoriasis is consistent with a T helper (TH) 1 profile (ie predominance of IL-2, IL-12 and interferon (IFN)-γ. In contrast, atopic dermatitis skin reveals a TH2 profile (IL-4, IL-5 and IL-10) (Table 2). These cytokine profiles may explain the relative under-representation of atopic dermatitis, asthma and urticaria – all TH2 diseases – in patients with psoriasis [4].

Genetic disposition (ie genotype) is important, but the psoriasis phenotype will manifest only in the context of a predisposing genotype and certain environmental triggers. Known triggers are shown in Table 3.

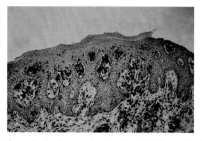

Fig. 7 Histology of plaque of psoriasis demonstrating T cell infiltrate in dermis and epidermis.

Table 2 Cutaneous cytokine imbalance in psoriasis and atopic dermatitis.

Psoriasis	Atopic dermatitis
TH1 cytokine profile:	TH2 cytokine profile:
IL-2	IL-4
IL-12	IL-5
IFN-γ	IL-10

IFN = interferon; IL = interleukin; TH = T helper.

Table 3 Trigger factors for psoriasis.

- Infection
  - β-haemolytic streptococcus
  - HIV
- Drugs
  - Lithium
  - β-adrenergic blockers
  - Anti-malarials
  - NSAIDs
  - Withdrawal of glucocorticosteroids
- Stress
- Hormonal
  - Post-partum
- Alcohol
- Skin trauma
  - Köbner phenomenon

NSAID = non-steroidal anti-inflammatory drug.

☐ MANAGEMENT OF PSORIASIS

For most purposes, psoriasis is a chronic unremitting disease, although probably 20% of patients experience temporary spontaneous remissions. Management needs to be a contract between physician and patient. It is important to ascertain individual patients' agenda for treatment: why do they want treatment now, and to what extent are they willing to go to achieve improvement. Recent studies have demonstrated that only 14% of patients consider current treatments for psoriasis to be effective, while 39% of patients do not comply with treatment [5]. Patients need educating as regards their expectations, in that treatments are suppressive and not curative, the goal being to improve psoriasis to the extent that it does not interfere with daily activities. Unfortunately, diets are unhelpful, but lifestyle changes such as reducing alcohol intake are often beneficial.

Approaches to management (Table 4) can be divided into:

☐ first-line, primary care-based, topical therapy (70% of patients), and

☐ second-line, hospital-based therapies, which include phototherapy, inpatient management and systemic therapies [6,7].

This review will highlight recent and probable future changes in practice, but not provide an exhaustive list of available therapies.

First-line therapies

Most current first-line therapies are effective only if applied assiduously (ie compliantly), but their use is largely hampered by cosmetic unacceptability (eg coal tar, dithranol and most ointment preparations). The two most recent innovations in topical therapy are the introduction of topical analogues of vitamin D3

Table 4 The management of psoriasis.

First-line (GP)	Second-line (hospital)
Emollients	Phototherapy
	UVB
Keratolytics	Photochemotherapy
	Psoralens & UVA
Coal tar	Inpatient/day treatment centre
Dithranol	Phototherapy and topical
Vitamin D3 analogues	Methotrexate
Topical corticosteroids	Systemic retinoids – acitretin
Topical retinoids	Cyclosporin
	Hydroxyurea

GP = general practitioner; UV = ultraviolet.

(calcipotriol and tacalcitol) and third-generation retinoids (tazarotene). Vitamin D3 analogues have rapidly achieved first place in the armamentarium of primary care-based therapy; they are moderately effective, more cosmetically agreeable than coal tar or dithranol, and can be used on a long-term chronic basis. The only side effect is some local irritation of uninvolved skin. Caution is therefore required if used in the flexures and in amounts higher than recommended; for example, more than 100 g a week of calcipotriol can cause hypercalcaemia. Tazarotene is locally effective, but more irritating than vitamin D3 analogues. Both categories of drug normalise the abnormal epidermal keratinocyte proliferation and differentiation seen in psoriasis.

Second-line therapies

Recent innovations in second-line therapy include the use of narrow-band ultraviolet (UV) B and safer regimens of cyclosporin.

Ultraviolet light

Broad-band UVB (290–320 nm) is a widely used adjunctive therapy for psoriasis and the mainstay of day-treatment centre management in combination with topical coal tar or dithranol. The 311–313 nm wavelength band of UVB is known to be the most potent for clearing psoriasis, and such narrow-band UVB cabinets are available. Unlike broad-band UVB, narrow-band UVB is effective as monotherapy for treatment of plaque psoriasis, and may be as good as psoralens plus UVA (PUVA) in this regard. It remains to be ascertained whether narrow-band UVB is subject to the same long-term sequelae as PUVA (ie photoageing and skin cancer).

Cyclosporin

One of the most effective systemic therapies for psoriasis treatment is cyclosporin. Cyclosporin is a noted T cell-targeted immunosuppressant, and its efficacy in clearing psoriasis was one of the key factors in determining the role of T cells in this disease [8]. Low-dose cyclosporin (3–5 mg/kg/day) will clear over 80% of cases of psoriasis within 12 weeks, usually considerably sooner. Unfortunately, long-term chronic use is contraindicated because of fears about hypertension and renal impairment. In an attempt to mitigate the potential nephrotoxicity of cyclosporin, it is now most often used in shorter-term (maximum 12 weeks) intermittent courses. This approach can be repeated several times a year and appears to be safer than continuous chronic use.

Relapses unresponsive to topical therapy can be treated either by further courses of cyclosporin or by rotating to another second-line treatment: the so-called rotational therapy (Fig. 8). Most second-line approaches to the treatment of psoriasis are associated with some form of toxicity, and rotational therapy is a method of minimising risk to individual organs (eg kidney from cyclosporin, skin from PUVA, liver from methotrexate, etc).

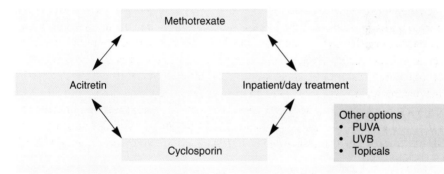

Fig. 8 Rotational therapy for psoriasis (PUVA = psoralens plus ultraviolet (UV) B).

☐ FUTURE THERAPIES

The future management of psoriasis will depend on an enhanced understanding of its molecular genetics, pathomechanisms, and psychosocial disability (Table 5). An appreciation of molecular genetics and the genes responsible for the psoriatic process opens the way for genotyping subgroups of psoriasis according to treatment response (pharmacogenetics). Thus, it may be possible to categorise patients according to the therapy likely to be most effective for them as individuals: for instance, methotrexate-responsive or cyclosporin-responsive. This would be an economical way of targeting therapy.

T cell targeting

Figure 9 illustrates all the current approaches in either clinical trials or clinical practice that target T cell function in psoriasis. The most promising area is that of co-stimulatory or accessory molecule blockade, inhibiting binding of the ligands responsible for providing activation signals between T cell and antigen-presenting

Table 5 Future developments in psoriasis management.

- Improved vitamin D3 and retinoid analogues
- T cell targeting
  - blockade of co-stimulatory molecules
  - inhibition of T cell proliferation
  - inhibition of T cell/endothelial cell binding
- Cytokine switching
  - IL-10
- Psychological symptom management
- Oral tolerance
- Photodynamic therapy

IL = interleukin.

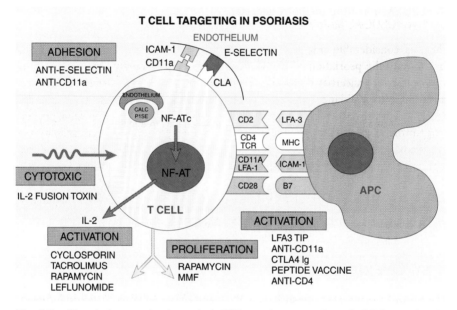

Fig. 9 T cell-targeted approaches in psoriasis (APC = antigen-presenting cell; CALC = calcineurin phosphatase; CLA = cutaneous lymphocyte associated antigen; ICAM = intercellular adhesion molecule; IL = interleukin; LFA = lymphocyte function associated antigen; MHC = major histocompatibility complex; MMF = mycophenolate mofetil; NAFT = nuclear factor of activated T cells; TCR = T cell receptor).

cell (APC). One such approach is the use of LFA3TIP, a fusion protein of immunoglobulin G_1 with LFA-3 which blocks binding of LFA-3 on APC to T cell CD2, thereby preventing T cell activation. Early phase I and II studies with LFA3TIP indicate marked efficacy in treatment of chronic plaque psoriasis if administered at relatively low doses intravenously once a week for 12 weeks. Once cleared, a significant number of patients remain clear for up to nine months. The safety profile for this compound appears good, with only transient falls in peripheral CD45RO T cell counts.

Cytokine switching

Cytokine imbalance within plaques of psoriasis, with overproduction of TH1 cytokines and the relative scarcity of concurrence of atopic dermatitis (TH2 disease) and psoriasis, suggests that restoration of normal cytokine homeostasis could be used to treat psoriasis. Such an approach has been used successfully in the treatment of atopic dermatitis in which subcutaneous systemic administration of IFN-γ (a TH1 cytokine) improves this skin disease. Early clinical trials attest to the utility of this approach: either direct injection of a TH2 cytokine (IL-10) into plaques or systemic administration of IL-10 via subcutaneous injection produces significant improvement in psoriasis [9]. Interestingly, some treatments already in use for the management of psoriasis may also work in part by local cytokine switching (eg vitamin D3 analogues).

☐ PSYCHOSOCIAL MANAGEMENT

There is considerable interest in the role played by stress in inducing and/or maintaining the psoriatic process. Up to 60% of our patients report that stress is responsible for exacerbating psoriasis, with most of their daily psychosocial stress attributable to avoidance coping [10]. As part of an overall package of care for patients with psoriasis, we have introduced a psychological symptom management programme as an adjunct to regular pharmacological treatment. The programme consists of six, weekly two-hour group sessions educating patients about psoriasis, cognitive behavioural management, stress management and relaxation techniques. Using this approach, psoriasis patients' overall clinical severity is significantly reduced as compared to regular treatments alone not only at the end of the course but also six months later. This suggests that patients can maintain control of their disease by using such an educational package.

☐ CONCLUSIONS

The management of psoriasis should be no different from that used in other chronic diseases such as asthma, and of necessity incorporates a multidisciplinary approach.

Further developments will undoubtedly involve T cell targeting, peptide vaccination approaches, and novel ways of delivering phototherapy such as photodynamic therapy. Whatever treatments are introduced are likely to be dictated by an enhanced understanding of fundamental basic mechanisms in psoriasis, coupled with an appreciation of individual patients' agenda for treatment.

REFERENCES

1   Finlay AY, Coles EC. The effect of severe psoriasis on the quality of life of 369 patients. *Br J Dermatol* 1995; **132**: 236–4.
2   Stern RS. Psoriasis. *Lancet* 1997; **350**: 349–53.
3   Griffiths CEM, Voorhees JJ. Psoriasis, T cells and autoimmunity. *J R Soc Med* 1996; **89**: 315–9.
4   Henseler T, Christophers E. Disease concomitance in psoriasis. *J Am Acad Dermatol* 1995; **32**: 982–6.

5   Richards HL, Fortune DG, O'Sullivan TM, *et al*. Patients with psoriasis and their compliance with medication. *J Am Acad Dermatol* 1999; **41**: 581–3.

6   Gawkrodger DJ. Current management of psoriasis. *J Dermatol Treat* 1997; **8**: 27–55.

7   Greaves MW, Weinstein GD. Treatment of psoriasis. *N Engl J Med* 1995; **332**: 581–8.

8   Ellis CN, Gorsulowsky DC, Hamilton TA, *et al*. Cyclosporine improves psoriasis in a double-blind study. *JAMA* 1986; **256**: 3110–6.

9   Asadullah K, Sterry W, Stephanek K, *et al*. IL-10 is a key cytokine in psoriasis. Proof of principle by IL-10 therapy; a new therapeutic approach. *J Clin Invest* 1998; **101**: 783–94.

10   Fortune DG, Main CJ, O'Sullivan TM, Griffiths CEM. Quality of life in patients with psoriasis: the contribution of clinical variables and psoriasis-specific stress. *Br J Dermatol* 1997; **137**: 755–60.

☐ SELF ASSESSMENT QUESTIONS

1   Psoriasis may be triggered by:
  (a) β-haemolytic streptococcus
  (b) Propranolol
  (c) Lithium
  (d) Thyroxine
  (e) Milk

2   Key cytokine components of a psoriatic plaque are:
  (a) Interferon-α
  (b) Interleukin (IL)-2
  (c) Transforming growth factor-β
  (d) IL-4
  (e) IL-12

3   Chronic plaque psoriasis:
  (a) Female preponderance
  (b) Majority of cases present before age 40
  (c) Psoriatic arthritis in approximately 7% of cases
  (d) Nail involvement is rare
  (e) Genetic locus on chromosome 6p

4   First-line treatment of chronic plaque psoriasis:
  (a) 70% of cases treatable with first-line therapy
  (b) Vitamin D2 analogues are the mainstay of topical therapy
  (c) Tazarotene is a third-generation retinoid
  (d) The main side effect of psoralens plus ultraviolet (UV) A (PUVA) therapy is nephrotoxicity
  (e) 54% of patients consider current treatments effective

5   Second-line treatment of chronic plaque psoriasis:
  (a) Narrow band UVB (311–313 nm) is a promising treatment
  (b) Cyclosporin is effective only in treatment of pustular psoriasis
  (c) Targeting of co-stimulatory molecules such as CD1a is a promising approach
  (d) The autoantigen in psoriasis is collagen
  (e) IL-10 administration can improve psoriasis

ANSWERS

1a	True	2a	False	3a	False	4a	True	5a	True
b	True	b	True	b	True	b	False	b	False
c	True	c	False	c	True	c	True	c	False
d	False	d	False	d	False	d	False	d	False
e	False	e	True	e	True	e	False	e	True

The hidden epidemic of basal cell carcinoma

Richard J Pye

□ INTRODUCTION

Priorities, debate and databases for malignancies focus on those diseases that are commonly fatal and do not usually include indices of morbidity. As a result, skin cancer has tended to become synonymous with malignant melanoma in the eyes of the media and in many medical publications. Whilst this is entirely appropriate, given the death rate in younger people, it obscures a huge burden of disease and associated morbidity with non-melanoma skin cancers; that is, squamous cell carcinoma (SCC) and basal cell carcinoma (BCC). BCC is the most common cancer worldwide in white populations and, although it rarely metastasises, the majority of the lesions involve the head and neck, an important cosmetic area. In managing these patients, not only does cure need to be considered but also the cosmetic and functional consequences of treatment. This chapter concerns recent developments in the understanding and management of BCC.

□ INCIDENCE

True incidence is difficult to measure in a disease characterised by a high background prevalence and multiple new primary tumours in a single patient. A pool of undiagnosed lesions makes incidence data vulnerable to change with education and publicity campaigns. Treatment is often destructive, with no material submitted for histology. The size of the epidemic in countries such as Australia means that even epidemiological studies pose financial considerations. It is also unclear whether all multiple new primary tumours should be registered or only the first tumour. Since it is a multiple tumour disease, perhaps each patient should be registered to establish the incidence and the effect of health education programmes and, in addition, each new tumour be registered separately to measure workload.

These problems have meant that accurate and comparable data from various regions or countries have been difficult to obtain. In Australia, countrywide household market surveys of men and women over the age of 14 years have revealed age-standardised BCC incidence rates per 100,000 of 849 for men and 605 for women [1]. Other studies in geographically defined settings in Australia have shown comparable results, except in Nambour, a subtropical community in Queensland, where the age-standardised rates per 100,000 in 18–69 year olds were 2,074 for men and 1,579 for women [2].

The variation worldwide is high and, whilst much can be explained by ultraviolet radiation exposure, the aetiology is clearly more complex than had previously been supposed [3].

In the UK, the age-standardised rates per 100,000 are lower at 112 for men and 54 for women [3], although in East Anglia it has more than doubled over the last decade (Fig. 1). These data, taken from the East Anglian Cancer Registry, include only the first tumour. All subsequent tumours in an individual are discounted, although the incidence of second and subsequent tumours is high, possibly up to 50%, most of them occurring in the first year after the initial diagnosis [4]. This suggests that current registration data grossly underestimate the workload involved in the treatment and follow-up of these patients.

BCC occurs from the age of 15 years upwards, but is more common in an older population. The greying/ageing of our population suggests that the incidence will continue to rise. This represents a significant workload which has not been fully recognised in the planning of future service developments.

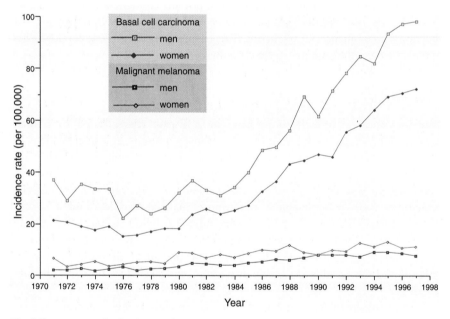

Fig. 1 European standardised rates of basal cell carcinoma (upper curves) and malignant melanoma (lower curves) in East Anglia, 1971–1997.

☐ BIOLOGY

The age-standardised incidence of BCC is much higher in white populations than in those with darker skins living in the same climate. Childhood migrants tend to acquire the incidence rate of the population they join, whereas those migrating in adult life show a risk midway between those of their adopted country and their country of origin. Individuals whose skin burns and who either never tan or tan poorly (skin phototypes I and II) are more at risk from BCC than those who always tan and rarely if ever burn (skin phototypes III–VI).

The precise relationship between cumulative dose of solar radiation and BCC risk is unclear. For example, in truncal areas the incidence of BCC is much higher than that of SCC, although these areas are not generally sun-exposed. The risk of BCC is increased by severe sunburn in childhood and by increased recreational sunlight exposure, particularly in childhood and adolescence. However, beyond a certain level of exposure, the risk of BCC does not increase further: thus, unlike SCC, the risk of BCC is not dose related [5,6].

These data suggest that the risk factors are similar to those for malignant melanoma. Health promotion messages should take this into account and target young people, parents and those caring for small children.

☐ GENETICS

In 1965, Gorlin described an autosomal dominant syndrome (now referred to as naevoid basal cell carcinoma syndrome (NBCCS)) in which patients have typical facies (bossing of skull and hypertelorism), developmental (skeletal) abnormalities and postnatal tumours (BCCs, which occur at an early age or in greater numbers than sporadic cases, and medulloblastoma). Within families, there is marked variation in expression of developmental abnormalities, age at onset of the BCCs, and the number of tumours.

Linkage analysis localised the gene to chromosome 9q22.3-3.1. A likely candidate was the human homologue of Drosophila segmental polarity gene, *Patched*. Several studies have now shown *Patched* to map to the NBCCS locus on chromosome 9q22.3, and mutations have been found in these patients and in patients with sporadic tumours.

The transmembrane protein *Patched* is a receptor for the morphogene *Sonic hedgehog*. *Sonic hedgehog/Patched* signalling involves another transmembrane protein, *Smoothened*, and its intracellular effectors, including the proto-oncogene *Gli* family. It is now well established that *Patched* is a tumour suppresser gene and is important in a number of human tumours [7]. Animal models show BCC-like tumours and/or developmental abnormalities associated with *Sonic hedgehog, Patched, Smoothened* and *Gli* family gene abnormality [8]. This signalling pathway is now emerging as an important regulator of oncogene transformation.

A number of patients with sporadic disease have 10 or more new primary tumours without any obvious risk factors. If studies show these individuals to have consistent gene abnormalities, their families may require genetic screening.

☐ TREATMENT

The diagnosis and treatment of many BCCs is based upon clinical judgement. Where there is doubt about the diagnosis, a biopsy may be of value and, in addition, provide information about the histological subtype of the tumour [9].

Surgical excision is the treatment of choice for well-defined, solid, cystic and superficial BCCs (Figs. 2 and 3). The extent of the tumour is a matter of clinical judgement, but cure rates of 95% and 93% at five and 10 years, respectively, are widely reported. Surgical margins vary, but the only detailed histological study suggests that a margin of 4 mm is required to produce these cure rates in tumours less than 20 mm in size [10]. Surgical margins are sometimes compromised around the eye and central face, leading to a higher recurrence rate.

Ill-defined, micronodular, infiltrating and sclerosing tumours have tumour edges that are difficult if not impossible to define (Figs. 4 and 5) and may extend to 15 mm beyond the clinical edge. There are no convincing data to suggest that surgery changes the morphology of tumours. Assuming adequate primary excision, recurrent tumours may have a mixed histology with a small infiltrating area that accounts for the recurrences. Both ill-defined and recurrent tumours require a different treatment strategy. Accurate histology reflecting all the margins seems to be essential to achieve cure. None of the reported range of histological techniques is ideal [11], but Mohs' micrographic surgery is probably the best as it allows review of the margins and same-day closure of the defects. Frederick Mohs first described this technique of horizontal sections in 1941, and it has been subsequently refined using frozen sections [12].

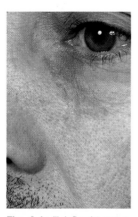

Fig. 2 Typical nodular basal cell carcinoma.

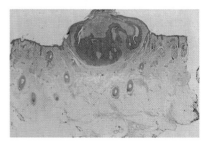

Fig. 3 Photomicrograph of a nodular basal cell carcinoma, showing the tumour to be well defined.

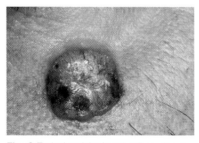

Fig. 4 An ill-defined tumour, for which even the diagnosis may pose a problem.

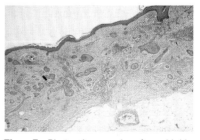

Fig. 5 Photomicrograph of a highly infiltrative and micronodular basal cell carcinoma. Nodules of tumour are similar in size to adnexae.

This technique is best performed under a local anaesthetic. Obvious tumour is debulked and, with a scalpel at 45° to the surface, a saucer-shaped excision is made to include the under surface and the entire epidermal margin. The tissue is then divided into sections, mapped and the edges colour coded to help with orientation. Each specimen is inverted so that the entire under surface and skin edge can be cut horizontally (Fig. 6). The sections are read by the operator, and the process repeated until the margins are clear. Repair is undertaken by either the operator or a reconstructive surgeon (Fig. 7(a)–(d)).

The operator needs to be trained in dermatopathology, surgery and reconstructive surgery. It is also essential that the operator is part of a team including technicians, dermatopathologists, plastic and occuloplastic reconstructive surgeons, and radiotherapists.

A number of advantages are conferred by Mohs' micrographic surgery (Table 1). Tumour can be accurately defined and the direction of the tumour spread identified, avoiding the need for 'blind' wide excision. This will often conserve tissue and

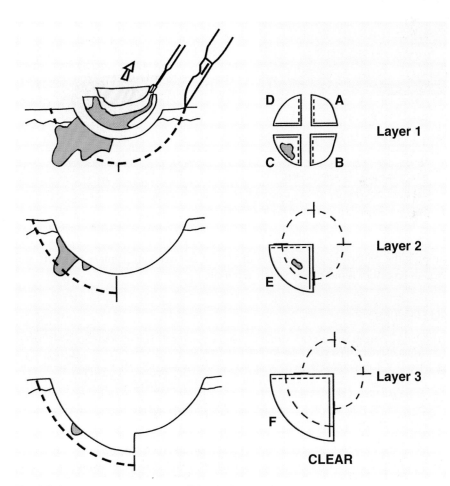

Fig. 6 A diagram showing the stages of Mohs' micrographic surgery.

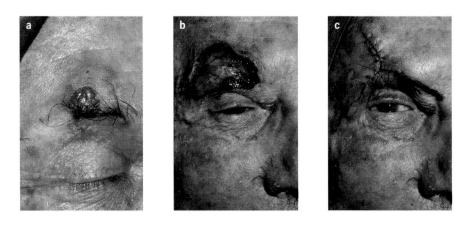

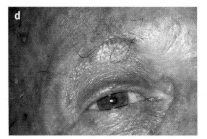

Fig. 7 (a) A patient with a mixed nodular and infiltrative basal cell carcinoma in the right eyebrow; **(b)** after two layers of Mohs' micrographic surgery all tumour has been removed; **(c)** immediate repair; **(d)** follow-up at four months

Table 1 Indications for Mohs' micrographic surgery.

- Micronodular, infiltrating and sclerotic basal cell carcinomas of the central face and periorbital area, especially in young patients
- Recurrent tumours, particularly those with an infiltrating history
- Tumours bigger than 20 mm on the head and neck

simplify the repairs. High cure rates of 99% at five years in primary tumours and 96% in recurrent tumours are widely reported.

REFERENCES

1   Marks R, Staples M, Giles GG. Trends in non-melanocytic skin cancer treated in Australia: the second national survey. *Int J Cancer* 1993; **53**: 585–90.
2   Green A, Battistutta D, Hart V, *et al.* Skin cancer in a subtropical Australian population: incidence and lack of association with occupation. The Nambour Study Group. *Am J Epidemiol* 1996; **144**: 1034–40.
3   Stern RS. The mysteries of geographic variability in non-melanoma skin cancer incidence. *Arch Dermatol* 1999; **135**: 843–4.
4   Karagas MR. Occurrence of cutaneous basal cell and squamous cell malignancies amongst those with a prior history of skin cancer. *J Invest Dermatol* 1994; **102**: S10–3.
5   Zanetti R, Rosso S, Martinez C, *et al.* The multicentre South European Study 'Helios'. I: Skin characteristics and sunburns in basal cell and squamous cell carcinomas of the skin. *Br J Cancer* 1996; **73**: 1440–6.

6   Rosso S, Zanetti R, Martinez C, *et al.* The multicentre South European Study 'Helios'. II: Different sun exposure patterns in the aetiology of basal cell and squamous cell carcinomas of the skin. *Br J Cancer* 1996; **73**: 1447–54.

7   Hahn H, Wojnowski L, Miller G, Zimmer AM. The patched signalling pathway in tumorigenesis and development: lessons from animal models. *J Mol Med* 1999; **77**: 459–68.

8   Murone M, Rosental A, deSauvage F J. Hedgehog signalling transduction: from flies to vertebrates. *Exp Cell Res* 1999; **253**: 25–33.

9   Telfer NR, Colver GB, Bowers PW. *Guidelines for the management of basal cell carcinoma.* London: British Association of Dermatologists, 1999.

10 Wolf DJ, Zitelli JA. Surgical margins for basal cell carcinoma. *Arch Dermatol* 1987; **123**: 340–4.

11 Rapini RP. Comparison of methods for checking surgical margins. *J Am Acad Dermatol* 1990; **23**: 288–94.

12 Shriner DL, McCoy DK, Goldberg DJ, Wagner RF Jr. Mohs' micrographic surgery. Review. *J Am Acad Dermatol* 1998; **39**: 79–97.

Key Points

▷ The incidence of basal cell carcinoma (BCC) is increasing at an alarming rate and it is the most common cancer in the UK

▷ Public health messages must be carefully targeted to the 'at risk' groups: fair skinned children and young adults

▷ Sun care should be encouraged, as should the avoidance of the noonday sun, the wearing of protective hats and clothing, and the use of sunscreens with a sun protection factor of 15

▷ As in malignant melanoma, the risk of 'flash frying' needs to be stressed

▷ Genetically 'at risk' individuals may be identifiable in the next few years. This will require a genetic screening programme, and patients will need careful counselling and support

▷ Treatment should be undertaken by suitably trained individuals, with Mohs' surgeons more widely available and perhaps in all major teaching hospitals

▷ Each patient with a BCC will require long-term careful follow-up by trained staff since up to 50% will develop one or more subsequent tumour

▷ The epidemic of BCC is beginning to have a profound effect on the departments of dermatology and plastic surgery around the country, and appropriate long-term planning needs to be undertaken

☐ SELF ASSESSMENT QUESTIONS

1   The effects of the sun:
   (a) Basal cell carcinoma (BCC) is more common in skin phototypes I and II
   (b) High childhood exposure is an important risk factor
   (c) BCC, like squamous cell carcinoma, is related to the cumulative dose of ultraviolet radiation
   (d) As in malignant melanoma, 'flash frying' and sunburn are important risk factors
   (e) Sunscreen protects against malignant melanoma but not against BCC

2   Non-melanoma skin cancer:
   (a) BCCs never metastasise

(b) BCC is the most common cancer in the UK

(c) Like malignant melanoma, BCC is more common in women

(d) It is rare for patients to have a second primary BCC

(e) Demographic changes will lead to a lower incidence of BCC

3 Genetics of basal cell carcinoma:
   (a) *Patched* is a tumour suppresser gene
   (b) *Patched* gene abnormalities are present in naevoid BCC syndrome (NBCCS)
   (c) Patients with NBCCS are at risk from medulloblastoma
   (d) *Patched* and *Sonic hedgehog* may be important signalling pathways for tumours other than BCC
   (e) *Patched* was originally identified in the bluebottle

4 Mohs' micrographic surgery:
   (a) 'Mohs' stands for 'maximum obtainable histological sections'
   (b) Mohs' is a system for obtaining complete histological sections of all tumour margins
   (c) Is the treatment of choice for nodular BCC
   (d) Is the treatment of choice for infiltrating tumours of the central face
   (e) Leads to unnecessary large defects

ANSWERS

1a True	2a False	3a True	4a False
b True	b True	b True	b True
c False	c False	c True	c False
d True	d False	d True	d True
e False	e False	e False	e False

Refining the management of HIV: the impact of recent therapies, drugs in development and new diagnostics

Graeme Moyle

The goal of all medical interventions is to prolong life and improve quality of life. In persons with HIV infection, given the available agents, this appears best achieved with combinations of potent antiretroviral drugs maximally to suppress viral replication (often called highly active antiretroviral therapy (HAART)), preferably to below the limits of a sensitive assay of HIV quantification. This generally facilitates at least partial immune restoration. Guidelines for the treatment and management of HIV infection have been developed in a number of countries in Europe, as well as in Australia and the US [1–4]. The British HIV Association (BHIVA) guidelines include a detailed discussion of their recommendations [5].

The guidelines attempt to represent the current state of knowledge but, as HIV/AIDS is a rapidly evolving medical field, it is inevitable that new data will change therapeutic choices and preferences. The expansion of drugs to treat HIV infection from only one in 1987–1992 to over 15 in 2000 has led to substantial increases in the complexity of HIV disease management. For this and other reasons, some guidelines recommend that only 'experts', people dealing with HIV infection essentially full-time, should manage HIV disease.

☐ DISEASE MARKERS

CD4 cell counts and plasma HIV-1 RNA (viral load (VL)) are used as markers of HIV disease in both clinical trials and clinical practice. Favourable changes in these markers, a decline in plasma HIV-1 RNA and increases in CD4 cell counts are the key means by which response to therapy is assessed. The dynamic range of these tests varies (VL: 50 copies/ml to over 500,000, CD4: 0 cells/µl to over 1,000). Additionally, VL tests show variability of about 0.3 $\log_{10}$ and CD4 counts by up to 25%. Diurnal, hormonal, and infection or vaccination related variation may increase the biological variation of the tests.

The relative importance and meaning of changes in surrogate markers in response to therapy may have different implications in early versus late disease. In advanced disease, the CD4 cell count is of greater prognostic significance than VL, whereas in early disease the reverse is true [6]. Most large controlled clinical trials in which it has been possible to assess the value of surrogate markers have been performed in patients whose CD4 cell counts were 200–500 cells/μl. In this situation, relatively transient falls in VL can produce a sustained increase or stabilisation in CD4 cell count, yet still influence the rate of development of clinical events two or three years later. Whether the value of treatment at the extremes of the CD4 cell count range, in particular during primary HIV-1 infection, is as great as in the populations studied requires further clarification.

The value of the availability of disease marker tests in accelerating drug approval and enabling disease staging is considerable, but such accelerated approval has led to relatively limited data being available on the long-term efficacy and safety of medications. For long-term survival, the suppression of VL over many years is likely to be important. However, most recent antiretroviral therapy studies are designed to examine short-term disease marker changes obtained in response to therapy (for the US, accelerated approval is generally 24 weeks), and subsequently to assess how well results are sustained to 48 weeks. Few studies include long-term monitoring of patients; most are terminated at 48 weeks or, at best, 72 weeks.

Furthermore, it is becoming clear that sequential therapy may be needed for long-term control of the disease. A particular combination may produce the best initial decline in VL which is also sustained for the longest period, but that same combination may preclude the use of a subsequent therapy either because of the emergence of a virus strain cross-resistant to other drugs of the same class or because of overlapping toxicity. Studies evaluating long-term strategies for sequential therapy, not simply initial therapy tactics, are only just beginning. The rapid changes in treatment paradigms through increasing numbers of drugs and improved sensitivity of disease marker tests have also added complexity to the attempts to answer these questions through database analyses.

New tests to evaluate HIV disease or guide treatment decisions are focusing on qualitative results rather than just on quantification. Virologically, resistance tests assessing either genotype or viral phenotype are increasingly available; their use is supported by three randomised clinical trials and the recommendations of guideline panels. More experimental is the potential to assess lymphocyte function and response to mitogens and antigens as a means of evaluating the function of the immune system, the benefits of therapy and the need for prophylactic medications. This type of testing is currently limited to a small number of laboratories; it is both costly and time-consuming, but is likely to become more automated and more widely available in the future.

☐ GETTING STARTED

The decision to start treatment requires, first and foremost, the consent and 'buy-in' of the patient. Commencing therapy is often a move from 'wellness' into the sick role, and the willingness to cross this Rubicon must be individualised and supported. The point at which a carer may move from suggesting the patient does not currently need therapy to one in which treatment should be considered, and then to the point of recommending therapy initiation represents a shifting in the balance of risk of therapy versus the risk of no therapy. Ultimately, part of that balance is that, whilst it is easier to keep a well person well than to make a sick person better, therapy in an asymptomatic person risks making that person feel worse. Actuarial analyses providing 3, 6 and 9 years' risk of AIDS or death, based on current CD4 and VL are available to assess risk [6]. Fewer data are available on what may be the risk of therapy over these periods. In general, a risk of less than 10% of disease progression over three years is considered to favour deferment of therapy, while a risk above 20% is a recommendation for therapy. The three groups of treatment-naïve patients for whom treatment guidelines are available are those with:

☐ primary HIV infection

☐ asymptomatic HIV infection, and

☐ symptomatic HIV disease/AIDS.

The recommendations of the BHIVA are summarised in Table 1.

The available drug classes act on two of the essential viral enzymes, reverse transcriptase (RT) and protease. Nucleoside analogue RT inhibitors are based on modifications of the natural purine or pyrimidine nucleotides. These agents act as both competitive inhibitors of RT and chain terminators of the growing HIV DNA chain. Non-nucleoside RT inhibitors act through attachment to a hydrophobic binding site adjacent to the RT catalytic site and thus disrupt enzyme function. Protease inhibitors (PI) bind competitively in the active site of HIV protease. This enzyme is a homodimer which is markedly dissimilar to human aspartic proteases. *In vivo* data indicate that HIV PIs have a wide therapeutic index with no relevant potential for inhibition of human aspartic proteases.

Table 1 When to start treatment: summary of British HIV Association recommendations [5].

HIV infection	Surrogate markers	Recommendation
Primary		If treatment considered, start as soon as possible, preferably within 6 months of acquiring HIV
Asymptomatic	CD4 count >500 cells/μl Any VL	Defer treatment
	CD4 count 350–500 cells/μl VL <30,000 copies/ml	Defer treatment
	CD4 count 350–500 cells/μl VL >30,000 copies/ml	Consider treatment or defer and monitor at least 3-monthly
	CD4 count 0–350 cells/μl Any VL	Treat
Symptomatic		Treat

VL = viral load.

☐ CHOOSING AND USING ANTIRETROVIRALS

The pivotal role of adherence in the success of antiretroviral therapy has been clearly demonstrated [7,8]. Characteristics predictive of poor adherence differ between studies, but generally include:

- ☐ psychological and psychiatric problems
- ☐ social and financial difficulties, and
- ☐ regimen complexities (eg food dependence, frequency of dosing).

Specific to HIV infection is the concern that taking of medication may accidentally lead to unmasking of HIV status to persons to whom the patient does not wish to disclose.

In real life, missing doses is most commonly due to simple forgetfulness and to drug toxicity, particularly upper gastrointestinal problems. Adherence is potentially more difficult in asymptomatic patients who may lack the reinforcement of an improved sense of well-being to stimulate regular pill-taking. For these patients, their first HIV-related symptoms may in fact be side effects from treatments which they have been told will help them.

These considerations have led to shifts in prescribing patterns – particularly in initial treatment regimens – to drugs with simple dosing schedules and low tablet volumes. With agents that are more difficult to administer, such as HIV PIs, the harnessing of pharmacokinetic interactions is now widely used to address variability in exposure and convenience of administration issues.

The value of performing resistance tests prior to commencing therapy, or at presentation with HIV, in guiding initial therapy has not been examined. However, this is widely considered in resource-rich environments. Data, mostly from continental Europe, the US and Australia, suggest that 10% or more of people presenting with primary HIV infection have acquired a virus resistant to at least one agent [9,10]. Interpretation of polymorphisms in resistance samples or natural variation in viral sensitivities, which have no influence on response to therapy, makes use of these tests at this time particularly challenging.

The British and US guidelines generally favour the use of two nucleosides plus either a (boosted) PI or a non-nucleoside RT inhibitor (NNRTI). Triple nucleoside approaches are currently under evaluation. They have advantages in terms of few drug interactions and low tablet volume, but more activity data are needed in persons with high VL. The recommendations in the UK guidelines are shown in Table 2.

☐ FAILURE TO ACHIEVE OR SUSTAIN VIRAL SUPPRESSION

Failure to achieve or sustain viral suppression may be secondary to:

- ☐ initiation of an insufficiently potent combination
- ☐ poor drug pharmacokinetics in an individual
- ☐ poor adherence, or
- ☐ viral resistance.

Table 2 Choice of initial therapy: summary of British HIV Association recommendations [5].

HIV infection	Regimen	Recommendation	Advantages	Disadvantages
Primary	Clinical trial	Recommended		
	HAART	Consider		
	No therapy	Consider		
Chronic	2NAs + PI*	Recommended	RCT evidence with clinical end-points	Toxicity common
			Evidence of efficacy in late disease	High pill burden
			Long-term follow-up	Drug interactions
	2NAs + 2PIs**	Recommended	Easier adherence	No clinical end-point data
			Better pharmacokinetics	Fewer comparative surrogate marker data
				Possible increased toxicity & drug interactions
	2NAs + NNRTI	Recommended	Equivalent or superior efficacy in surrogate marker trials at 72 weeks	No clinical end-point data
			Easier adherence	Lack of surrogate marker data in late disease
			Less known toxicity than PI-containing regimen	Shorter follow-up
				Little evidence of immune reconstitution
				Single mutations may lead to cross-class resistance
	3NAs††	Under evaluation	Spares PIs & NNRTIs	No clinical end-point data
			Fewer drug interactions	Short-term surrogate marker data only
				Less effective at high VL

* Hard-gel saquinavir should not be used as the sole PI. There are fewer data concerning use of saquinavir soft-gel in this context than for other PIs.
** Primary reason for combining PIs is to improve pharmacokinetics. Suggested regimens: low-dose ritonavir (ie 100–400 mg) with saquinavir, indinavir or amprenavir.
† Recommended NNRTIs are efavirenz or nevirapine. In one controlled trial, efavirenz was as effective in patients with VLs >100,000 copies/ml as in those with <100,000 copies/ml. There are fewer data from controlled trials to address this issue for nevirapine.
†† May be suitable for patients with VL = 100,000 copies/ml. Two regimens have been studied: abacavir + lamivudine + zidovudine and stavudine + didanosine + lamivudine.
HAART = highly active antiretroviral therapy; NA = nucleoside; NNRTI = non-nucleoside reverse transcriptase inhibitor; PI = protease inhibitor; RCT = randomised controlled trial; VL = viral load.

Viral rebound is usually defined as a VL above 50 copies/ml beyond 24 weeks, although this time point may be too soon in those who commence therapy above 100,000 copies/ml. Despite apparent virological rebound, individuals who maintain low VLs on therapy do not seem to progress in the short term, and the CD4 count may neither fall nor continue to rise. However, the longer that viral replication continues in the presence of drug selection pressure, the greater the likelihood that resistance will develop. For some drugs (eg 3TC or NNRTIs), a mutation at one position in the RT gene can cause high-level resistance. Thus, if viral replication is shown to be persisting, and other options are available which are likely to enable more complete viral suppression, therapy should be changed. Because of the known technical problems with VL tests, when a patient shows a rise in VL just above the detectable limit it should be rechecked within 2–4 weeks to confirm rebound.

In general, a good virological response is mostly likely to be obtained when as many of the drugs as possible in the regimen are changed. The minimum recommendation is to use resistance testing, and to include at least one new nucleoside analogue and at least one agent from an unused drug class. Interpretation of data from second-line and 'salvage' therapy is limited due to the heterogeneity of patients included in completed studies. What is clear, however, is that three-drug therapy does not appear to be adequate in the majority of patients given second-line therapy, and that regimens containing five or more drugs may be needed in people who have received all available drug classes.

☐ TREATMENT MONITORING

The potential to perform therapeutic drug monitoring, particularly of PIs, is currently being evaluated at a number of treatment centres. Response to these agents is known to be dose-related, and it may be possible in a so-called 'salvage' circumstance to overcome viral resistance through increased drug exposures. More data on ideal drug concentrations in the different circumstances are now required to assess the potential of therapeutic drug monitoring.

☐ NEW DRUGS FOR HIV

Given the problems with managing HIV disease in patients known to have multidrug-resistant virus, there remains an urgent need both for new drugs from available or established drug classes and for novel therapeutic approaches.

New drugs from available or established drug classes

Several new PIs are in development, most notably:

☐ Lopinavir (ABT-378/r), a PI designed to be active against most ritonavir – and indinavir-resistant viruses (the pharmacokinetic enhancer ritonavir is included in the formulation to enable twice daily dosing), and

☐ BMS-232,632 which is likely to be the first once daily PI.

☐ Tipranavir, a novel agent which does not rely on the peptidomimetic structure used in current agents, and hence it may be active against a wide range of viruses resistant to current PIs. More detailed pharmacology studies are needed before this drug advances into larger studies.

A similar range of new NNRTIs, with improved pharmacology and some potential for activity against NNRTI-resistant virus, is also in development. Among the nucleoside analogues, FTC has the potential for once daily use, and also possesses activity against hepatitis B.

The nucleotide tenofovir is the first agent in this class not to be associated with proximal tubule dysfunction, and additionally retains activity in the presence of at least some nucleoside analogue resistance.

However, many of these agents represent improved variations on a theme, and may not represent optimal therapies for all multidrug-resistant viruses.

New agents have been identified which inhibit HIV binding to either CXCR4 or CCR5 co-receptors, prevent viral fusion with susceptible human cells or block viral integrase. Many of them are, however, only in phase 0 development at present. The most advanced of these new classes is T-20, a peptide fusion inhibitor. Whilst requiring twice daily subcutaneous dosing (at present), this agent has demonstrated 1.5 $\log_{10}$ VL reductions in multidrug-experienced patients. It was shown in a single-arm phase II extension study that these responses may be durable in combination with a conventional 'salvage' regimen. Back-up compounds, possibly with activity against T-20 resistant virus and with improved pharmacology, are also being evaluated in phase 0.

Novel therapeutic strategies

Adjunctive therapies in development include therapeutic vaccines and immune modulators. The immune system cytokine interleukin-2 is now in clinical end-point studies, and has been shown to lead to impressive rises in CD4 cell numbers without perturbing viral control in treated individuals. Data demonstrating that these rises represent acceleration of immune restoration remain to be obtained.

☐ CONCLUSIONS

Treatment of HIV now requires expert management in conjunction with sophisticated back-up, including facilities to test VL, CD4 cell count and viral resistance. In the future, more detailed assessment of immune function and possibly therapeutic drug monitoring are likely to be widely used. The complexity of therapy in an individual increases with each viral rebound, and in many cases involves the use of considerable polypharmacy and the manipulation of drug exposures through the harnessing of complex drug interactions. An array of new drugs is in development, but many of those likely to emerge from current clinical programmes represent improved versions of currently available therapeutic classes.

REFERENCES

1   Delfraissy JF, *et al.* Prise en charge thérapeutique des personnes infectées par le VIH: recommandations du groupe d'experts. France: Flammarion, 1999.

2   Smith D, Whittaker B, Crowe S, *et al. Antiretroviral therapy for HIV infection: principles of use (standard of care guidelines).* HIV/AIDS clinical trials and treatments advisory committee booklet. Australia: NHMRC, 1997.

3   Carpenter CC, Fischl MA, Hammer SM, *et al.* Antiretroviral therapy for HIV infection in 1998: updated recommendations of the International AIDS Society-USA Panel. *JAMA* 1998; **280:** 78–86.

4   Centers for Disease Control and Prevention. Report of the NIH Panel to define principles of therapy of HIV infection and guidelines for the use of antiretroviral agents in HIV-infected adults and adolescents. *MMWR* 1998; **47:** 1–91.

5   The BHIVA Guidelines Writing Committee. *The British HIV Association guidelines for antiretroviral treatment of HIV seropositive individuals.* www.aidsmap.com.

6   Mellors JW, Munoz A, Giorgi JV, *et al.* Plasma viral load and CD4+ lymphocytes as prognostic markers of HIV-1 infection. *Ann Intern Med* 1997; **126:** 946–54.

7   Paterson D, Swindells S, Mohr J, *et al.* How much adherence is enough? A prospective study of adherence to protease inhibitor therapy using MEMSCaps. *6th Conference on Retroviruses and Opportunistic Infections.* Chicago, 1999: Abstract 92.8.

8   Demasi R, Tolson J, Pham S, *et al.* Self-reported adherence to HAART and correlation with HIV RNA: initial results with the Patient Medication Adherence Questionnaire. *6th Conference on Retroviruses and Opportunistic Infections.* Chicago, 1999: Abstract 94.

9   Perrin L. Transmission of drug-resistant HIV. *6th Conference on Retroviruses and Opportunistic Infections.* Chicago, 1999: Abstract S35.

10 Little S, Daar E, Keiser P, *et al.* The spectrum and frequency of reduced antiretroviral drug susceptibility with primary HIV infection in the United States. *6th Conference on Retroviruses and Opportunistic Infections.* Chicago, 1999: Abstract LB-10.

☐ SELF ASSESSMENT QUESTIONS

1   Available antiretroviral drug classes include:
(a) Nucleoside analogues
(b) Integrase inhibitors
(c) Protease inhibitors (PIs)
(d) Fusion inhibitors
(e) Interleukins

2   Viral load tests:
(a) Have natural variability of approximately $0.3 \log_{10}$
(b) Can be use for HIV-1 and -2
(c) Results may be higher after infection
(d) Provide prognostic information
(e) Have a dynamic range of 0–500 copies/ml

3   Suggestions in the British guidelines for second-line therapy include:
(a) Use resistance test where available
(b) Include at least one new drug class
(c) Avoid pharmacokinetic interactions between PIs
(d) Consider 'booster' drugs like hydroxyurea

4   Ritonavir:
   (a) May be used as an antiretroviral
   (b) May be used as a pharmacokinetic enhancer of other PIs
   (c) 600 mg twice daily is the minimal amount needed to boost other PIs
   (d) Must be dosed separately from lopinavir (ABT-378)

5   Available protease inhibitors:
   (a) Are peptidomimetic
   (b) Include efavirenz and nevirapine
   (c) Cannot be combined with non-nucleoside reverse transcriptase inhibitors
   (d) May have favourable pharmacokinetic interactions when combined
   (e) Involve low tablet loads

ANSWERS

1a True	2a True	3a True	4a True	5a True
b False	b False	b True	b True	b False
c True	c True	c False	c False	c False
d False	d True	d True	d False	d True
e False	e False			e False

Food poisoning

Hugh Pennington

'It must be something I ate' is one of the most frequently heard aetiological statements. It occupies this rank because it is often true. Gastrointestinal (GI) nfectious diseases are still common in Britain, even at the beginning of this new millennium [1]. (Ref. 1 provides an excellent general review containing a good deal of technical and public health data not brought together elsewhere in such a readable format.) This is reason enough for this chapter. However, there are other, equally good, reasons for considering these diseases at this time: they bridge the gap between 'bogs and drains' Victorian medicine and state-of-the-art molecular biology in particularly interesting ways. To understand them properly, we have to think in population terms as well as considering the management of the individual patient. GI infectious diseases demonstrate that epidemiology works in real time. The fact that one of the pathogens, *Escherichia coli* 0157, falls into the category of 'newly emerging pathogens' makes us realise that evolution can throw up new unpredictable challenges even in long established fields of medical practice.

What is food poisoning? The government's Advisory Committee on the Microbiological Safety of Food defines food poisoning as:

any disease of an infectious or toxic nature caused by or thought to be caused by the consumption of food or water

It encompasses a range of conditions caused by a variety of different agents including:

- [ ] bacterial infections (eg *Salmonella, Campylobacter*)
- [ ] pre-formed bacterial toxins (eg botulism)
- [ ] other biological toxins (eg paralytic shellfish and scombrotoxin poisoning)
- [ ] viral infections (eg small round structured viruses (SRSVs))
- [ ] other parasitic infections (eg protozoa), and
- [ ] toxic chemicals (eg heavy metals).

☐ FOOD POISONING STATISTICS

The Communicable Disease Surveillance Centre of the Public Health Laboratory Service publishes quantitative data weekly in its Communicable Disease Report on the amount of food poisoning in England and Wales. A recent summary of laboratory reports (Table 1) shows the provisional position at the end of 1999. Before examining their impact, consideration must be given to their significance. Like most health statistics, these numbers do not accurately reflect the burden of disease. Laboratory reports have at present no statutory basis. Their main problem is that they refer only to cases which present themselves to a doctor, who then successfully investigates them bacteriologically. This is a minority of patients in the case of food poisoning and, until recently, the size of this minority has been estimated only by guesswork. The main utility of laboratory data is that they demonstrate changes in the incidence of different infections over time. This measure is affected by alterations in laboratory practice, such as improvements in the sensitivity of tests, and by changes in the pattern of referral of samples for testing. The size of these effects is unknown because there is no way of directly estimating them. Nevertheless, the robustness of laboratory reports as an indicator of disease is much better than notifications. Although statutory, the latter are almost worthless, being part of an information system for infectious diseases which needs root and branch reform. Major weaknesses are undernotification or uneven notification, and a complete lack of reference to causative agents.

The Infectious Intestinal Disease study [3] is a recently completed major investigation into aetiology in England. Its detailed report has not yet been published, but those results that are available show that current statistics underreport the incidence of disease, by a few-fold for bacterial infection and by many-fold for viruses.

This chapter will focus on the four commonest and most important causes of food-borne illness:

- ☐   *Campylobacter*

- ☐   *Salmonella*

- ☐   *E. coli* 0157, and

- ☐   small round structured viruses(SRSV).

Table 1 Common gastrointestinal infections, England and Wales, laboratory reports for 1999 (from [2]).

Pathogen	No. of reports
Campylobacter	54,994
Salmonella	17,000*
Escherichia coli 0157	1,102[†]
Rotavirus	14,965
SRSV	2,005

* provisional
[†] verocytotoxin producing isolates
SSRV = small round structured virus.

Rotavirus is an important intestinal infectious disease, but it is hardly ever spread by food and so will not be discussed further.

☐ CAMPYLOBACTER

Campylobacter jejuni [4] is the commonest cause of acute bacterial enteritis in the UK. (Ref. 4 is a well focused account with emphasis on unsolved problems, out of date in only a few respects.) *Campylobacter spp* occur naturally in the intestines of a wide range of wild and domesticated animals and birds, and can be found in inland and coastal waters as a result of faecal contamination by animals and sewage discharge. Human infections arise from direct contact with animals or through contact with naturally contaminated raw or undercooked food products such as poultry and other meats. Contaminated untreated milk has caused several large outbreaks. However, such occurrences are rare and the majority of infections are sporadic. The source of infection in most cases remains unidentified.

Infection has been established in a volunteer with a dose of 500 organisms taken in a glass of milk. A low infectious dose is consistent with the high attack rates observed in water-borne and milk-borne outbreaks of infection.

An estimate of the incubation period calculated from 'point-source' outbreaks and volunteer experiments is three days, with a range of 1.5–4 days. It has been said that abdominal pain lasts longer and is more severe in *Campylobacter* enteritis than in *Salmonella* enteritis. It may also precede the onset of diarrhoea and, if severe, the patients (usually young adults) may be admitted to hospital with suspected appendicitis. The onset of diarrhoea, with liquid bile-stained stools, is often abrupt. Resolution occurs spontaneously after a few days. The most frequent complication is reactive arthritis, which affects about 1–2% of patients. Serological evidence of recent *Campylobacter* infection has been reported in 14–38% of patients with the Guillain-Barré syndrome.

☐ ESCHERICHIA COLI O157

E. coli O157 infections cause a range of illnesses in humans [5]. This strain is an *E. coli* clone differing from those normally found in the human gut by possessing additional virulence factors, including:

- ☐ the expression of one or more verocytotoxins (potent Shiga-like toxins), and

- ☐ a pathogenicity island: this is a large block of DNA coding for multiple factors including:

  - – intimin, an outer membrane protein (coded by the *eae* gene) involved in the intimate attachment of bacteria to enterocytes and subsequent effacement of microvilli, and

  - – the *tir* protein, which is translocated into host enterocytes to act as the receptor for intimin.

Other *E. coli* serotypes (0111, 0261) have also been described as causing haemorrhagic colitis and the other complications associated with *E. coli* 0157 infections, but they have not been important – so far – in the UK. A proportion of infections is asymptomatic. Clinical manifestations include:

☐ mild diarrhoea

☐ haemorrhagic colitis

☐ the haemolytic uraemic syndrome (HUS), and

☐ thrombotic thrombocytopaenic purpura (TTP).

Haemorrhagic colitis consists of inflammation of the large bowel, with severe bloody diarrhoea. It occurs in about half of all cases, and may require hospitalisation. Symptoms usually resolve within two weeks.

HUS presents as a combination of anaemia, acute renal failure and low platelet count, which may be accompanied by fever. A minority (2–3%) of those with *E. coli* 0157 infection go on to develop HUS; this is more likely in children under five years and the elderly. HUS is the commonest cause of acute renal failure in children in the UK. Its onset is usually preceded by diarrhoea, often about a week earlier. Dialysis may be required during the acute phase. Although the progress is generally good in children, a minority of patients develop long-term sequelae, such as hypertension and end-stage renal failure.

TTP is characterised by fever with skin and central nervous system involvement, and is thought to be due to the aggregation of platelets in various organs. The incubation period is about three days. Most cases commonly present as diarrhoea accompanied by severe abdominal cramps, and vomiting may occur. There may be permanent brain damage.

E. coli 0157 exists in a wide range of animals (wild, farmyard and domestic) and even birds. Its main reservoir is the rumens and intestines of cattle, and possibly sheep. Animal manure or slurry can be a source of environmental or water contamination, and can directly contaminate food such as vegetables. It seems likely that there can be animal to animal infection/re-infection. There is good evidence that it is transferred to animal carcasses through contamination from faecal matter during the slaughter process. Outbreaks, particularly in the USA, have been associated with the consumption of rare hamburgers. Outbreaks have also been attributed to other meats, milk, cheese and apple juice. In a large Japanese outbreak, radishes were a possible source of the infection. The vehicle for most cases of infection, however, remains unknown.

The organism survives well in frozen storage. It is killed by heating but survives if food is not properly cooked. If appropriate hygiene measures are not taken, there can also be cross-contamination between raw meat carrying the organism and cooked or ready-to-eat foods. It is relatively tolerant to acidic conditions (compared, for example, with *Salmonella*).

Human infection may occur as a result of direct contact with animals carrying the organism, from contamination from their faeces or through consumption of contaminated food or water. It may also spread directly from person to person as a result of poor hygiene practices, which allow faecal-oral spread. The latter is a particular potential problem in institutions such as nursing homes, day-care centres or hospitals, and in places where pre-school children meet. Outbreaks have occurred in these circumstances. The role of asymptomatic food handlers in outbreaks is unclear, but may be important in light of the low infectious dose, which can be as low as 10–100 organisms.

☐ SALMONELLA

The *Salmonella* group includes over 2,200 different serotypes of closely related bacteria. A short incubation period of 6–48 hours (usually 12–36 hours) is followed by the onset of classical food poisoning symptoms and signs: diarrhoea, abdominal pain and vomiting, usually with fever. *S. enteritidis* Phage Type 4 has been of particular concern in recent years because it is able to contaminate egg contents following infection of chicken reproductive tissues. There was a big increase in *S. enteritidis* food poisoning in the late 1980s and early 1990s, and it was the main driving force behind the overall upward trend in *Salmonella* cases during this time. Large doses of *Salmonella* are usually required for human infection, but this varies with serotype and can be low if the organism is contained in foods such as chocolate, cheese and salami. Minimal infective doses also vary with age and health; in the young they are very low.

   S. typhimurium DT104 has also caused concern in recent years because of its resistance to a range of antibiotics (ampicillin, chloramphenicol, streptomycin, sulphonamides and tetracycline) [6]. *S. typhimurium* DT104 infections in humans also increased during the 1990s. Outbreak investigations implicated a wide range of food products as vehicles, reflecting the prevalence of these bacteria among farm animals and poultry. A number of cases have also occurred in people caring for livestock (particularly calves), suggesting a possible occupational risk to farm staff.

☐ SMALL ROUND STRUCTURED VIRUSES

SRSV gastroenteritis occurs throughout the year [7]. Following a dose-dependent incubation period of 15–50 hours, clinical symptoms develop rapidly (fever, malaise, abdominal cramps, projectile vomiting, diarrhoea). The virus spreads easily from person to person by the faecal/oral route. Environmental contamination and spread by vomit (hand to mouth, via contaminated surfaces, and by aerosol) occur frequently. Spread by contamination of food by food handlers may also occur. Excretion of SRSVs occurs throughout the symptomatic period (usually 24–48 hours) and for at least two days after recovery. The infectious dose in SRSV infection is thought to be as little as 10–100 virus particles, which accounts for explosive outbreaks.

☐ TREATMENT OF FOOD POISONING

Uncomplicated cases in previously healthy persons not at the extremes of age nearly always resolve spontaneously and specific treatment by antibiotics is unnecessary.

Indeed, there is evidence that antibiotics may prolong the duration of excretion of *Salmonella* organisms, and with *E. coli* 0157 may be associated with the development of HUS. Erythromycin has been used for severe *Campylobacter* infections. Dehydration sometimes needs active management. Renal insufficiency in HUS may require dialysis, but no specific treatment for this condition has been shown to affect its course or to prevent TTP.

☐ AETIOLOGICAL DIAGNOSIS OF FOOD POISONING

The identification of the causative organism in faeces (or vomit for SRSV) is by far the most secure way of making an aetiological diagnosis. Bacterial culture allows a precise identification to type or subtype – a crucial step in the investigation of outbreaks and in the tracking of the source of the organisms. SRSV cannot be cultured, and electron microscopy for virus identification is still widely used although polymerase chain reaction is playing an increasing role. The serotyping of *Salmonella* isolates gives useful information and can be supplemented by phage typing, which is also used to subgroup *E. coli* 0157 isolates. High-resolution molecular typing methods are used in outbreaks of both these organisms and of *Campylobacter* to establish whether the causative organism is coming from a point source. Pulsed field gel electrophoresis, which analyses genome fragments produced by rare-cutter restriction enzymes, is the method of choice.

☐ FOOD POISONING IN 2000

What is the current position? There is one major piece of good news (Fig. 1). The fall in the number of reports of salmonellosis that started after a peak in 1997 has continued in a satisfactory way. The provisional total for 1999 of just over 17,000 cases represents a fall of 34% from the 1998 total of 23,728 cases; it is slightly more than half the 1997 figure of over 32,500, and is the lowest figure since 1986. It is reasonable to suppose that improvements in hen house hygiene, coupled with the vaccination of poultry, are responsible. Major falls have not, however, been recorded for *Campylobacter* and *E. coli* 0157. The number of laboratory reports for the latter rose from 902 in 1998 to 1,102 in 1999. *Campylobacter* figures fell only from 58,059 to 54,994 cases.

The UK Food Standards Agency

The starting position for the new UK Food Standards Agency, which begins operating in 2000, is that it inherits a policy for *Salmonella* that seems to be working well – that of eliminating the pathogen at source. For *E. coli* 0157 and *Campylobacter* there is still a long way to go. The best that can be said, in general, for attempts to control these pathogens by improvements in slaughterhouses, meat processing, butchers' shops, catering establishments and food hygiene is that they are containing the problem rather than solving it.

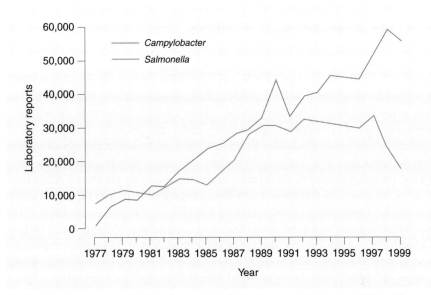

Fig. 1 Laboratory reports of selected gastrointestinal pathogens in England and Wales (*Sources:* Public Health Laboratory Service (PHLS) *Salmonella* data set and laboratory reports to the Communicable Disease Surveillance Centre of the PHLS).

☐ WHAT NEEDS TO BE DONE?

Food poisoning demands attention because:

☐ it is common (mostly now due to *Campylobacter*)

☐ it can cause very severe illness with significant mortality rates (mostly following *E. coli* 0157 infections), and

☐ it is preventable (recent successes with *Salmonella* are showing the way).

Many outstanding questions remain:

1 The source of the organism is unknown in the overwhelming majority of *Campylobacter* infections.

2 We do not know how to prevent or specifically treat HUS that follows *E. coli* 0157 infections. The verocytotoxins VT1 and VT2 produced by the organism are thought to be involved, but the detailed pathogenetic mechanisms are not understood.

3 We do not know how to get rid of *E. coli* 0157 from cattle. This organism appeared in the UK only in 1983, and had never been detected anywhere in the world before the late 1970s. It is now becoming a significant issue because, as knowledge about *E. coli* 0157 builds up, it seems that the spread of the organism directly from animals or from the environment may be more important than previously thought.

4   We have no idea why human *E. coli* 0157 infections are more common in Scotland than anywhere else in the world.

☐ THE POLITICS OF FOOD POISONING IS DRIVEN BY ITS BIOLOGY

In the year in which the new UK Food Standards Agency starts work any account of food poisoning would be incomplete without some discussion of why the government moved to establish such a body. To do this, the political importance of food safety needs consideration. There is a paradox here. Roughly speaking, for every person recorded as suffering from food poisoning one dies of coronary heart disease. Yet legislators have bent all their efforts to preventing the former rather than the latter. Why is this? Clearly, the state has a major role in protecting public safety. The public constantly exerts pressure for this to be done effectively. Not unreasonably, there is an expectation that food consumed in a restaurant or bought in good faith in a shop should not cause acute illness a day or two later. Outbreaks have a particular resonance, which causes them massively to influence public opinion and drive policy. Coronary heart disease does not cause outbreaks and, as a result, suffers as a health issue.

Central Scotland *Escherichia coli* 0157 outbreak

Events that took place during the Central Scotland *E. coli* 0157 outbreak in November and December 1996 provide a vivid illustration as to why food poisoning can have such an impact [8]. To date, it stands as one of the largest outbreaks worldwide in terms of mortality (21 associated deaths) and the largest in Europe in the number of human infections (503 cases, with 279 confirmed microbiologically).

The outbreak was made up of several separate but related components, one of which was the church hall incident. From time to time Wishaw Old Parish Church holds a special lunch for old and frail members of the parish. On 17 November 1996, the 74 people who attended were served cooked beef stew (later shown to contain the organism) with puff pastry. They started to fall ill two days later, 45 became infected, 17 were admitted to hospital, and eight died (aged 69–83 years). Only three of those who died had suffered from previous conditions likely to exacerbate a GI infection.

Events as dramatic as these make it easy to understand why food poisoning – and food safety in general – so often occupies centre stage!

REFERENCES

1   *Safer eating. Microbiological food poisoning and its prevention.* London: Parliamentary Office of Science and Technology, 1997.

2   Common gastrointestinal infections. Annual summary. *CDR Weekly*, 14 January 2000: **10**.

3   Wheeler JG, Sethi D, Cowden JM, *et al.* Study of infectious intestinal disease in England: rates in the community, presenting to general practice, and reported to national surveillance. *Br Med J* 1999; **318**: 1046–50.

4   Advisory Committee on the Microbiological Safety of Food. *Interim report on Campylobacter.* London: HMSO, 1993.

5   Kaper JB, O'Brien AD (eds). *Escherichia coli 0157:H7 and other Shiga toxin-producing E. coli strains.* Washington, DC: ASM Press, 1998.

6   Advisory Committee on the Microbiological Safety of Food. *Report on microbial antibiotic resistance in relation to food safety.* London: The Stationery Office, 1999.

7   Advisory Committee on the Microbiological Safety of Food. *Report on foodborne viral infections.* London: The Stationery Office, 1998.

8   The Pennington Group. Report on the circumstances leading to the 1996 outbreak of infection with *E. coli* 0157 in Central Scotland, the implications for food safety and the lessons to be learned. Edinburgh: The Stationery Office, 1997.

☐ SELF ASSESSMENT QUESTIONS

1   Food poisoning:
   (a) Is statutorily notifiable
   (b) Is over-reported in national statistics
   (c) Is commonly caused by rotaviruses
   (d) Is commonly caused by *Campylobacter*
   (e) Has become much commoner in the last two decades

2   *Campylobacter:*
   (a) Is the commonest bacterial cause of gastrointestinal infectious disease
   (b) Is associated with the Guillain-Barré syndrome
   (c) Is commonly found in shellfish
   (d) Commonly causes food poisoning outbreaks
   (e) Is commonly found on uncooked poultry meat

3   *Escherichia coli* 0157 infections:
   (a) Have a higher complications rate in children aged 5 and under
   (b) Can have a high mortality rate in the elderly
   (c) Lead in a minority of cases to the haemolytic uraemic syndrome
   (d) Are rarely spread person-to-person
   (e) May lead to severe and permanent brain damage

4   Small round structured viruses:
   (a) Can spread readily by the aerosol route
   (b) Cause explosive outbreaks
   (c) Cause projectile vomiting
   (d) Are always spread by food
   (e) Can be rapidly diagnosed by ELISA tests

5   The use of antibiotics:
   (a) May prolong *Salmonella* infections
   (b) May increase the incidence of the haemolytic uraemic syndrome following *E. coli* 0157 infections
   (c) In animals has led to the development of resistance in *Salmonella typhimurium*

(d) May be required to treat systemic infections caused by *Salmonella* or *Campylobacter*

(e) Is associated with the reactive arthritis that sometimes follows *Campylobacter* infections

ANSWERS

1a True	2a True	3a True	4a True	5a True
b False	b True	b True	b True	b True
c False	c False	c True	c True	c True
d True	d False	d False	d False	d True
e True	e True	e True	e False	e False

The current drug scene

John Henry

☐ INTRODUCTION

Drug misuse is having an increasing effect on many aspects of society. The 'rave' and club scene have seen a variety of substances promoted as dance drugs; cannabis use is widespread, and addictive drugs such as heroin and cocaine have made a major impact, even though they may be initially promoted as 'recreational'. Although harm limitation messages attempt to minimise the immediate and long-term dangers to health, drug use now has many medical and social consequences. Because of the frequency and intensity of use, many drug users end up as patients, often with unusual symptoms and syndromes. Today's physician therefore needs to be aware of the acute and long-term complications of drug misuse at all levels, from the casual user who experiences complications to the addict with major medical and social problems. It is also necessary to have a grasp of the steps to be taken in managing the clinical problems which occur. This chapter provides an update on some of the commoner substances misused and situations encountered.

☐ OPIOIDS

Opioid misuse is the most common drug problem in Britain at present. Although it may start by being 'recreational', it soon becomes addictive: two weeks of regular use is sufficient to lead to addiction, with withdrawal symptoms if the drug is abruptly discontinued. Opioids, including heroin, may also be used to counteract the 'comedown' following the use of drugs such as ecstasy, and heroin may also be injected together with cocaine to minimise the 'crash' that immediately follows cocaine use. The main illicit opioid is heroin (diamorphine), and the strength of street supplies can vary from 10–90% purity. The most important feature of opioids is that they can depress respiration by slowing it; this is the usual reason why people die of opioid toxicity. In any individual, this effect is dose-dependent. Another major feature of the opioids is the degree of tolerance which occurs. The initial dose of pure heroin required to produce euphoria is 10 mg or less, but the average user attending a dependence clinic will be taking 750 mg of street heroin per day. There can thus be an escalation of dose by up to ten-fold as tolerance and dependence develop. Methadone is the favoured drug for opioid replacement therapy, but can similarly be toxic in overdose. The *British National Formulary* recommends a starting dose of 10–20 mg per day, but a

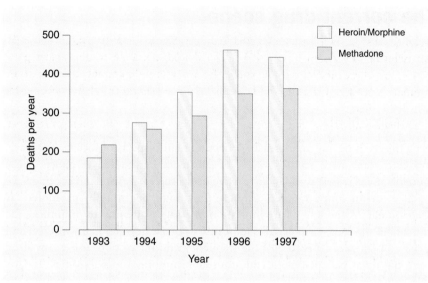

Fig. 1 Deaths involving heroin and methadone (Office for National Statistics, England and Wales 1993–1997).

dose as low as 30 mg might prove fatal for a non-dependent individual. The 'recreational' use of methadone derives entirely from supplies which have started as legitimate prescriptions.

Management of opioid overdose

The patient with an opioid overdose will usually have the typical signs of depressed consciousness, pinpoint pupils and slowing of respiration. The most important measure is to ensure that the airway is patent and that respiration is adequate. Cardiopulmonary resuscitation may be needed if respiration is inadequate or if a pulse cannot be felt. Mouth to mouth or bag and mask ventilation will be required if the patient is apnoeic or breathing slowly or irregularly. Naloxone is a highly effective antidote. A dose of 1–2 mg intravenously (IV) will usually reverse the signs of opioid toxicity within a minute, thus providing confirmation of the diagnosis of opioid toxicity as well as putting the patient's life out of immediate danger. However, the effect does not last long, so that further doses or an infusion may be needed. The patient should be restrained from absconding immediately in case of collapse a few minutes later as the effect of naloxone wears off. The benefits of naloxone are obvious and the risks are low. Adverse effects are uncommon; in 453 cases in which naloxone was administered to heroin-dependent patients, the incidence of complications was 1.3%. These included immediate violence, pulmonary oedema, convulsions and asystole [1].

Other complications of opioid overdose include pneumonia due to aspiration of vomit or inability to clear secretions, rhabdomyolysis due to pressure on muscles, and compartment syndromes also due to prolonged pressure while comatose.

☐ COCAINE

Cocaine is well known for its medicinal use as a local anaesthetic, but has recently become increasingly popular in Britain as an abused substance. Its pharmacological properties include inhibition of reuptake of dopamine and norepinephrine at nerve terminals, a tendency to thrombosis by making platelets more 'sticky', and a local anaesthetic effect.

The hydrochloride salt is usually snorted as lines of powder, producing an intense 'rush' due to blockade of dopamine reuptake at critical sites in the central nervous system. However, use of cocaine may also result in confusion, paranoia, hallucinations, aggression and violence. The other major pharmacological effect of cocaine, blockade of norepinephrine reuptake, leads to widespread vasoconstriction and hypertension. The combined action of these properties can lead to seizures, cerebrovascular accidents, palpitations, chest pain and myocardial infarction (MI). Chest pain is the commonest reason for attending hospital after the use of cocaine, and a recent study suggested that MI is 23 times more likely following the use of cocaine [2]. In some cases there are ST segment abnormalities which resolve. The patient needs to be observed for 12 hours in case an MI should develop.

Prolonged use of cocaine may also lead to depression or paranoia and violent, antisocial behaviour, including homicide and suicide. Because of its powerful vasoconstrictor effect, snorting cocaine hydrochloride causes damage to nasal membranes and the nasal septal cartilage. The repeated stresses on the cardiovascular system lead to accelerated atheroma, and data from the USA indicate that long-term users are likely to have an increased incidence of MI.

☐ CRACK

Crack cocaine is crystalline free base cocaine which is taken in the form of small crystals or 'rocks' which are vaporised by flaming a rock with a cigarette lighter and drawing the resultant vapour directly into the lungs by inhalation. It is believed to have more intense effects than cocaine hydrochloride and, in addition to the systemic effects and complications of cocaine use, causes local damage to the airways and lungs. Crack cocaine thus produces a further set of potential complications which may range from thermal injury to the airways to foreign body inhalation. Users tend to cough black sputum and may develop chest pain due to tracheal damage. Pneumothorax or pneumomediastinum may occur, and a sudden decrease of pulmonary oxygen transfer leading to hypoxia and shortness of breath may also occur, known as 'crack lung'.

Cocaine excited delirium

Many of the clinical features of cocaine toxicity became apparent during the epidemic of cocaine in the USA during the 1980s [3]. Long-term, regular cocaine users may develop a sudden severe disturbance of temperature regulation, followed by disturbed behaviour, collapse and death. Although rare, this syndrome is well recognised in the USA and Canada, and cases now occur in Britain. The user will feel that he is becoming hot, may try to cool himself with water, tear off his clothes and go out into the open. His behaviour becomes increasingly paranoid and bizarre and the police are frequently called to restrain the individual, who may then collapse and die (Table 1).

Table 1 Features of excited delirium.

Phase	Clinical	Behavioural
1 Hyperthermia	Rise in body temperature Profuse sweating	Attempts to cool body Removes clothes Goes into the open
2 Delirium	Paranoid behaviour Dilated pupils	Shouting Thrashing Violence Unexpected strength
3 Respiratory arrest	Collapse Breathing stops	Loss of strength
4 Death	Cardiorespiratory arrest	

Management of cocaine toxicity

Although there is no specific antidote for cocaine, there are several effective measures for controlling the manifestations of toxicity. Physical restraint should be avoided where possible. A high inspired oxygen concentration should be provided, and IV diazepam. This reduces cerebral excitation, prevents agitation, hallucinations and violence, and will also reduce blood pressure, so diazepam should be considered as the first-line agent. After this, nitrates can be used to reduce blood pressure. Aspirin should be given to the patient with chest pain to counter the prothrombotic effects of cocaine and prevent MI. Calcium antagonists may be useful if arrhythmias predominate, but beta-blockade should not be used in case it produces paradoxical alpha-mediated vasoconstriction.

☐ AMPHETAMINE SULPHATE

Amphetamine sulphate is widely used for its euphoriant effect. At low doses it increases wakefulness and can prevent accidents caused by drowsiness. Recreational use leads to prolonged wakefulness, impaired judgement and concentration, a sensation of rapid passage of time (hence its street name 'speed'), a tendency to repetitive behaviour and suppression of hunger and tiredness. Tolerance occurs, but addiction is uncommon.

Diagnostic testing

An ECG should be carried out as a screen for hyperkalaemia and cardiac dysrhythmias. A urine sample should be tested for blood and, if positive, be examined for the presence of red blood cells. A positive dipstick test in the absence of red blood cells strongly suggests early rhabdomyolysis, and aggressive IV hydration is indicated. Electrolytes and creatine phosphokinase should also be measured to screen for rhabdomyolssis and early renal insufficiency. A positive urine drug screen may confirm the clinical diagnosis in a patient with the above findings, and may help to define the duration of toxicity when either amphetamine or cocaine are suspected.

Management of amphetamine toxicity

Patients with evidence of drug use but without signs and symptoms of toxicity do not require any specific treatment other than a referral for drug counselling. Following stabilisation and satisfactory assessment of ABCs in a patient with potential amphetamine toxicity, physical and pharmacological restraints should be used as needed to prevent injury to the patient and others. Patients with agitation or autonomic instability should be sedated with a rapid, titratable IV benzodiazepine such as diazepam, lorazepam, or midazolam. Normalisation of vital signs may follow appropriate sedation with benzodiazepines or may require more specific therapy. Hypertension not responding to adequate sedation should be treated with a specific antihypertensive agent (considering the patient's age and probable baseline blood pressure). Phentolamine, a specific alpha-antagonist has been used successfully, especially for phenylpropanolamine toxicity: the initial dose can be 5 mg IV. Nitroprusside can also be used and may be more easily titrated. Beta-blockers should be avoided because they may lead to unopposed alpha-agonism and worsen hypertension. Patients with altered mental status, lethargy or depressed consciousness should have a computed tomography scan of the brain because both intracranial haemorrhage and infarction have been associated with amphetamine use.

☐ ECSTASY

The 'ecstasy' group drugs are amphetamine derivatives; the best known is 3,4-methylenedioxymethamphetamine (MDMA). These drugs are usually taken by mouth and their effects tend to be similar – they show no clear clinical or toxic differences. However, the contents of tablets sold as ecstasy vary widely. While some contain MDMA, others may contain amphetamine sulphate, caffeine, ketamine, LSD or mixtures of these substances in differing amounts. MDMA was widely used in the USA in the 1980s, but there were few reports of serious toxicity. The drug then came to Britain, where it has tended to be used as a dance drug at parties and 'raves'. In the early 1990s this led to a number of cases of severe and fatal hyperthermia [4]. This syndrome can be explained on the basis of the use of ecstasy as a rave drug (Table 2).

Hyperthermia

The hyperthermic patient usually presents with a history of ecstasy ingestion, usually followed by continuous dancing for several hours, leading to collapse or convulsions.

Table 2 Reasons for the acute hyperthermic and hyponatraemic effects of MDMA.

Reasons for hyperthermia	Reasons for hyponatraemia
• Prolonged exertion, warm environment	• Harm limitation message 'drink fluids'
• Amphetamine-like effect – disregard for body signals (thirst, exhaustion) – promotes repetitive activity	• Amphetamine-like effect – dry mouth and throat – repetitive behaviour
• Mood enhancing effect – euphoria – feeling of energy	• Mood enhancing effect – reduced inhibitions – impaired judgement
• Serotonergic effect – increased muscle tone, heat production	• Serotonergic effect – reduced renal response to water load (SIADH)

MDMA = 3,4-methylenedioxymethamphetamine.

Examination shows dilated pupils, sweating (though in severe cases this may have ceased), a marked sinus tachycardia (rates of 140–160 beats per minute are not uncommon), hypotension, and core temperature of 39–42°C. Cases such as this represent an acute medical emergency.

Management of ecstasy-induced hyperthermia

Once a high core temperature has been confirmed, one litre of 0.9% saline should be given immediately without waiting to measure central pressure. If this brings down the pulse rate and raises the blood pressure, a further litre can be given, after which the central venous pressure should be measured and further fluids given as required. The fluid replacement usually enables thermoregulation by sweating and vasodilation without the need for active cooling. Since severe hyperthermia reduces the calcium requirement for excitation-contraction coupling, further heat production may occur even in the absence of exertion once the patient has developed hyperthermia. This can be prevented by administration of dantrolene, which acts as a calcium antagonist at the level of the sarcolemmal membrane. This drug is indicated if the core temperature is above 39°C, but restoring fluid volume remains the first priority.

Ecstasy-induced hyponatraemia

Another problem seen in ecstasy users is acute hyponatraemia, with mute states, headache and vomiting secondary to excessive fluid ingestion. The problem here is that ecstasy causes secretion of antidiuretic hormone (arginine vasopressin), so that excess fluid leads to fluid overload because the kidneys do not respond. Severe symptoms may develop with plasma sodium levels of 130 mmol/l or above, and the urine is inappropriately concentrated, with raised osmolality due to excessive production of antidiuretic hormone (Table 2). In most cases, stopping all fluid input and providing supportive care is all that is required, but in severe cases IV mannitol, diuretics, or hypertonic saline may be indicated.

Other problems which may occur in ecstasy users include acute renal failure due to rhabdomyolysis, hepatitis (probably due to an idiosyncratic immunological response), cerebrovascular accidents and acute psychiatric disturbances.

Although there have been several reports of patients developing psychiatric illness, the proportion of ecstasy users who develop long-term psychiatric complications, such as psychosis, depression, anxiety and panic attacks, is unknown. Recent reports indicate that memory is affected in people who have used the drug intermittently for a couple of years. Longer-term use might lead to severe memory impairment [5].

☐ KETAMINE

Ketamine has a history of legitimate use as a dissociative anaesthetic for use in animals and humans. It is now widely used as a club drug, and has also been sold in tablet form as ecstasy. It may be snorted as lines of powder, but may also be smoked or taken by injection. 'Out of body' sensations and hallucinatory states are common and, although users may enter a drowsy, dreamy state, confusion, aggression and violence may occur. The pupils are usually widely dilated, and the patient may be sweating. Mild pyrexia is common. The most effective antidote for agitation or hallucinations is diazepam. Effects usually last about an hour, but may persist for 48–72 hours, particularly when the drug has been snorted.

☐ GAMMA HYDROXYBUTYRATE

Gamma hydroxybutyrate, known as GHB, GBH, Liquid X and Liquid E, has been used as a body building substance, diet supplement, anaesthetic agent and sedative. However, recently it has become a drug of abuse, as it produces an alcohol-like euphoric intoxication.

Overdose may lead to confusion, dizziness, drowsiness, nausea, vomiting and coma. Muscle tremors and spasms may occur and patients are often hypothermic. A fatal outcome is unlikely and management is supportive.

It is sold as a liquid, capsules or powder and tastes like seaweed. Gamma butyrolactone, a precursor which is metabolised to GHB, is also increasingly being used. Regular users may experience withdrawal symptoms on discontinuation.

☐ ALKYL NITRITES ('POPPERS')

Amyl nitrite is a volatile yellow liquid whose main use in the past was to relieve the pain of angina pectoris. It is provided in fragile glass ampoules which are crushed or 'popped' in the fingers and inhaled. It is one of the alkyl nitrites which are volatile liquids that are rapidly absorbed via the lungs; butyl nitrite and propyl nitrite are more commonly abused. When inhaled, they relax smooth muscle and lower blood pressure. Vasodilation of the cerebral vessels causes an increase in intracranial pressure and produces an euphoric effect which lasts about a minute. The peripheral vasodilation results in palpitations, skin flushing, hypoxia and dizziness, while the euphoric effect is experienced as a brief 'high'. Headaches are a frequent side effect and may persist for several hours after inhalation. The 'high' from alkyl nitrites is increased when combined with alcohol, which may explain why they are widely sold clandestinely in pubs.

Clinical manifestations of nitrite intoxication develop rapidly and depend on the route of exposure. Acute inhalation may result in hypotension and tachycardia within minutes. However, inhalation of high concentrations may also produce transient hypertension and bradycardia. Ingestion produces similar symptoms with the addition of nausea and vomiting. Excessive inhalation or ingestion may produce methaemoglobinaemia, and fatalities have occurred as a result of severe methaemoglobinaemia, but only after ingestion. Activated charcoal (50 g adult, 1 g/kg child) should be given within one hour of ingestion. Asymptomatic patients should be observed for a minimum of two hours post ingestion. If the patient is symptomatic, methaemoglobin levels should be measured. A patient who is cyanosed should be given oxygen in high concentrations; however, cyanosis occurs at a methaemoglobin concentration of 15%, which may not represent severe poisoning.

☐ LSD AND PSILOCYBE MUSHROOMS

LSD (lysergic acid diethylamide) is the best known hallucinogenic substance. The dose is small (50–200 μg), and is usually impregnated on paper squares which are ingested, though it is sometimes sold in small tablets ('microdots'). There is a high degree of tolerance to LSD, so that the drug is not taken on a regular basis and addiction does not occur.

Psilocybe similanceata (magic mushrooms) are small brown mushrooms whose psychoactive ingredients, psilocybin and psilocin, produce effects similar to LSD but which are usually shorter-lived and milder. It takes over 30 mushrooms to produce a hallucinogenic 'trip'. The effects of LSD usually begin within 30–60 min and resolve within 4–6 hours, or longer after a high dose. The effects produced depend on the state of mind of the user. Pleasant visual distortions are sought after, but the experience may be disturbing (a 'bad trip') and can lead to erratic or violent behaviour. Laboratory confirmation of LSD and psilocybe exposure is possible, but many laboratories do not have sufficiently sensitive assays to identify LSD in a urine screen. The clinical diagnosis is based on the history and physical examination.

Management

Physical restraint may be necessary to prevent harm to the patient, attendants or others. Any hallucinating or disturbed patient should be nursed in a quiet, dimly lit environment, and should be addressed by one member of staff, who tries to 'talk down' the patient in reassuring tones. Talking to another person in front of the patient may fuel paranoid thoughts and precipitate violent behaviour. Intravenous diazepam or haloperidol may be necessary as a means of pharmacological restraint.

□ CANNABIS

Cannabis is usually smoked, and sometimes ingested. About 10–15% of the population are now cannabis users, therefore the medical profession needs to know about its medical effects apart from the potential medical uses. Some patients with conditions such as multiple sclerosis and rheumatoid arthritis smoke cannabis because it relieves their symptoms. However, there is currently no licensed medical cannabis preparation in Britain apart from nabilone which is licensed for the relief of nausea in patients receiving anti-cancer medication. This topic has recently been reviewed by the British Medical Association [6].

Although Fig. 2 suggests that about 15 deaths per year are currently associated with cannabis use, it is highly probable that death was due to other drugs taken in these cases. Most people who use cannabis experience a relaxed, euphoric state, described as being 'stoned'. Although cannabis overdose is unlikely to be fatal, heavy use and overdose are likely to lead to agitation, hallucinations and paranoid behaviour. The Diagnostic and Statistical Manual of the American Psychiatric Association includes a wide range of cannabis use disorders and cannabis-induced disorders [7]. Its diagnostic criteria for cannabis intoxication (Table 3) help the physician to identify the clinical features of recent overdose or heavy use. The effects on the cardiovascular system can lead to dizziness and hypotension; tachycardia is a common feature, and the pink conjunctivae are characteristic and a useful diagnostic sign. The effects on reaction time and skilled activities can lead to accidents. Users are often unaware of the impairment, which may last up to 24 hours [8].

Although many short-term effects are clearly demonstrable, long-term effects are still debated. Since cannabis is usually smoked, it is to be anticipated that in time

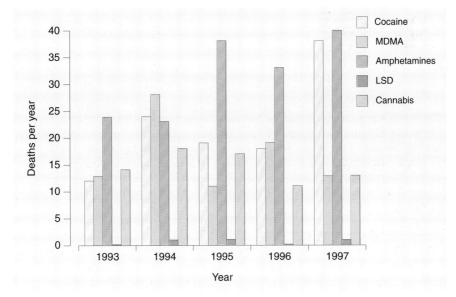

Fig. 2 Drug deaths other than from opioids (Office for National Statistics, England and Wales 1993–1997).

Table 3 Diagnostic criteria for cannabis intoxication [7].

(a) Recent use of cannabis
(b) Clinically significant maladaptive behavioural or psychological changes (eg impaired motor co-ordination, euphoria, anxiety, sensation of slowed time, impaired judgement, social withdrawal) that developed during, or shortly after, cannabis use
(c) Two (or more) of the following signs, developing with two hours of cannabis use: • conjunctival injection • increased appetite • dry mouth • tachycardia
(d) Symptoms are not due to a general medical condition and are not better accounted for by another mental disorder

many users will experience the effects of chronic cigarette smoking, including bronchogenic carcinoma, chronic obstructive airways disease and MI. Although it is clear that cannabis can produce hallucinations and psychotic states, there is debate as to whether cannabis use leads to schizophrenia. However, there does appear to be a clear association between cannabis use and the subsequent development of schizophrenia. The most widely cited report studied almost 50,000 Swedish army recruits and found a relative risk of 2.4 for all users of cannabis compared with non-users, while the relative risk was 6.0 for those who had used cannabis on 50 occasions or more [9].

REFERENCES

1   Osterwalder JJ. Naloxone. Intoxications with intravenous heroin and heroin mixtures – harmless or hazardous? A prospective clinical study. *Clin Toxicol* 1996; **34**: 409–16.

2   Mittleman MA, Mintzer D, Maclure M, *et al.* Triggering of myocardial infarction by cocaine. *Circulation* 1999; **99**: 2737–41.

3   Wetli CV, Fishbain DA. Cocaine-induced psychosis and sudden death in recreational cocaine users. *J Forensic Sci* 1985; **30**: 873–80.

4   Henry JA, Jeffreys KJ, Dawling S. Toxicity and deaths from 3,4-methylenedioxymethamphetamine ('ecstasy'). *Lancet* 1992; **340**: 384–7.

5   Gouzoulis-Mayfrank E, Daumann J, Tuchtenhagen F, *et al.* Impaired cognitive performance in drug free users of recreational ecstasy. *J Neurol Neurosurg Psychiatry* 2000; **68**: 719–25.

6   British Medical Association. *Therapeutic uses of cannabis*. London: Harwood Academic Publishers, 1997.

7   American Psychiatric Association. *Diagnostic and Statistical Manual*. IVth edn. Washington: APA, 1994.

8   Leirer VO, Yesavage JA, Morrow DG. Marijuana carry-over effects on aircraft pilot performance. *Aviat Space Environ Med* 1991; **62**: 221–7.

9   Andreasson S, Allebeck P, Engstrom A, Rydberg U. Cannabis and schizophrenia. A longitudinal study of Swedish conscripts. *Lancet* 1987; **ii**: 1483–6.

☐ SELF ASSESSMENT QUESTIONS

1   Cannabis:
    (a) Is harmless when smoked
    (b) Causes tachycardia
    (c) Is strongly linked with depression
    (d) Suppresses appetite
    (e) Can cause hallucinations

2   MDMA (ecstasy):
    (a) Is commonly injected
    (b) Is mostly taken at clubs and parties
    (c) Can lead to hyponatraemia
    (d) Is a major cause of drug related deaths
    (e) Can produce exertional heat stroke

3   Intravenous injection of illicit drugs:
    (a) Is associated with hepatitis A transmission
    (b) Is the most toxic route of admission
    (c) Is the preferred route for cocaine
    (d) Can lead to right-sided endocarditis
    (e) Development of hepatitis C can be prevented by vaccination

4   Cocaine:
    (a) May cause hallucinations
    (b) Chest pain is a common feature of toxicity
    (c) Cocaine hydrochloride is known as crack
    (d) May cause hyperthermia
    (e) Propranolol is the drug of choice for cocaine toxicity

5   Heroin addiction:
    (a) Is the main cause of drug related deaths in Britain
    (b) Tolerance is uncommon
    (c) Overdose causes rapid shallow respiration
    (d) Naloxone is an effective treatment for addiction
    (e) Methadone replacement therapy is curative

ANSWERS

1a False	2a False	3a False	4a True	5a True
b True	b True	b True	b True	b False
c False	c True	c False	c False	c False
d False	d False	d True	d True	d False
e True	e True	e False	e False	e False

New imaging techniques: positron emission tomography

Tim Fryer

□ INTRODUCTION

Positron emission tomography (PET) facilitates quantitative *in vivo* investigation of regional physiology, biochemistry and pharmacology. It is the most specific and sensitive means for quantitatively imaging molecular pathways and molecular interactions *in vivo*. PET provides information that complements the anatomical information obtained by X-ray computed tomography (CT) and magnetic resonance imaging (MRI). Medical imaging using positrons was first proposed 50 years ago and PET was first implemented 25 years ago, inspired by the discovery of CT. PET was initially used almost exclusively as a research tool in the assessment of various neurological and cardiac disorders. However, the past decade has seen the greatest expansion in the clinical use of PET, as its diagnostic utility and cost-effectiveness in a wide range of disease states, particularly oncology, has been demonstrated. PET is now regarded as the gold standard technique in the diagnosis of various oncological, neurological and myocardial diseases, and in the assessment of their response to therapy. Furthermore, the recent development of high-resolution small animal scanners allows PET to study *in vivo* animal models of human disease and fundamental biology, such as gene expression and therapy. Consequently, PET is expected to play an important role in the preclinical development of therapeutic pharmaceuticals, in addition to its current role in clinical trials.

□ FUNDAMENTAL PRINCIPLES OF POSITRON EMISSION TOMOGRAPHY

PET involves the administration of a positron-emitting tracer (radiopharmaceutical), followed by detection of the photons that result from positron-electron annihilations within the subject, using a PET scanner. Tomographic image reconstruction techniques, broadly similar to those used in CT, are then used to produce a 3D image of the radiopharmaceutical's distribution. Kinetic modelling techniques can then be used on the image and accompanying blood data to produce quantitative parametric maps of, for example, blood flow or pharmaceutical binding potential.

Positron emission tomography radiopharmaceuticals

As positron emitters do not exist in nature, they must be manufactured. The key positron emitters are produced by bombarding stable nuclei with positively charged ions using a particle accelerator (cyclotron). The cost of a cyclotron, approximately £1 million, and the building costs to house it are two of the reasons why PET is an expensive imaging modality.

Three of the most important positron emitters used in PET are carbon-11 (^{11}C), nitrogen-13 (^{13}N) and oxygen-15 (^{15}O). Molecules labelled with these positron emitters, for example H$_2$^{15}O, have the same pharmacological properties *in vivo* as the non-radioactive versions. This facilitates quantitative imaging and is one of the major advantages of PET over standard nuclear medicine tomographic imaging (SPECT). The short half-life of these PET radionuclides (^{11}C, 20.4 min; ^{13}N, 10.0 min; ^{15}O, 2.1 min) is advantageous in terms of both the signal-to-noise ratio of the acquired data for a given radiation risk to the patient, and the ability to perform multiple scans in one imaging session. However, key disadvantages are that radiosynthesis must be rapid, it is not possible to acquire useful images long after radiopharmaceutical administration and, most importantly, it is not feasible to transport these radionuclides to sites remote from their production.

The other key positron emitter is fluorine-18 (^{18}F), which can be used as a replacement for the hydroxyl group in key molecules. The longer half-life of ^{18}F (109.7 min) relative to the radionuclides mentioned above facilitates transportation of ^{18}F-labelled tracers to sites remote from a cyclotron. This, together with its proven diagnostic ability in a multitude of diseases, is why [^{18}F]fluorodeoxyglucose (FDG), an analogue of glucose, is currently the most widely used PET tracer. A detailed review of PET radiopharmaceuticals is given by Tewson and Krohn [1].

Data acquisition and image reconstruction

The data collected by a PET scanner (Fig. 1) correspond to detection of temporally coincident photon pairs. These photon pairs are produced when positrons, emitted from the administered positron-emitting radiopharmaceutical, annihilate with electrons naturally present in the body. The positrons usually travel about 1mm in the tissue prior to annihilation, and the photons travel virtually back-to-back to conserve the near-zero momentum of the electron-positron system at the time of

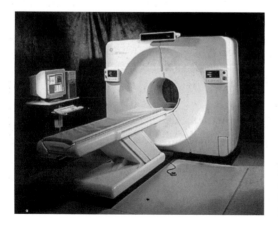

Fig. 1 The GE Advance positron emission tomography scanner (courtesy of GE Medical Systems, Milwaukee, USA).

annihilation. However, the standard assumption made in PET is that the point of positron emission lies on the line joining the detection points of the two photons (Fig. 2). A cylindrical configuration of detectors collects data sufficient for tomographic reconstruction of a quantitative (after data corrections) 3D image of the distribution of radiopharmaceutical. A more detailed discussion of the fundamental physics of PET can be found in a recently published book [2].

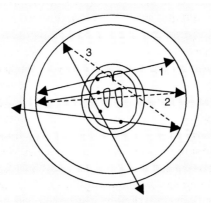

Fig. 2 Photon events detected in positron emission tomography: true (1), scattered (2) and random (3); quantitative imaging requires corrections for types 2 and 3.

Relative to CT and MRI, PET images have low signal-to-noise and poor resolution (ca 5 mm) (Fig. 3). The limited resolution reduces detectability of small lesions, and quantification of tracer concentration is compromised in structures with dimensions less than approximately twice the image resolution; this is known as the partial volume effect. Anatomical imaging can be used to ameliorate this effect. The next generation of PET scanners, currently in the prototype stage, will provide better signal-to-noise and resolution (ca 2.5 mm). These scanners may facilitate significantly more sensitive whole-body oncology imaging than is currently possible.

In most cases where the desired result of the PET scan is a quantitative map of a physiological or pharmacological parameter, blood samples must be taken during

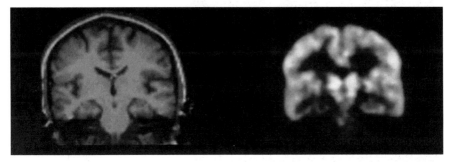

Fig. 3 Co-registered coronal magnetic resonance and [18F]fluorodeoxyglucose-positron emission tomography images.

PET data acquisition to ascertain blood radioactivity concentrations. In some cases, the radioactivity in the blood due to metabolites of the administered radiopharmaceutical must also be measured.

Data analysis

PET data analysis can be qualitative (ie visual inspection), semi-quantitative and quantitative. Visual diagnosis, the most common form of data analysis in clinical PET, can be improved in certain cases if PET is co-registered to an anatomical image (CT or MRI) and information from both modalities is utilised; this technique is generally known as image fusion.

One common semi-quantitative approach used is standardised uptake value (SUV) in FDG oncology, where the uptake in a tumour is normalised to the injected activity per unit weight or surface area. The aim of using SUV is to produce a reliable measure of tumour glucose metabolism using a single image without blood sampling, which can then be used to differentiate benign from malignant disease, and to assess the response to therapy. The reliability of SUV has been questioned, particularly for obese patients and those with diabetes mellitus.

To illustrate quantitative data analysis, consider FDG imaging. As FDG is not fully metabolised, it can be characterised by a three-compartment model with four rate constants (Fig. 4). In many tissues, the levels of glucose-6-phosphatase are low and FDG approximates a bound tracer ($k_4 \rightarrow 0$) whose tissue concentration tends to a plateau. In these circumstances, a single plateau image in conjunction with *a priori* rate constants and a dynamic blood curve (input function) can be used to quantify FDG uptake. Alternatively, the rate constants can be determined by acquiring

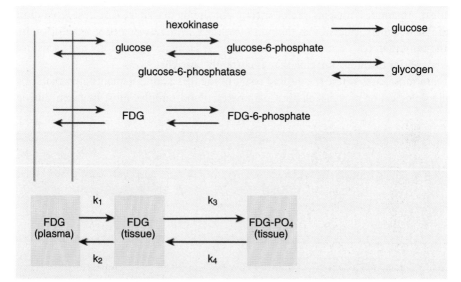

Fig. 4 Metabolic pathways of [^{18}F]fluorodeoxyglucose (FDG) and the three-compartment kinetic model for FDG (PO$_4$ = phosphate).

dynamic PET and blood data, and fitting the data to the compartmental model. To convert FDG uptake or rate constants into glucose metabolism, a conversion factor known as the *lumped constant* must be known. For highly metabolised tracers, such as [^{11}C]thymidine, a cell proliferation marker, the kinetic modelling can become highly complex and more than one scan may be required in order to separate the tracer from its radioactive metabolites.

Regional quantitative information can be obtained by performing the kinetic modelling with regions of interest (ROI) or by superimposing ROI on parametric images. However, parametric images are being increasingly analysed using statistical parametric mapping, traditionally used to localise activation sites in brain mapping experiments, to produce a map displaying deviation from normality.

☐ CLINICAL APPLICATIONS

Oncology

Glucose metabolism

The most common PET scan currently performed is assessment of tumour glucose metabolism using [^{18}F]FDG. This is based on the finding that, in general, neoplastic cells use more glucose than normal cells. Although this phenomenon is not fully understood, malignant transformation of some cell lines is associated with increased cellular activity of hexokinase, reduced activity of glucose-6-phosphatase and a greater concentration of glucose transporter proteins. The hypoxic environment found in many tumours may also contribute to enhanced FDG uptake. However, the variable uptake of FDG by benign tissues such as muscle and inflammatory cells can limit the specificity of FDG-PET [3].

FDG imaging has been applied to a wide range of tumours, notably lung, brain, head and neck, lymphoma, colorectal, melanoma, breast, sarcoma, oesophageal, pancreatic, ovarian, cervical and testicular (Fig. 5). The diagnostic uses of FDG are listed in Table 1.

FDG imaging is very helpful in specific situations where CT has known limitations, such as differentiation of recurrence and scar tissue (Table 2). A detailed,

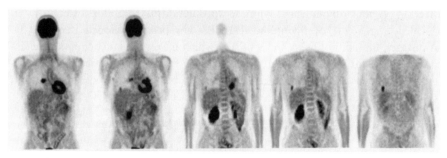

Fig. 5 Coronal whole-body [^{18}F]fluorodeoxyglucose (FDG)-positron emission tomography images reveal lung metastases for a patient with testicular cancer. Excretion of FDG leads to high image intensity in the kidneys and bladder (courtesy of the Institute of Nuclear Medicine, UCLH Trust Hospitals and UCL, London).

Table 1 Diagnostic uses of [^{18}F]fluorodeoxyglucose.

- Differentiation of benign and malignant lesions
- Staging
- Grading
- Guidance for biopsy
- Detection of recurrent disease
- Differentiation of recurrence from scar tissue
- Monitoring response to therapy

Table 2 Studies comparing the diagnostic accuracy [%] of [^{18}F]fluorodeoxyglucose (FDG)-positron emission tomography (PET) and computed tomography (CT).

Study	No.	CT	PET	PET+CT
Lymph node staging in NSCLC	105	64	85	90
Recurrence of colorectal cancer	49	63	93	–
Detection of pancreatic cancer	79	80	95	–
Staging oesophageal carcinoma	38	45	74	82
Recurrence of lymphoma	44	48	98	–

NSCLC = non-small cell lung cancer.

recent review of the applications of FDG in oncology is given in two articles by Delbeke [4,5].

Cell proliferation

[^{11}C]thymidine has been used as a PET tracer of the incorporation of thymidine, a nucleotide precursor, into DNA, and thus as a non-invasive measure of cellular proliferation. Analysis of [^{11}C]thymidine images is complicated as it is rapidly metabolised, producing radiolabelled metabolites that cannot be incorporated into DNA. Despite this, recent work has indicated that a kinetic model exists which can quantitate thymidine flux into DNA, and [^{11}C]thymidine has been used to assess the effect of various thymidylate synthase (proliferation) inhibitors. Recently, an ^{18}F-labelled analogue of thymidine, [^{18}F]FLT, has been developed that has the advantages, first, of not being metabolised (which makes the kinetic modelling less complex than for [^{11}C]thymidine) and, secondly, that it can be used at PET sites remote from a cyclotron. This tracer may prove to be one of the most important in the future of oncology PET due to its improved specificity over FDG.

Amino acid uptake

Radiolabelled amino acids have proven useful in imaging the enhanced amino acid uptake in tumours, especially brain tumours, but also lymphoma, lung tumours and breast cancer. The most common amino acid tracer is [^{11}C]methionine (MET) but this tracer is limited to centres with a cyclotron due to its short half-life. The desire for an ^{18}F-labelled amino acid analogue has recently culminated in the synthesis of [^{18}F]fluoroethyl-L-tyrosine (FET).

Hypoxia

Tumour hypoxia influences response to treatment and may also play a role in tumour aggressiveness and propensity to metastasise. Over 15 years ago, misonidazole, an azomycin-based radiosensitiser, was found to link to cellular molecules at rates inversely proportional to intracellular oxygen concentration. [^{18}F]fluoromisonidazole (FMISO) has proven useful in assessing hypoxia in human tumours; one study using FMISO detected hypoxia in 97% of the tumours investigated. It has been used to assess tumour hypoxia before treatment and during fractionated radiotherapy. More recently, [^{18}F]fluoroetanidazole (FETA) and [^{18}F]EF1 have been developed, whose main advantage over FMISO is that they are less readily metabolised. [^{64}Cu]ATSM may prove to be a more sensitive marker of hypoxia than FMISO.

Receptor imaging

The majority of breast cancers are hormone dependent, and oestrogen receptor (ER) status of the tumour is an important prognostic factor. The value of being able quantitatively to assess ER status has led to the development of [^{18}F]fluoroestradiol (FES), an oestrogen analogue with a high affinity for ER+ tissue. FES has been successfully used to image ER+ breast cancers, which are less aggressive than ER– cancers and more likely to respond to hormonal therapy; it is highly sensitive (93%) in detecting ER+ metastases and assessing their response to tamoxifen. However, FES-PET cannot be used to diagnose breast cancer because ER– and benign lesions cannot be distinguished.

Pharmacokinetics of anti-cancer drugs

By radiolabelling anti-cancer drugs, PET offers the possibility of quantitatively assessing their delivery, uptake and metabolism. Examples include [^{18}F]fluorouracil, used in the treatment of liver metastases, and [^{11}C]temozolomide which has found some utility in glioma and melanoma. Interestingly, the *in vivo* pharmacokinetics of temozolomide have also been assessed by labelling it with ^{13}C and using MRI. The sensitivity per gram of tracer was a million times higher with PET due to the very low tracer-to-background signal in MRI [6].

Gene therapy

The gene therapy approach investigated most extensively by PET to date is the enzyme/prodrug system herpes simplex virus, thymidine kinase/ganciclovir (HSV*tk*/GCV). The radiolabelled HSV*tk* substrates [^{18}F]fluoromethylguanine (FHPG) and [^{18}F]fluoroganciclovir (FGCV) have both been used to image HSV*tk* expression in tumours [7]. These studies are in their early stages, confined to animals.

Brain imaging

Brain mapping

Neuronal activation produces marked regional increases in blood flow. Consequently, blood flow PET, usually using $H_2^{15}O$, has been used in brain mapping studies. A bolus of tracer is administered whilst a cognitive task is being performed. Both normal volunteers and patients have been assessed. As well as fundamental brain research, activation studies are sometimes performed prior to neurosurgery to delineate the spatial extent of important cognitive areas. Only qualitative blood flow results are required, so functional MRI is rapidly taking over from PET for brain mapping studies as it offers superior temporal and spatial resolution, better signal-to-noise and eliminates the risk from ionising radiation.

Dementias

PET studies of dementia have revealed patterns of hypometabolism and, in some dementias, reductions in blood flow. Most studies have been aimed at Alzheimer's disease (AD), for which FDG-PET has been found to be the most sensitive technique for early diagnosis. In fact, PET can detect metabolic changes in pre-symptomatic patients, particularly in the posterior cingulate, and consequently it can be used to assess response to therapy in the early stages of the disease. For various dementias, hypometabolism in the temporoparietal regions tends to correlate with the severity of the disease. In AD, PET has indicated that this hypometabolism is due both to tissue loss and to reduced synaptic activity. A reduction in density of serotonin 5HT-2A receptors in the later stages of AD has been found.

FDG-PET can be used to differentiate the dementias from each other and from other conditions such as depression, based on the spatial pattern of hypometabolism (Fig. 6).

Movement disorders

Most PET studies of movement disorders have looked at Parkinson's disease (PD) and, to a lesser extent, Huntington's disease (HD). PD is associated with striatal dopaminergic dysfunction, which has been assessed using [18F]fluoro-L-dopa (FDOPA), a marker of levodopa metabolism into dopamine. FDOPA uptake is

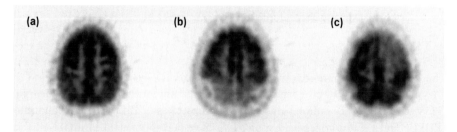

Fig. 6 Transaxial [18F]fluorodeoxyglucose images for **(a)** normal, **(b)** Alzheimer's disease, and **(c)** unilateral Pick's disease.

significantly bilaterally reduced in the putamen and, to a lesser extent, in the caudate contralateral to any PD movement impairment. However, assessment of metabolic changes in the basal ganglia and thalamic areas using FDG may be the most sensitive means of differentiating early PD from other syndromes that mimic PD. Both FDG and FDOPA have been used to assess the success of therapy through implantation of embryonic tissue containing dopamine-producing cells. Dopamine receptor D_2 binding, assessed using the antagonist [¹¹C]raclopride, is increased in the putamen of PD patients contralateral to the most affected side. The reduction of raclopride binding after administration of levodopa correlates with drug-free scores of disability.

In HD, there is a reduction in metabolism and D_1 and D_2 binding in the striatum, with caudate hypometabolism correlating well with functional status. The combination of FDG and [¹¹C]raclopride is found to provide accurate diagnosis of HD in asymptomatic gene carriers.

Psychiatric disorders

The underlying pathology and response to therapy of psychiatric disorders has been assessed by examination of blood flow and synaptic neurotransmission, particularly the dopamine pathway. Findings in schizophrenia, the most widely studied disorder, include blood flow patterns that correlate with psychomotor poverty, disorganisation, hallucinations and reality distortion. A whole array of PET ligands and radiolabelled drugs, particularly antipsychotics and psychostimulants, has been used to assess neuroreceptor status and the action potential of therapeutic drugs. These studies have indicated that the binding of certain neuroleptics is higher than empirically predicted. Consequently, lower doses of medications such as haloperidol can be used, reducing side effects. Recent developments include tracers used to examine post-receptor intracellular signal transduction.

Epilepsy

PET has predominantly been used in interictal studies of focal epilepsy due to the short half-lives of the tracers involved. In both neocortical and temporal lobe epilepsy, decreased binding of [¹¹C]flumazenil, an antagonist for benzodiazepine receptors, has been found to be a more sensitive and specific measure than hypometabolism revealed by interictal FDG which is, in turn, more sensitive than MRI. In addition, flumazenil is more accurate than FDG at localising the spatial extent of the epileptic focus prior to resection. Ictal FDG studies indicate a diffuse increase in metabolism, but the temporal resolution is not adequate to define the focus of activity. Imaging ictal activity is more feasible using SPECT with long-lived blood flow tracers that are extracted from the blood on the first pass.

Brain trauma

PET can provide valuable information on brain physiology after acute brain injury through its ability to image regional cerebral blood flow (CBF), cerebral oxygen metabolism ($CMRO_2$), oxygen extraction fraction and glucose metabolism. For instance, PET has indicated that unless intracranial pressure is very high, hyperventilation promotes ischaemia rather than diminishes it. This contradicts previous medical practice. PET is also being used to assess the diagnostic utility of bedside monitoring systems, such as transcranial Doppler ultrasound and cerebral probes.

A recently published review [8] gives further details on some of the above neurological applications of PET.

Stroke

In acute stroke patients, PET has revealed three main focal CBF-$CMRO_2$ patterns: reduced CBF and $CMRO_2$, reduced CBF but normal $CMRO_2$, and increased CBF and normal $CMRO_2$. The first and last of these patterns predict poor and good outcome, respectively. For the second pattern (intermediate severity), the volume of ischaemic penumbra revealed by PET has a greater prognostic accuracy than neurological scores.

Cardiology

Myocardial viability

Viable myocardium is that which exhibits improved systolic function after coronary revascularisation. Differentiation of viable and non-viable myocardium is of critical importance in assessing which patients with coronary artery disease (CAD) and left ventricular dysfunction will benefit from revascularisation.

Various PET protocols have been used to assess myocardial viability. The most common is to compare regional myocardial perfusion and metabolism using a blood flow tracer (usually $H_2^{15}O$ or $^{13}NH_3$) and FDG, respectively. Regions showing a concordant decrease in blood flow and metabolism are generally classified as infarcted and irreversibly injured, whereas regions with normal or increased metabolism, despite a perfusion defect, are considered ischaemic and viable. The assessment of metabolism in the myocardium is complicated due to the various substrates used to support oxidative metabolism. This limitation applies to fatty acid metabolism imaging using, for example, [^{11}C]palmitate, as well as FDG. Attempts to circumvent this include using standardised FDG imaging conditions, for example, the hyperinsulinaemic eugly-caemic clamp method, and tracers which give a measure of total oxidative metabolism: [^{11}C]acetate, which is oxidised in the tricarboxylic acid cycle, and oxygen gas ($^{15}O_2$). Certain studies have indicated that acetate imaging is a better predictor of viability than FDG; a comparison of techniques used to assess viability is given in Fig. 7.

Myocardial blood flow

PET measurement of myocardial blood flow, usually using $H_2^{15}O$ or $^{13}NH_3$, has been used in the diagnosis of various cardiac disorders. In patients with CAD, blood flow under rest conditions can be preserved up to a 95% stenosis, but hyperaemic

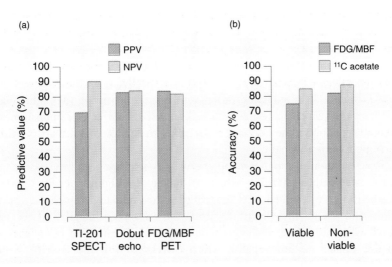

Fig. 7 Comparison of techniques used to assess myocardial viability: **(a)** multicentre trial results [9], **(b)** single-centre comparison of [¹⁸F]fluorodeoxyglucose (FDG)/myocardial blood flow (MBF) and [¹¹C]acetate positron emission tomography (PET) for dysfunctional myocardium [10] (Dobut echo = dobutamine echocardiography; NPV = negative predictive value; PPV = positive predictive value; SPECT = single-photon emission computed tomography).

response diminishes above approximately 40% stenosis and vanishes around 80%. Consequently, in combination with a stress agent, PET diagnosis of CAD is highly accurate (typical figures for ¹³NH₃: sensitivity 94%, specificity 97%). In the absence of significant CAD, coronary vasodilator reserve (CVR), the ratio of hyperaemic blood flow to that at rest, provides information on the function of the coronary microcirculation. CVR is globally reduced in primary and secondary left ventricular hypertrophy, indicating coronary microvascular dysfunction that may contribute to the development of myocardial ischaemia. Blood flow imaging can also be used to differentiate hypertrophic cardiomyopathy from secondary left ventricular hypertrophy (higher resting and hyperaemic blood flow) and physiological left ventricular hypertrophy (higher hyperaemic blood flow).

Hypoxia

Imaging of myocardial hypoxia is an alternative approach to imaging blood flow and/or metabolism in the diagnosis of ischaemia. Several *in vitro* and animal *in vivo* studies have shown the potential of [¹⁸F]FMISO (see above) for direct detection of viable ischaemic myocardium. However, other studies indicate that sensitivity to transient ischaemia (myocardial stunning) may be limited.

Autonomous nervous system

Dysfunction of the autonomic nervous system underlies a number of myocardial disorders. PET has been used to investigate these changes by assessing the status of myocardial receptors such as those of the β-adrenergic system which are involved in the control of heart rate, and the rate and force of cardiac contraction. The most notable PET ligands are ^{11}C-labelled CGP12177, GB67, MQNB and PK11195, which have been used to investigate β-adrenergic, α-adrenergic, muscarinic acetylcholine and peripheral-type benzodiazepine receptors, respectively. Key findings with these ligands include a 50% reduction in left venticular β density in idiopathic dilated cardiomyopathy, which correlated well with impaired contractile responsiveness to intracoronary dobutamine infusion, and a diffuse reduction of β density in primary hypertrophic cardiomyopathy.

Characterisation of the presynaptic nervous system has been investigated using ^{11}C]hydroxyephedrine (HED), which is subject to highly specific uptake in sympathetic nerve terminals, ^{11}C]epinephrine to evaluate sympathetic vesicular function and ^{11}C]phenylephrine to assess the enzymatic integrity of the nerve terminal. Clinical findings include a reduction in HED retention in patients with idiopathic dilated cardiomyopathy, which correlated with the severity of heart failure, and a significant reduction in the distribution volume of HED in patients with hypertrophic cardiomyopathy.

Further details on some of the above applications of PET in cardiology can be found in the review article by Bergmann [11].

Other positron emission tomography studies

The applications of PET imaging outside the main areas of oncology, neurology and cardiology include blood flow imaging in orthopaedic conditions, assessing inflammatory processes through uptake of FDG or ^{11}C]PK11195 by macrophages, and differentiation of lung infection from rejection in post-transplant patients.

☐ COST-EFFECTIVENESS OF CLINICAL POSITRON EMISSION TOMOGRAPHY

One reason why the clinical use of PET has been somewhat delayed has been doubts over its cost-effectiveness. How the situation has evolved can be ascertained by the reimbursement policies of American medical insurance agencies. For example, the

Table 3 Positron emission tomography (PET) studies covered by Medicare.

PET study	Year
Evaluation of coronary artery disease	1995
Evaluation of solitary pulmonary nodules	1998
Staging of non-small cell lung cancer	1998
Detection and localisation of recurrent colorectal cancer	1999
Staging and characterisation of lymphoma	1999
Evaluation of recurrent melanoma	1999

list of studies covered by Medicare (Table 3) has expanded as cost-effectiveness has been demonstrated. One American study on the management of patients with solitary pulmonary nodules indicated that PET could save $250 million per year based on the elimination of 20,000–30,000 unnecessary thoracotomies. Another study on pre-operative evaluation of recurrent colorectal cancer found that PET saved, on average, $3,800 per patient by avoiding unnecessary surgery.

However, the relatively high capital outlay and running costs are still limiting factors. Capital costs are significantly reduced if a PET centre operates without a cyclotron, and radiopharmaceuticals, such as [^{18}F]FDG, are purchased from an external supplier. However, the lack of a cyclotron precludes the use of the important short-lived positron emitters, ^{11}C, ^{13}N and ^{15}O. A further reduction in capital outlay can be made if an adapted nuclear medicine gamma camera is used rather than a dedicated PET scanner: the adaptation costs about 10% of the price of a dedicated scanner. These financial arguments have led to FDG oncology imaging with gamma camera PET (GCPET) systems becoming the fastest expanding sector of clinical PET, even though the diagnostic performance is known to be inferior to dedicated PET. Whether GCPET turns out to be a cost-effective option in terms of overall patient management remains to be seen.

☐ PHARMACOLOGICAL APPLICATIONS

The ability of PET to image pharmacokinetics (drug delivery and binding) and pharmacodynamics (physiological response to therapy) has made it a modality of interest to the pharmaceutical industry. The recent development of high resolution small animal PET scanners will see PET being used in the preclinical development of therapeutic pharmaceuticals, using animal models of human disease, in addition to its current role in early-stage clinical trials. A detailed discussion on the current and future uses of PET in pharmaceutical research has recently been published [12].

☐ CONCLUSIONS

PET is one of the most rapidly expanding imaging modalities. The research applications are aiding the fundamental understanding of disease processes and pharmaceutical development. In clinical use, compared to other techniques, PET can potentially lead to earlier, and/or more accurate, diagnosis and assessment of response to therapy for many disorders. There is increasing evidence of its cost-effectiveness in overall patient management, particularly in oncology. The future for PET looks bright.

REFERENCES

1   Tewson TJ, Krohn KA. PET radiopharmaceuticals: state-of-the-art and future prospects. *Semin Nucl Med* 1998; **28**: 221–34.

2   Bendriem B, Townsend DW. *The theory and practice of 3D PET*. Dordrecht: Kluwer Academic, 1998.

3   Bakheet SM, Powe J. Benign causes of 18-FDG uptake in whole body imaging. *Semin Nucl Med* 1998; **28**: 352–8.

4   Delbeke D. Oncological applications of FDG PET imaging: brain tumors, colorectal cancer, lymphoma and melanoma. *J Nucl Med* 1999; **40**: 591–603.

5   Delbeke D. Oncological applications of FDG PET imaging. *J Nucl Med* 1999; **40**: 1706–15.

6   Jones T. The role of positron emission tomography within the spectrum of medical imaging. *Eur J Nucl Med* 1996; **23**: 207–11.

7   Hustinx R, Eck SL, Alavi A. Potential applications of PET imaging in developing novel cancer therapies. *J Nucl Med* 1999; **40**: 995–1002.

8   Iacoboni M, Baron J-C, Frackowiak RSJ, *et al*. Emission tomography contribution to clinical neurology. *Clin Neurophys* 1999; **110**: 2–23.

9   Bonow RO. Identification of viable myocardium. *Circulation* 1996; **94**: 2674–80.

10   Gropler RJ, Geltman EM, Sampathkumaran K, *et al*. Comparison of C-11 acetate with fluorine-18-fluorodeoxyglucose for delineating viable myocardium by positron emission tomography. *J Am Coll Cardiol* 1993; **22**: 1587–97.

11   Bergmann SR. Cardiac positron emission tomography. *Semin Nucl Med* 1998; **28**: 320–40.

12   Fowler JS, Volkow ND, Wang GJ, *et al*. PET and drug research and development. *J Nucl Med* 1999; **40**: 1154–63.

□ SELF ASSESSMENT QUESTIONS

1   Fundamentals of positron emission tomography (PET):
   (a) PET can provide quantitative information on *in vivo* physiology, biochemistry and pharmacology
   (b) PET uses radioactive tracers
   (c) Magnetic resonance imaging (MRI) is a more sensitive tracer technique than PET
   (d) The resolution of PET images is better than MRI and computed tomography (CT)
   (e) Calculation of standardised uptake value requires blood sampling

2   PET in oncology:
   (a) [¹⁸F]fluorodeoxyglucose (FDG) is the most common PET tracer used for tumour imaging
   (b) [¹⁸F]FDG is taken up only by tumours
   (c) CT is better than PET at differentiating scar from tumour recurrence
   (d) [¹¹C]methionine is a more accurate tracer for detecting glioma than [¹⁸F]FDG
   (e) Image fusion of PET and CT can provide more accurate diagnosis than PET or CT alone

3   Brain PET imaging:
   (a) Functional MRI is replacing PET for brain mapping studies
   (b) PET can detect Alzheimer's disease earlier than any other technique
   (c) PET is the method of choice for ictal epilepsy imaging
   (d) PET is used to image ischaemia in stroke and head trauma
   (e) PET blood flow imaging is unable to differentiate different psychiatric disorders

4   Cardiac and other PET imaging:
   (a) [¹⁸F]FDG/myocardial blood flow (MBF) PET is significantly superior to stress echocardiography in the diagnosis of viable myocardium

(b) [^{11}C]acetate PET appears to be more accurate at detecting viable myocardium than [^{18}F]FDG/MBF PET

(c) PET blood flow imaging is an accurate technique for diagnosing coronary artery disease

(d) PET is being used to investigate synaptic dysfunction in cardiac disorders

(e) Inflammation cannot be imaged using PET

5   Miscellaneous:

(a) PET has no utility in pharmaceutical development

(b) Small animal PET scanners are being used in fundamental research, such as gene therapy

(c) A cyclotron is required on-site in order to use ^{15}O-labelled tracers

(d) Gamma camera PET provides superior information than PET

(e) PET is an expensive technique but can be cost-effective in overall patient management

ANSWERS

1a True	2a True	3a True	4a False	5a False
b True	b False	b True	b True	b True
c False	c False	c False	c True	c True
d False	d True	d True	d True	d False
e False	e True	e False	e False	e True

Advances in patient monitoring

Paul Beatty

The objective of patient monitoring is 'to identify trends and prevent untoward events'. This definition implies that patient monitors should include repeated observations, predict events giving adequate warning time, and make diagnostic information available to the clinician. In this instance, the term 'diagnostic' includes not only diagnostic in the sense of indicating the medical condition of the patient but also any specific information about the situation. For example, a breathing system fault monitor might simply warn the anaesthetist that a failure in a breathing system has occurred, but a design that would suggest the *type* of failure, thus reducing the time to fix the fault, would be much better. Stating what fault has occurred is also a diagnostic function.

Patient monitoring comes in all sorts of shapes and sizes. Clinical observations such as the colour or texture of skin are just as much a patient monitor as anything else. However, in the context of this chapter patient monitoring will be taken to mean continuous monitoring of the patient's physiological variables by electronic instruments (eg ECG, cardiac output, etc).

It is worth noting that, in a sense, patient monitoring is a screening procedure, not a specific diagnostic test. Thus, as with all screening procedures, to be effective it needs to be as widely applied as possible and become part of the routine of clinical practice. Simply inventing a new physiological measurement is not enough; an instrument that makes that measure available as a monitor at an economic cost is also required. This means that advances in patient monitoring are often driven more by the cost of a new technology and its availability through activity in other fields than by direct activity by those interested in patient monitoring *per se*. Figure 1 (derived from information obtained by reviewing advertisements in anaesthesia journals) shows the growth in the number of features available in anaesthesia patient monitors over the last 30 years (a 'feature' means a measurement or derived measurement displayed by the monitor).

The expansion in the number of features available in the years 1980–95 occurred when instrument design became dominated by microprocessor computer technology developed for other industries. This enabled manufacturers to add new features to instruments at low marginal cost.

The historical trend in patient monitoring has been for new monitors to become:

☐   more powerful due to new technology, particularly computing power

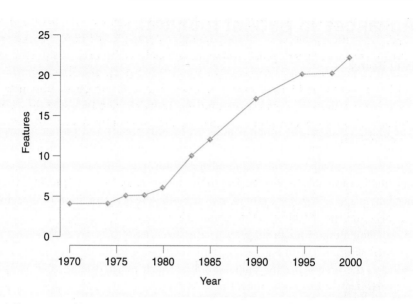

Fig. 1 The number of features available in top of range anaesthesia patient monitors 1970–2000.

☐   more user friendly by using that power to control screens etc, and

☐   smarter and smaller/more portable by exploiting trends in electronic design.

Relatively few genuinely new monitoring principles have appeared. However, where they have appeared, since these address unsolved questions, they are important.

☐ NEW MEASURES

Depth of anaesthesia

The problem of awareness under anaesthesia and the need to develop a monitor of the adequacy or depth of anaesthesia have produced two monitors, both now available as clinical instruments. Bi-Spectral Index (BIS) [1] analyses EEG to obtain an index of depth of anaesthesia (0 fully asleep to 100 fully awake). BIS seems to be a measure that considers higher cortical functions; it is not a pure EEG monitor, but includes a component of frontalis EMG activity that has been used in the past during anaesthesia. An alternative method using respiratory sinus arrhythmia (RSA) [2] looks at modulation by anaesthesia of this spontaneously occurring non-pathological arrhythmia at the brain stem level. Good correlation between RSA and changes in anaesthetic agent in specific centres in the brain has been shown using positron emission tomography (PET).

Gastric tonometry

In intensive care, systems for gastric tonometry show promise as a monitor of multiple organ failure (MOF). The primary value determined by gastric tonometry is gastric PCO_2 (notation $PgCO_2$) which is used to estimate the gastric mucosal PCO_2. In a normal situation, $PgCO_2$ approximates to arterial PCO_2. An increase in $PgCO_2$ (regional hypercapnia) indicates an imbalance between the production of CO_2 (metabolism) and its removal (perfusion) (see Fig. 2). The gastric mucosa is an early victim of blood flow redistribution, so it is hoped that gastric tonometry will be an early indicator of inadequate mucosal perfusion, and thence of the deranged tissue metabolism which appears to play a critical role in the development of sepsis and MOF [3].

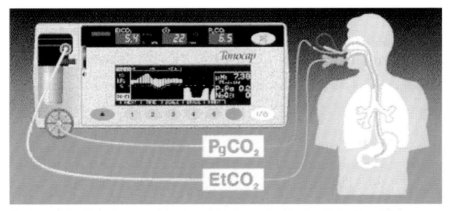

Fig. 2 A schematic of the measurement of gastric tonometry (courtesy Datex-Ohmeda).

Functional electrical impedance tomography in the brain

Probably the most exciting technique at present being assessed for feasibility is the use of electrical impedance tomography (EIT) for monitoring functional changes in the brain. EIT, a non-invasive method of imaging tissue by measuring differences in resistance or capacitance, is not a new technique. Current at high frequency is injected into the slice to be imaged, using an array of electrodes around the slice. Pairs of electrodes are used sequentially to inject the current, and for each pair all other pairs are used to measure the induced voltages. When all possible injection pairs and measurement pairs have been used, an image is reconstructed based on electrical resistance or capacitance in a way mathematically analogous to image reconstruction in a computed tomography scanner. Recently, a group at University College London [4] demonstrated that when electrodes were applied directly to the dura of the brain, images of visually evoked changes could be demonstrated (Fig. 3). The schematic on the left of the figure shows the placement of the ring electrode used on the surface of a rabbit's brain. The bar above the sequence of right-hand images shows when a visual stimulus was applied. The stimulus causes an activation of the visual cortex of the rabbit.

EIT is, in principle, non-invasive and cost-effective compared to PET or functional magnetic resonance imaging, and can be performed on a hospital ward. Systems that can make measurements in intact skull are essential as the basis of a

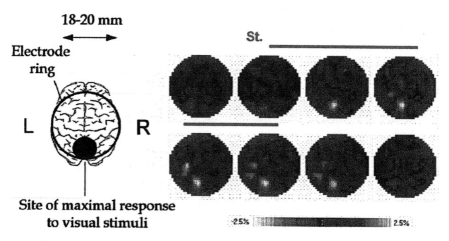

18-20 mm

Electrode ring

L   R

Site of maximal response to visual stimuli

St.

-2.5%   2.5%

Fig. 3 Visual evoked changes in rabbit brain [4] (courtesy Physiological Measurement, IOPP).

viable monitor of brain function. The resistance of the skull, which is relatively high, imposes severe sensitivity limitations. However, calculations of the required sensitivity for measurements of this type in intact skull suggest that this sort of monitor is viable [5].

□ ADVANCES IN 'USER FRIENDLY' DESIGN

The issue of making an instrument more 'user friendly' is not just a matter of convenience for clinicians but probably the most important challenge in instrument design relevant to patient safety. Table 1 shows figures of critical incidents (effectively near miss accidents) observed during training of anaesthetists in an anaesthesia simulator [6]. The results from this study are unusual only in that, since it was a simulator, it was in fact possible to separate fixation error, the concentration by the operator on a single aspect of the scene to the neglect of other important aspects, from other forms of human factors' error (HFE). The overall rate of HFE error is typically 86.4% of all critical incidents observed [7]. Detailed examination of these and other results indicates that about half the HFEs are concerned with monitoring equipment or other devices on which information is displayed. This far outweighs all other forms of instrument influenced incidents. Reducing HFE by

Table 1 Critical incidents occurring during anaesthesia simulation.

Cause of critical incident	%
Human factors' error	65.9
Fixation error	20.5
Unknown cause	10.6
Equipment failure	3.0

better instrument design is thus the single most important safety issue now faced by designers. While anaesthesia is the area of monitoring most studied in respect of HFE, the psychological and ergonomic literature indicates that similar rates of HFE would be expected in all similar environments such as intensive care and high dependency.

Research has concentrated on improving display design in this context. There is a growing awareness that displays for monitoring require different characteristics from those intended for control of, for instance, drug administration. Monitoring displays require good 'at a glance' characteristics to maximise the pre-attentive information obtained by the clinician from the display. This pre-attentive information has been shown in other safety critical complex environments to be critical in helping operators anticipate developing incidents. Polygon displays are one possible design for ergonomic monitoring displays.

A polygon display developed in Aberdeen [8] for use in the intensive care unit for the monitoring and detection of septic shock is shown in Fig. 4. The normal values of these variables lie on the polygon so, if all the values are normal no triangles will be seen. If the value is below normal, the triangles extend inside the polygon and, if above normal, outside. The triangles can also be colour coded for severity. In a polygon display, it can be judged at a glance how far the patient is away from the normal. The shape of the resulting display and its distortion from a regular shape become characteristic of the type of problem – diagnostic, in fact. Polygon displays have appeared on anaesthesia equipment, but have yet to become common practice on a wide range of patient monitoring instruments.

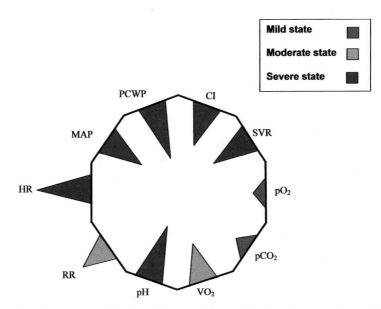

Fig. 4 Polygon display for monitoring septic shock (CI = cardiac index; HR = heart rate; MAP = mean arterial pressure; pCO_2 = partial pressure of arterial carbon dioxide; PCWP = pulmonary capillary wedge pressure; pH = acidity; pO_2 = partial pressure of arterial oxygen; RR = respiration rate; SVR = systemic vascular resistance; VO_2 = oxygen uptake).

□ SMARTER MONITORS

The fall in the cost of computer power has enabled instrument manufacturers to put advanced analysis tools, including those using artificial intelligence, into even the smallest of instruments. Figure 5 shows an ambulatory ECG monitor that incorporates diagnostic artificial intelligence and is intended for use by general practitioners (GPs). The instrument is used as a screening tool by the GP for further referral. It is attached to a patient who is reporting symptoms consistent with cardiac arrhythmia, and the patient is seen again 24 hours later. The unit records unusual cardiac events and classifies them into diagnostic classes using an artificial neural network. In trials in several GP surgeries, the device gave a diagnostic success rate of 96% against a recognised gold standard (compared with 91% by a panel of cardiologists on the same cases). The device cut the referral rate to a cardiologist from 92% to 48% and saved patients 6–8 weeks' delay in obtaining an outpatient examination at the hospital.

The way in which such systems are designed can be illustrated by one of our own projects, an intelligent breathing system failure alarm, which also uses a neural network analyser. The majority of critical incidents due to equipment failure in anaesthesia are related to breathing systems. One of the standard methods by which anaesthetists are taught to identify a failure is the shape of the capnograph tracing. Characteristic faults have characteristic capnograph shapes. Several groups have devised monitoring systems that detect and diagnose breathing system failure, but they have tended to be specific to a given manufacturer's anaesthesia machines and have involved expensive transducers because they need to be calibrated accurately. We wondered if it would be possible to cut costs and make a universal alarm by considering only the shape of wave forms obtained at the mouthpiece of the breathing system during failures and normal operation. From three wave forms, pressure, flow and the capnogram measured at the patient connector, for a range of

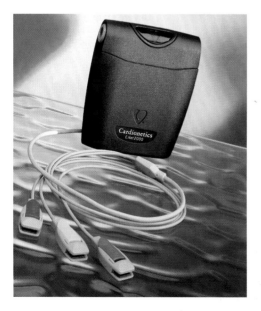

Fig. 5 Cardionetics C.Net 2000 Smart ambulatory ECG monitor (courtesy Cardionetics).

simulated failures and normal breathing, single breath waveforms were extracted and projected on to 1 × 1 squares regardless of amplitude or breathing rate, effectively reducing them to their fundamental shapes. The only pre-processing was to filter the waves and use a flat-line detector to plot all values at zero in cases where signals went to a flat line in failure mode. The waveforms for normal breathing and with a fault are shown after segmentation in Fig. 6.

These waveforms were then sampled and a neural network classifier strained to identify the failure types. The results for unseen data on single breaths after inducing a fault (Table 2) compare well with other systems, such as the Utah Anesthesia Workstation which gave an overall correct classification rate of 86.9% for 13 failure modes in spontaneous ventilation with a circle breathing system [9].

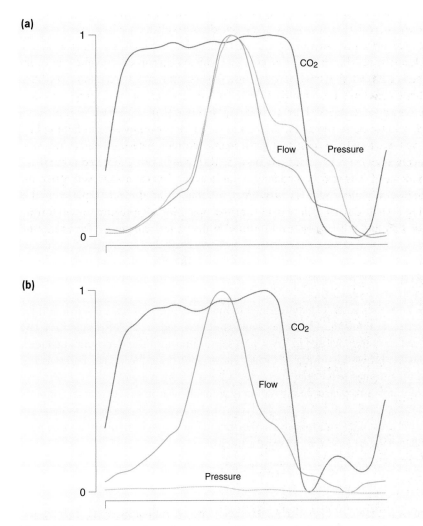

Fig. 6 (a) Segmented waveforms in normal breathing with no fault. **(b)** Segmented waveform with expiratory tubing disconnected (CO_2 = carbon dioxide).

Table 2 The results on unseen failures for the Manchester system during simulated spontaneous ventilation on an Ohmeda Enclosed Afferent Reservoir breathing system.

Actual	N	D1	D2	D3	D4	L1	L2	L3	Total
				Predicted					
Normal (N)	31					1			32
Disconnection at mouthpiece (D1)		17							17
Disconnection at Y piece (D2)			11						11
Disconnection of expiratory tubing (D3)				13					13
Disconnection of fresh gas supply (D4)					7				7
Leak at mouthpiece (L1)	1					14			15
Leak in expiratory tubing (L2)							13		13
Leak in inspiratory tubing (L3)					1			10	11
Total	32	17	11	13	8	15	13	10	119

	%		%			%
Classification rate	97.5 ± 2.8	Sensitivity	98.9	False −ve rate	1.1
Specificity	96.9	False +ve rate	3.1	False alarm rate	1.2

☐ SMALLER PORTABLE MONITORS

The last stage of development of a method, which usually takes place after the technique has become well established, is the miniaturisation of the instruments used. Pulse oximetry has been one of the great success stories of patient monitoring in the last 15 years. Its widespread introduction into anaesthesia is credited with a significant reduction in the severity, if not the frequency, of hypoxic incidents. Almost certainly, any anaesthetist in Europe or the US not using one could be considered negligent. Pulse oximetry is now entering the miniaturisation stage of instrument development.

Fig. 7 shows a completely integrated monitor intended for use on wards and for short-term monitoring. The unit contains all the required electronics in a few integrated circuits contained in a two-part sensor housing. The electronics include a pulse quality processing unit. The display shows SpO_2% and heart rate, and switches on and off automatically when applied or removed from a finger.

In monitors like this, miniaturisation is probably near its practical and economic limit. Whilst smaller units are possible, display size and other practical problems set minimum sizes in given applications. Further, designs much smaller than this pose constructional problems that increase unit cost.

☐ WHAT OF THE FUTURE?

Barring the emergence of a completely new technology, the process of incremental advance based on improved digital processing power at reducing cost will continue. There will be the usual steady trickle of new methods, but human factors' design

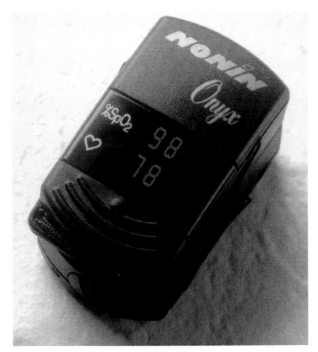

Fig. 7 The Nonin *Onyx* pulse oximeter.

issues and the diffusion of monitoring out of the hospital into primary care and the home will see most development.

Human factors' areas

In the human factors' areas, there may be devices like that shown in Fig. 8. This is a head-mounted display, a similar design of which was the subject of a preliminary study in 1990 [10]. It represented an attempt to address the difficulty in anaesthesia that monitor screens are often behind the anaesthetists when they are attending to the patient. The device was placed at the bifocal point of the dominant eye of the user so as not to obscure forward vision. It was connected by cable to the monitors and displayed a table of the monitored values. It was tested on a group of anaesthetists, most of whom were sympathetic to its use although they wanted standard displays not a table of values. Head-mounted display technology has improved since that study, and this sort of radical approach to design is now more feasible.

Monitoring out of hospital

Migration of monitoring out of the hospital has been illustrated in one or two of the devices considered here. A review of the manufacturers' literature shows that wireless systems and other ambulatory instruments are increasing in number and

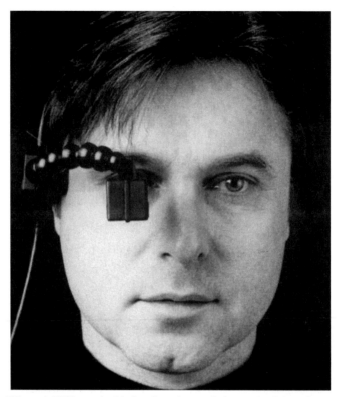

Fig. 8 Liquid Image's MI Monocular Display. A modern equivalent to the 'Private Eye' head-mounted display used by Block [10].

forming important parts of the overall monitoring environment in the wider hospital, if not out on the streets. Pressures like the ageing population requiring physiological monitoring at home, the opportunity to reduce capital costs in hospital building, and the availability of better equipped and flexible GP units, will ensure this trend continues. Patients will probably also prefer it.

However, more monitoring requires patients (or their carers), who are not clinically trained, to apply sensors to themselves to connect to those monitors. This needs to be made as easy as possible. What about a garment to apply the sensors rather than electrodes and leads? The Georgian Technical Institute's Wearable Mother Board is one such garment (Fig. 9). Woven into this sensile garment is a network of optical cables to which transducers such as ECG or respiratory impedance monitors are clipped. It was designed for the US military, and intended to be light, comfortable and resistant to sweat even when the wearer was active in battle. The idea behind this design was that if the person was hit, the entry and exit point of the bullet would be detected by the optical cabling acting as an impact sensor. The subsequent state of the person could then be assessed for triage before undertaking the hazardous procedure of retrieval. The project has been discontinued by the military but, if this could be done for soldiers, are such smart garments a tool for taking monitoring further out into the community?

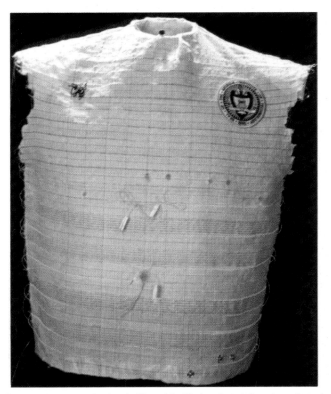

Fig. 9 The Georgian Technical Institute's Wearable Mother Board (courtesy Georgian Technical Institute).

□ CONCLUSION

We will continue to see a few new monitors. Those that are developed will depend on computer power. The trend to smaller units will continue. Instruments will become smarter and smarter thanks to the increased computer power. In short, there will be monitors everywhere!

REFERENCES

1   Rampil I. A primer for EEG signal processing in anesthesia. *Anesthesiology* 1998; **89**: 980–1002.

2   Pomfrett C. RR intervals and the depth of anaesthesia. In: Cashman JN (ed). *Recent advances in anaesthesia and analgesia*. Churchill Livingstone: London, 1995: Ch 6, 89–105.

3   Bennett-Guerrero E, Panah MH, Bodian CA, *et al.* Automated detection of gastric luminal partial pressure of carbon dioxide during cardiovascular surgery using the Tonocap. *Anesthesiology* 2000; **92**: 38–45.

4   Holder DS, Rao A, Hanquan Y. Imaging of physiologically evoked responses by electrical impedance tomography with cortical electrodes in the anaesthetized rabbit. *Physiol Meas* 1996; **17** (Suppl 4A): A179–86.

5   Towers CM, McCann H, Wang M, *et al.* Simulation of EIT for monitoring impedance variations within the human head. In: Holder D (ed). *Proceedings of the British Electrical Impedance Tomography Conference, 1999*. London: British EIT Conference, 1999.

6   DeAnda A, Gaba DM. Unplanned incidents during comprehensive anesthesia simulation. *Anesth Analg* 1990; **71**: 77–82.

7   Cooper JB, Newbower RS, Kitz RJ. An analysis of major errors and equipment failures in anesthesia management: a consideration for prevention and detection. *Anesthesiology* 1984; **60**: 34–42.

8   Green CA, Logie RH, Gilhooly KJ. Aberdeen polygons: computer displays of physiological profiles for intensive care. *Ergonomics* 1996; **39**: 412–28.

9   Westenskow DR, Orr JA, Simon FH, *et al.* Intelligent alarms reduce anesthesiologist's response time to critical faults. *Anesthesiology* 1992; **77**: 1074–9.

10 Block FE, Yablok DO, McDonald JS. Clinical evaluation of the 'heads-up' display of anesthesia data. *Int J Clin Monit Comput* 1995; **12**: 21–4.

☐ SELF ASSESSMENT QUESTIONS

1   The principles and development of monitoring:
(a) Monitoring aims at identifying trends and preventing untoward events
(b) All real patient monitors are electronic instruments
(c) The cost and availability of new technology are often more important in the development of new monitors than the invention of new measurements
(d) New measurements are important because they tend to address vital unsolved monitoring challenges
(e) The explosion in the number of features in anaesthesia instruments is due to the availability of cheap computing

2   Human factors' error in monitoring:
(a) Is the largest contributor to critical incidents during anaesthesia
(b) Associated with monitoring instruments contributes to less than 10% of critical incidents
(c) From optimal ergonomic performance, it is believed that displays intended for use in monitoring should be different from those intended for treatment control
(d) Polygon displays are suitable for control tasks
(e) Head-mounted displays may be a way for anaesthetists to see displays continuously

3   New patient monitors:
(a) Gastric tonometry measures CO_2 concentrations in the stomach in an attempt to give advance warning of the onset of multiple organ failure
(b) Electrical impedance tomography (EIT) is a method of constructing an image of a slice of the body using electrical resistance
(c) Bispectral index is a measure of neuromuscular relaxation during anaesthesia
(d) EIT changes in the visual cortex of rabbits have been demonstrated in response to visual stimuli
(e) The main fundamental obstacle to using EIT for examination of human brain functions is the resistance of the skull

4   Smarter, smaller monitors:
(a) Statistical classifiers such as neural networks have to be used in smart monitors to supply diagnostic results
(b) The use of smart monitors in primary care offers no improvement of service
(c) Cost falls when instruments are miniaturised
(d) Miniaturisation of instruments tends to be the last phase of instrument development
(e) Miniaturisation to the smallest possible size may be limited by practical problems such as display size

5   Future developments:
(a) Head-mounted displays in anaesthesia may be useful because the monitors are far from the patient.
(b) New trends pushing new monitor development will appear
(c) Migration of monitoring into the community is expected
(d) No new technologies will be required to make monitoring at home easier
(e) New monitors will be more expensive

ANSWERS

1a True	2a True	3a True	4a True	5a True
b False	b False	b True	b False	b False
c True	c True	c False	c True	c True
d True	d False	d True	d True	d False
e True	e True	e True	e True	e False

Decision support systems in medicine

Adrian Wilson

☐ CLINICAL DECISION MAKING

Using computers to support the clinical decision making process has been a goal of computer scientists, medical engineers and enthusiastic clinicians for more than three decades. Yet, despite a considerable investment in research, such systems have only recently had any impact in the clinical environment [1–3], which is perhaps surprising given the ubiquitous role computers play in many other professional activities. This chapter explores some of the reasons behind the slow acceptance of computerised clinical decision support systems, and suggests why emerging techniques in mathematical modelling and computer science could result in such support systems being more widely used in the clinical environment in the future.

Clinical decision making is characterised by the interpretation of symptoms, signs and the results of clinical investigations, for diagnosis, assessment of the patient's state or treatment planning. It is guided by nationally and locally defined standards and protocols of care, and is informed by a knowledge of disease processes, their diagnosis and the treatment options (Fig. 1). Clinical care is, however, not one decision but rather is characterised by repeated cycles of assessing the patient's state and delivering therapy. This view of clinical decision making can be applied at all levels of clinical care, from the family doctor's surgery through critical care environments in hospital. If computerised clinical decision support systems are going to be successful in the clinical environment, they must fit into this complex framework and present the support in a form that is readily understood by clinicians. All too often in the past, developers of clinical decision support systems have concentrated on complex data processing whilst paying only minimal attention to the needs of clinical users, and ignoring the potential for optimised data displays to support the clinical decision making process [4].

☐ HUMAN COMPUTER INTERACTION

Human computer interaction (HCI) is the name given to the way in which human beings interact with computers. Up to 10 years ago the majority of computer displays were text based, and the user was required to type in pre-learned commands in order to communicate with the computer. Today, computer displays are characterised by graphical direct manipulation user interfaces (GUIs) where options are selected from the screen with a pointing device. Such displays are intended to be intuitive where little or no learning is required. However, it is only

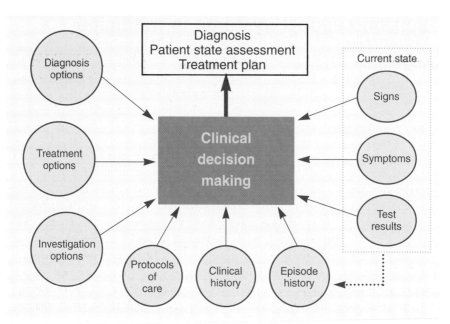

Fig. 1 Diagrammatic representation of the clinical decision making process showing the major data sources, together with the areas of knowledge against which these are evaluated.

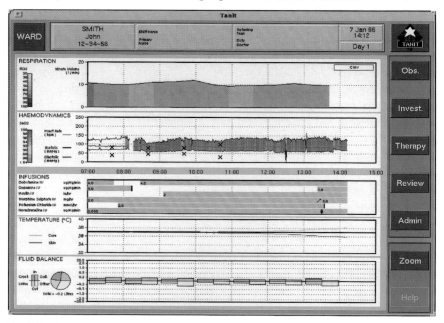

Fig. 2 The bedside screen for rapid assessment of a patient's state from an intensive care unit data management system. The height of the uppermost trace in the centre of the screen gives the minute ventilation, and the fill colour gives the FiO_2. In the next trace, the upper and lower bounds of the graph represent the systolic and diastolic systemic blood pressures, respectively, and the fill colour represents O_2sat. The bars beneath give the amounts and times of vasoactive drug therapy. The next graph gives the core and surface temperatures, while the bottom-most graph shows fluid input and output information partitioned on the basis of crystalloid and colloid.

necessary to look at the user interface of a modern word processor to see that considerable skill and knowledge are still required! Therefore, whilst GUI interfaces have simplified access to complex computer software, in their most general form they are not necessarily suitable for the clinical environment. An intuitive interface is required that offers only the options needed – and no more.

Professional activities can be characterised as 'tasks' taking place in 'contexts'. For example, prescribing a drug (the task) occurs on a ward during a ward round (the context). If computers are to support clinical activities effectively, the tasks and contexts must be analysed so that an optimised display is created where the clinician is presented with only the information needed to perform a specific task. Figure 2 shows the optimised display from an intensive care unit data management system designed to give an overview of the current state of the patient. Here, although the quantity of data is high, the display is devoid of unimportant or irrelevant data. The buttons down the right-hand side of the display allow navigation to other parts of the system on the basis of routinely performed tasks. The drug prescription screen (Fig. 3) from the same system provides another example of clinical decision support based on optimised displays. The upper pane on the left-hand side gives the therapy prescription. When a drug is selected, a recommended dose is displayed, absolute dose limits are set to support range checking, and the normalised dose is automatically calculated. The lower pane on the left-hand side of the screen gives

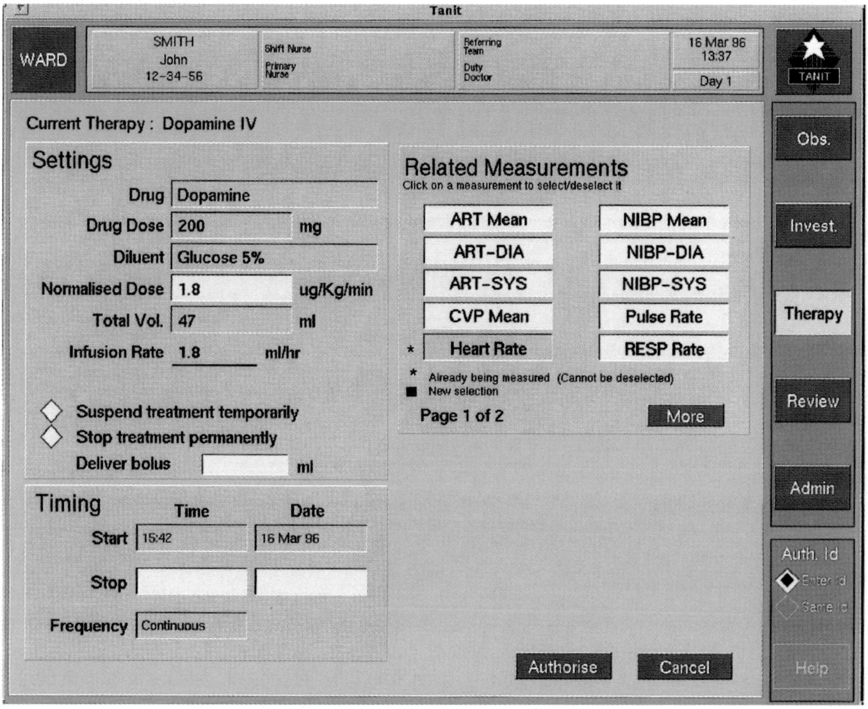

Fig. 3 Drug management screen from an intensive care unit data management system illustrating the use of optimal interfaces to support both tasks and protocols of care.

delivery timing information. The pane on the right-hand side of the screen displays the measurements which should be made during the administration of that particular drug to monitor both its direct effects and any possible side effects. These, together with the dose range information, are obtained from local protocols of care and the manufacturer's data sheet.

Such approaches are not only applicable to critical care environments. We have recently addressed the problem of trying to encourage evidence-based practice within a major teaching hospital. It was argued that in order to do this we would need to make the evidence readily available in the ward in close proximity to patients and their medical records. For this, we developed an interface designed to be used on a web browser on a ward which integrated reference material with a patient's medical record (Fig. 4). Although there is currently no direct link between the two, evaluations have shown that the optimised displays have improved the use of reference material in clinical decision making [5]. Producing optimised, task based displays, which are intuitive, easy to use and context sensitive, is a key step in gaining acceptance of computer technology in the clinical environment. This, in turn, is the first step to achieving acceptance of clinical decision support systems.

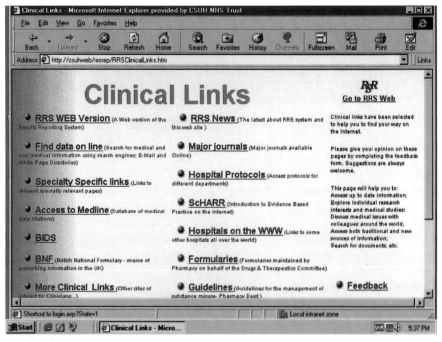

Fig. 4 A ward-based screen to encourage evidence-based medicine. 'RRS WEB Version' provides a navigation path to the results reporting system containing the clinical laboratory and nuclear medicine imaging results for patients in the hospital. The other entries provide navigation paths to a variety of reference material, including the major medical journals, bibliographic services and hospital protocols. For convenience, reference material is also indexed under 'Specialty Specific links'.

☐ CLASSICAL APPROACHES TO SUPPORT FOR CLINICAL DECISION MAKING

Once optimised displays have been achieved, the next stage is to use computers to process the complete data sets used in clinical decision making to produce results which further support clinical decision making. Many approaches have been proposed over the years but the majority are derived from three techniques:

☐ expert systems

☐ statistical inference, and

☐ pattern recognition techniques.

Expert systems

Expert systems are essentially rule based systems which consist of 'IF-THEN-ELSE' statements, which form the rules from which the technique gets its name. The technique was the basis of one of the earliest examples of a successful clinical decision support system, 'MYCIN' [6]. MYCIN helped the user select an appropriate antibiotic based on patient measurements entered through a text based interface. Expert systems work well for well defined problems such as the selection of antibiotics or identifying drug interactions, but they have proved less successful in supporting complex patient-specific clinical decision making tasks. All expert systems depend on obtaining the rules from human experts. Poor agreement between clinicians on which factors are most important in a particular clinical decision has led to large and complex rule sets which are difficult to maintain. In addition, as rule sets become large, interaction between the rules leading to ambiguities in the decision making process becomes a significant problem. For these reasons, expert systems for clinical diagnosis have not found widespread acceptance in the clinical environment. Even when such systems have been successful in the environment in which they were developed, they have not transferred well to other environments because differences in clinical opinion and protocols of care require differences in the rule sets. This lack of portability of diagnostic support systems based on expert system shells has been widely reported in the literature and has contributed to their poor acceptance clinically [7]. Recent reports, however, suggest that expert systems which report drug interaction at the time when a prescription is made, have proved of value in the clinical environment [2,3].

Statistical techniques

A second approach to processing data to support the clinical decision making process is to use statistical techniques to combine different signs, symptoms and therapeutic details to yield a probability of a particular diagnosis or of the success of a therapy. The seminal work in this regard is that of de Dombal [8] who developed a clinical decision support system for diagnosing acute abdominal pain. Using this work as an example of the technique, the probability that a specific sign, symptom or risk factor is associated with a specific disease process is determined according to

Bayes's theorem from retrospective data. This process is repeated for all the different signs, symptoms or risk factors associated with abdominal pain, and for all possible sources of that pain. To diagnose the cause of abdominal pain in an individual patient, the information for each sign, symptom or risk factor shown by that patient is entered into the computer system. The probability of the patient having each disease is then determined as the product of the probabilities for each of the patient's signs, symptoms or risk factors being associated with that disease. The diagnosis is then based on the disease which has the highest probability. This system was shown to work effectively in Leeds, where it was developed [8], but offered poor geographic portability since different social environments affect patterns of signs, symptoms and risk factors [9].

Pattern recognition techniques

The final sets of techniques available to support clinical decision making are those which perform pattern recognition – essentially looking for patterns in the signs, symptoms and results of clinical investigations related to a particular diagnosis or indicative that a particular therapeutic regimen should be pursued. Techniques in this category include [10]:

- genetic algorithms

- neural networks, and

- fuzzy logic.

Consider the application of pattern recognition techniques to the problem of diagnosing abdominal pain. All the signs, symptoms and risk factors associated with the diagnosis must first be identified by human experts. Values for these factors are obtained from retrospective patient data, together with an absolute diagnosis of the source of the pain. This is called the 'training set'. The training set is then used to 'train' the pattern recognition system to transform the signs, symptoms and risk factors presented into a diagnosis. Once trained, the system may be used to diagnose abdominal pain in an individual patient. The patient's signs, symptoms and risk factors are entered into the computer system, which then presents the user with a diagnosis.

Pattern recognition techniques, often involving complex computation, highlight a further problem with the introduction of clinical decision support systems into the clinical environment: traceability of decisions. With the requirement for increasing openness in clinical decision making and increasing pressure for a comprehensive audit of all clinical activities, it is essential that computer systems which support that process are also open to interrogation. This makes the pattern recognition techniques the most contentious of all since they provide 'black box' systems where the decision making process is complex and not open to simple inspection by the end users. Therefore, in their current form such techniques have a limited role in the clinical decision support systems of the future. Further work on the techniques themselves is needed to make the decision making process open to interrogation by end users.

Training set data

All pattern recognition techniques require 'training' on retrospective data and, as such, suffer similar problems of geographical portability to those techniques based on expert systems and statistical inference approaches. Both the statistical inference and pattern recognition techniques rely on high quality retrospective training set data to determine the relationships between the data entered and the resultant clinical decision. Herein lies their principal weakness. The problem of poor success in providing appropriate support is not inherent in the techniques themselves but rather in their dependence on the training sets. The extraction of retrospective data is currently done manually, which is time consuming, and patient data are often incomplete. Within the next few years, the majority of medical records will be in machine readable form. Data mining techniques applied to these should produce much larger and more robust training sets. The data mining techniques can also be used to generate rules automatically for decision support systems based on expert systems. Improvements in knowledge extraction and representation techniques will improve the support from expert systems. The advent of large volumes of patient data in a machine readable form will enable clinical decision support systems to be trained locally and automatically, overcoming many of the problems of portability and bias. However, biological variability will ultimately limit the performance of clinical decision support systems based on these techniques, as it does with human experts.

☐ MODELLING AND SUPPORT FOR CLINICAL DECISION MAKING

There is clearly a need to refine and extend the data processing techniques that have been used in the past, but there is also a need to look towards introducing techniques which are currently the subject of research into the clinical environment. With the advent of increasing computational power, modelling at levels between the cellular and the whole organ system becomes a practical possibility. One example of current research in this area allows the patterns of stress in metacarpophalangeal joint implants to be visualised in order to improve their design [11] (Fig. 5). Similarly, finite volume modelling can allow the study of fluid and gas flow through complex anatomical pathways, including the airways (Fig. 6), to investigate the effects of various disease processes or treatments. As yet, these techniques remain in research laboratories, but with increasing computer power and appropriate user interfaces they have a potentially vital role to play in clinical decision making in the future. As before, one of the key elements in moving such techniques from the research laboratory into the clinical environment is HCI. Figure 7 shows an instrumented glove which, linked to the skeletal model, produces an animated display of joint movements [12]. Currently, this is a tool for implant design and assessment, but in the future it may be possible for a pre-operative patient to wear the glove whilst a series of virtual implants are performed to identify the one which best suits that particular patient.

   In a second example (Fig. 8), a three-dimensional image of a heart is produced using virtual reality techniques. Such a display could be constructed from the spiral computed tomography scan of a patient with an electrical map of that patient's heart, superimposed in order to investigate a complex cardiac pathology.

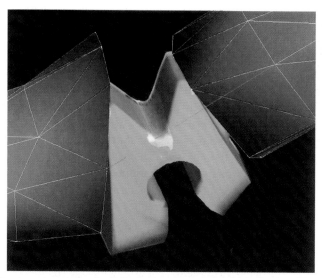

Fig. 5 A finite element analysis of a Sutter metacarpophalangeal joint implant. The areas of high stress (red) are the positions where the joints fail after implantation. These match with the failures found in clinical practice.

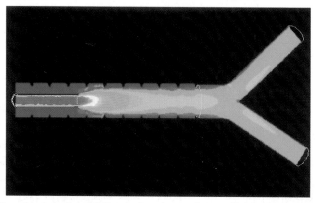

Fig. 6 A finite volume analysis of flow in the airway of an artificially ventilated patient during maximum inspiratory flow showing the position of the endotracheal tube and the cartilaginous rings on the 'ideal' airway. The diagram shows clearly the distribution of flow within the airway and the effect of unequal diameters below the bifurcation.

These are currently research activities, but they could become clinical decision support tools within a few years.

☐ CONCLUSIONS

Whilst research carried out in the past into clinical decision support systems has had little impact in the clinical environment, it must be remembered that medical records were maintained in paper form at the time when many of the systems described were developed. Within the next five years it is possible that the majority

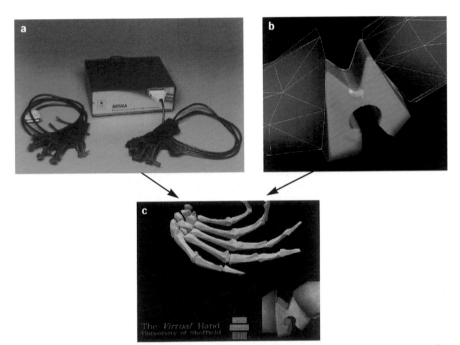

Fig. 7 An instrumented glove which measures finger movements **(a)**, coupled with the results of a stress analysis **(b)**, allows the construction of an animated skeletal hand **(c)**, with the prosthetic joint implanted in the index finger. An expanded image of the stress patterns in the prosthetic joint as it is flexed is also shown (lower right).

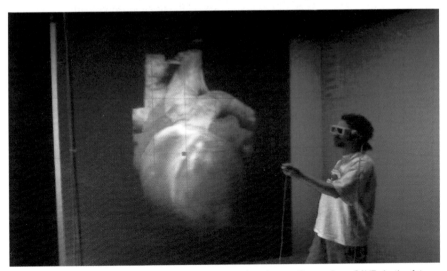

Fig. 8 An illustration of how the heart might appear in a four active surface CAVE. In the future, anatomical, mechanical and cellular models of the heart could be used to create a virtual organ which could then be displayed in this way. The virtual organ could be used to evaluate surgical procedures or to perform in-silico drug testing. (Printed with the kind permission of Professor N Avis, Centre for Virtual Environments, University of Salford. The virtual heart displayed uses anatomy data from Professor Hunter's group at the University of Auckland, into which the Oxford cardiac cellular models from Professor Noble's group in Oxford have been embedded.)

of medical records will be stored on computers. This, coupled with access to reference material available through the Internet, will allow the seamless integration of patient-specific and reference material to support evidence-based medicine. In addition, machine readable medical records will form a rich resource for training a new generation of clinical decision support systems. Many of the problems of the past have been due to problems in communication between those developing systems and the potential users. GUIs and virtual reality techniques can form the bridge between the two communities and provide new and effective displays to support clinical decision making. In itself, this will provide new challenges to those involved in research to process data to support clinical decision making. Thus, far from our current state of knowledge being the end of research into clinical decision support systems, it places us at the brink of an exciting new era in which clinical decision support systems can have a major impact on clinical care.

REFERENCES

1   Classen D. Clinical decision support systems to improve clinical practice and quality of care. *JAMA* 1998; **280**: 1360–1.
2   Shea S, Clayton D. Clinical decision support systems begin to come of age. *Am J Med* 1999; **106**: 261–2.
3   Effects of computer based clinical decision support systems on physician performance and patient outcomes: a systematic review. *JAMA* 1998; **80**: 1339–46.
4   Wilson AJ, Bowes CL, Holland J. Telematics and protocols of care in critical care environments. In: Gordon C, Christiansen J (eds). *Health telematics for clinical guidelines and protocols*. Amsterdam: IOP Press, 1994.
5   Goncalves S, Steele B, Franks C, Wilson A. Integration of information sources in a clinical environment. *Health Informatics J* 1999; **5**: 193–9.
6   Shortliffe EH, Davis R, Axline SG, *et al*. Computer-based consultations in clinical therapeutics: explanation and rule acquisition capabilities of the MYCIN system. *Comput Biomed Res* 1975; **8**: 303–20.
7   Ohayon MM. Validation of expert systems: examples and considerations. *Medinfo* 1995; **8**: 1071–5.
8   de Dombal FT, Leaper DJ, Staniland JR, *et al*. Computer-aided diagnosis of acute abdominal pain. *Br Med J* 1972; **2**: 9–13.
9   Adams ID, Chan M, Clifford PC, *et al*. Computer aided diagnosis of acute abdominal pain: a multicentre study. *Br Med J* 1986; **293**: 800–4.
10   Linkens DA, Nyongesa HO. Learning systems in intelligent control: an appraisal of fuzzy, neural and genetic control applications. *IEE Proc-Control Theory Appl* 1996; **143**: 367–86.
11   Penrose JMT, Williams NW, Hose DR, Trowbridge EA. An examination of one-piece metacarpophalangeal joint implants using finite element analysis. *J Med Eng Technol* 1996; **20**: 145–50.
12   Williams NW. The virtual hand. The Pulvertaft Prize Essay for 1996. *J Hand Surg Br* 1997; **22**: 560–7.

☐ SELF ASSESSMENT QUESTIONS

1   Computerised clinical decision support:
   (a) Is a recent phenomenon
   (b) Aims to support doctors in delivering patient care

(c) Has had little impact in the clinical environment
(d) Has had inadequate research funding
(e) Has a future with recent advances in computer technology

2   Human computer interaction:
(a) Analyses the way people interact with computers
(b) Has no role to play in clinical decision support on its own
(c) Analyses work activities in terms of tasks
(d) Aims to provide the user with screens offering a wide variety of options
(e) Is relevant only to critical care environments

3   Traditional approaches to clinical decision support:
(a) Mimic the way in which doctors think
(b) Use clinical experts to set the rules in rule based systems
(c) Mostly use retrospective analysis of case histories
(d) Provide flexible systems which are geographically portable
(e) Use artificial intelligence techniques to improve traceability of decisions

4   Modelling:
(a) Provides a potentially new approach to clinical decision support
(b) Can be used to study anatomical structures
(c) Cannot be used to support surgical decision making
(d) Can be used to perform in-silico drug testing
(e) Cannot be tailored to the individual patient

5   Future trends in clinical decision support:
(a) Depend on the availability of machine readable medical records
(b) Will be more complex for the user
(c) Require a massive increase in computer power
(d) Should produce systems which support traceability
(e) Should have a major impact on the clinical environment

ANSWERS

1a False	2a True	3a False	4a True	5a True
b True	b False	b True	b True	b False
c True	c True	c True	c False	c False
d False	d False	d False	d True	d True
e True	e False	e False	e True	e True

Artificial organs for renal therapy

Joseph P Barbenel and John D S Gaylor

The last decade has seen the development of a wide range of devices for implantation or extracorporeal use which can be described as artificial organs. This chapter will be limited to devices whose primary purpose is to modify the composition of the blood. The replacement of renal function by dialysis – the artificial kidney – is a well established and widely applied methodology and serves as a paradigm for such devices. Progress in artificial organs has depended upon the development and utilisation of new ideas in materials and design, coupled to better understanding of the medical and biological problems involved. Artificial organs function by physical mechanisms; these will be described in order to clarify the nature of the progress which has led to their development and future improvement.

☐ THE PRINCIPLES OF RENAL DIALYSIS

Chemical species to be removed

Molecules with a molecular weight up to about 58 kDa are cleared in the glomerular filtrate. Renal failure is accompanied by a gradual retention and increase in the plasma concentration of a large number of organic compounds. Some (eg urea, creatinine) are the metabolites of proteins, but a number of other larger molecules are also retained. The retention products are generally divided into those with:

☐ low molecular weight (≤300 Da) (eg urea (60.1 Da), creatinine (113.1 Da))

☐ middle molecular weight (300–12,000 Da) (eg peptides, β2-microglobulin), and

☐ high molecular weight (>12 kDa) (eg myoglobins).

The distinction between the small and middle molecules is not absolute, and some small molecules (eg hippuric acid (179.2 Da)) behave as if they were middle molecules because they are bound to plasma proteins. The exact nature of the middle molecules and their significance is a matter of some discussion [1].

General principles.

The principle of treating renal failure is the removal of some dissolved substances (solutes) from the blood by transport across a semipermeable membrane which separates the blood from an isotonic washing fluid, the dialysate (Fig. 1). The

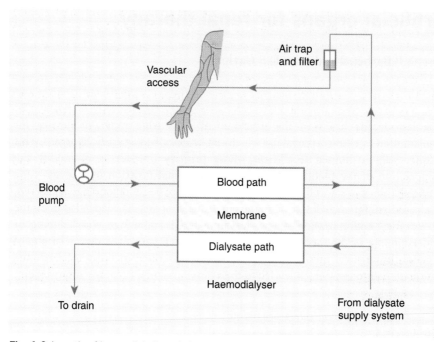

Fig. 1 Schematic of haemodialysis technique.

removal of solutes is achieved primarily by the transport mechanism of *dialysis*, while the removal of excess body water is achieved by another transport mechanism, *ultrafiltration*, which also removes some solutes. Consideration of the physical principles involved in both processes leads to a simple equation which can be written as:

$$\text{Mass transfer per unit area} = \frac{\text{driving force}}{\text{resistance to transport}}$$

The transfer of any solute can be characterised by its clearance, which is analogous to the glomerular clearance (K) in the kidney, defined as:

$$K = \frac{\text{solute transfer rate}}{\text{blood concentration at the device inlet}}$$

Dialysis

The driving force in the diffusion process which underlies dialysis is always a concentration difference. In dialysers, the driving force of solutes which can diffuse through the dialysis membrane is the high concentration of solutes in the blood relative to their concentration in the dialysate. Flow velocities of blood and dialysate are reduced in the vicinity of the dialysis membrane due to fluid friction. This effect, coupled with the diffusion process through the membrane, gives rise to solute concentration gradients near the membrane interfaces.

The diffusion path is thus divided into three segments representing the three fundamental elements of the dialyser: the membrane, the blood side and the dialysate side. The resistance to transport also has three components: the dialysis membrane, the blood and the dialysate.

The resistance of the dialysis membrane depends upon the solute considered. Small molecules diffuse through the membrane and encounter a lower membrane resistance than the large molecules. Whatever the molecular weight of the solute, thin homogeneous membranes have a lower resistance than thick ones. Resistance in the blood and dialysate is produced by the resistance to molecular motion of the solutes involved in the concentration gradients mentioned above. Blood and dialysate resistances are primarily influenced by the flow velocities and dimensions of the flow paths and, in contrast to the membrane resistance, are largely independent of solute molecular weight.

The total resistance from the blood to the dialysate is a sum of the resistances in each of the three components. For small molecules such as urea the three resistances are approximately equal but for larger molecules the membrane resistance becomes predominant. The blood concentration of solutes which do not diffuse through the membrane remains constant.

Ultrafiltration

The driving force in ultrafiltration is a pressure difference. Under the action of a pressure difference across the dialysis membrane, plasma water transfers from the blood into the dialysate stream. The water flux due to ultrafiltration also carries (convects) some solutes through the membrane. The rate of solute transfer depends on solute size and molecular weight, and also on the membrane pore size and thickness. The proteins which cannot pass through the membrane exert an osmotic pressure which opposes the applied hydrostatic pressure and produces a resistance to transport.

Combined effects of dialysis and ultrafiltration

In haemodialysers, blood and dialysate flow under pressure, often in opposite directions. At the blood inlet end, the pressure acting on blood is greatest, and on dialysate least. The concentration and pressure gradients lead to both dialysis and ultrafiltration from the blood. At the blood exit, the pressure gradient between blood and dialysate may be reversed relative to the entry conditions because the effect of blood viscosity is greater than that of dialysate viscosity. Ultrafiltration of water and solutes from dialysate into blood will occur and may transfer bacterial products and other pyrogens to the blood. Dialysis will also occur during ultrafiltration and it is impossible completely to separate the two processes in currently available artificial kidney devices.

☐ HAEMOFILTRATION

There are ultrafiltration membranes which transfer small and middle molecules at similar rates, unlike conventional dialysis membranes. These high flux membranes permit another form of therapy for renal failure, *haemofiltration,* and enable more efficient removal of higher molecular weight solutes. As with conventional ultrafiltration, the driving force is a pressure difference across the ultrafiltration membrane. In haemofiltration devices, the loss of water by ultrafiltration significantly increases the blood concentration of cells, plasma proteins and molecules which are too large to pass through the membrane. Cells and plasma proteins collect at the membrane surface and reduce the effective area of the membrane by blocking the membrane pores upon which ultrafiltration depends, thus producing a resistance to transport.

During haemofiltration, large volumes of filtrate are produced which have to be replaced. One method is to dispose of the filtrate and replace it with a substitution fluid which has a composition as close as possible to that of the normal extracellular fluid. This may be achieved by diluting the blood prior to ultrafiltration or by adding the fluid after filtration. The composition and quality of the fluid are critical, and the use of large quantities of substitution fluid may be expensive.

The composition of the glomerular filtrate in the kidney is altered by tubular secretion or adsorption. The composition of the ultrafiltrate produced by haemofilters can also be modified by treating it in a dialyser or with an adsorbent before returning the filtrate to the blood.

□ MATERIALS

Artificial kidneys contain a variety of materials, most of which are polymers. The choice of materials and the development of improved or novel materials have to satisfy the important criteria of blood-material interactions and transport properties.

Blood-material interactions

Exposure of blood to polymeric materials initiates deleterious changes in the blood (Fig. 2) [2]. Surfaces exposed to blood rapidly become coated by a wide range of plasma proteins which may become denatured or replaced by alternative materials (eg high molecular weight kininogen). The protein adsorption is followed by interaction with cells and with the coagulation, fibrinolytic and complement systems.

The coagulation cascade can be triggered by adsorbed high molecular weight kininogen which reacts with contact proteins in the plasma (eg factor VII or VI) or by direct interaction of platelets with surfaces. The coagulation cascade is amplified by self-perpetuating feedback mechanisms, and the end product is the generation of thrombin which converts circulating fibrinogen to fibrin and also produces irreversible platelet aggregation.

The contact of blood with artificial surfaces may also induce an immune response. A critical step is the process of complement activation via either the classical or alternative pathways.

Substances such as endotoxins which may be in the dialysate can also permeate across the membrane and initiate deleterious blood changes.

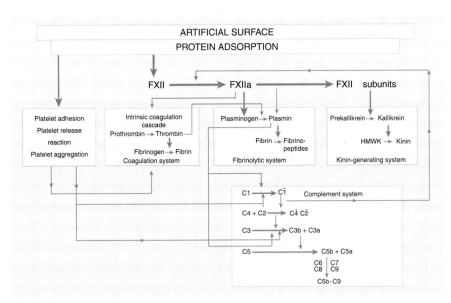

Fig. 2 Interactions that may occur following blood contact with artificial surfaces (C1, C2, etc = complement 1, 2, etc; FXII = factor XII; HMWK = high molecular weight kininogen) (from [2], with permission).

Transport properties

The choice of membrane material influences both which molecules can be transferred across it and the mechanism of transfer. Regenerated cellulose provides effective small-solute transport, but has the major drawback of limited capacity to transfer middle molecules which have become of increasing clinical importance. Synthetic membrane materials have been developed which contain very fine pores, allowing ultrafiltration of both small and middle molecules.

Currently used materials

The first dialyser, reported by Kolff and Berk in 1944 [3], had a dialysis membrane of regenerated cellulose sausage skin casings. This was associated with the occurrence of leucopenia in the early phase of haemodialysis, which was found to be due to leukocyte sequestration in the pulmonary capillaries following complement activation.

Although regenerated cellulose has disadvantages, it is relatively cheap and still accounts for 40–50% of all haemodialysis membranes. Complement activation is mostly produced by hydroxyl groups. Modified celluloses have been developed by replacing all or some of the hydroxyl groups to reduce blood-material interactions. These materials and synthetic membranes based on polycarbonate or polyacrylonitrile, often blended with other polymers, can be made into homogeneous films for dialysis. Synthetic thermoplastics such as polysulphones, polyamides and polyacrylonitrile can be fabricated into very thin membranes which contain very fine pores, allowing high rates of ultrafiltration.

Utilisation and device design

The principle of a haemodialyser is simple, requiring flow channels for blood and dialysate separated by a suitably supported membrane. The implementation of this principle has led to many dialyser models (currently over 400) which may be rather complex [4].

The most important design progress has been based on the development of membranes with improved transfer properties. However, there has been a steady decrease in the thickness of membranes. This further enhances their transfer properties, which reduces the area of membrane required to produce a specified efficiency of solute removal (Fig. 3). The most important advance has been the ability to fabricate the materials into hollow fibres, typically 0.2 mm internal diameter; this produces a high area of membrane contact relative to the volume of blood.

Fibres, initially produced from hydrophobic materials, have a complex structure (Fig. 4) characterised by one surface having a skin, typically a fraction of a micrometer thick, containing very fine micropores allowing ultrafiltration. The bulk of the membrane structure consists of larger interconnecting pores which provide mechanical support for the membrane on the inner surface. In addition to improving the transfer properties of the membrane, the hollow fibres have a built-in support system which simplifies the design and construction of haemodialysers.

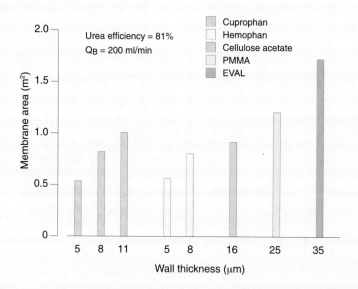

Fig. 3 Influence of hollow fibre wall thickness and membrane material on surface area required to achieve an 81% urea removal efficiency (Cuprophan = regenerated cellulose; EVAL = polyethylene/vinyl alcohol; Hemophan = derivatised cellulose; PMMA = polymethylmethacrylate; Q_B = blood flow rate).

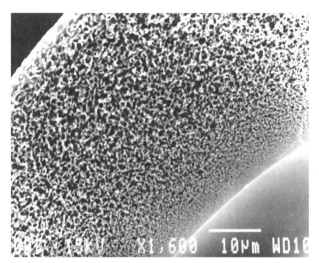

Fig. 4 Cross-section of the wall of a polysulphone hollow fibre for haemodialysis. The dense, rate-controlling layer at the fibre lumen surface (lower right-hand corner) is supported by a porous structure which increases in porosity towards the fibre outer surface (top left-hand corner).

☐ CLINICAL IMPLICATIONS

Progress in dialyser design means that current dialysers are both smaller and simpler to use than their predecessors and can more efficiently remove a wider range of solutes from the blood (Table 1, Fig. 5). There has been considerable discussion on how best to utilise improved dialyser performance clinically, which has led to the concept of the dialyser dose:

$$\text{dialyser dose} = Kt/V$$

(K = dialyser urea clearance; t = duration of dialysis; V = volume of body water in which the urea is distributed.) There appears to be little general agreement on what

Table 1 Clearance of urea, vitamin B12 (a marker solute for middle molecules) and β2-microglobulin (β2m) in dialysers with different membranes (modified from [5]).

Dialyser	Membrane	Surface area (m²)	Clearance (K)* (ml/min) Urea	Vitamin B12	β2m
Althin 135 SCE	Saponified cellulose ester	1.5	177	43	0
Hospal Filtral 16	Sulfonated PAN (AN69)	1.6	181	91	36
Baxter CA-210	Cellulose acetate (HE)	2.1	192	77	0
Baxter CT-190	Cellulose triacetate	1.9	192	137	39
Fresenius F80	Polysulphone	1.9	196	144	54

* K measured *in vitro* at 200 ml/min test-solution flow and 500 ml/min dialysate flow.
PAN = polyacrylonitrile; HE = high-efficiency.

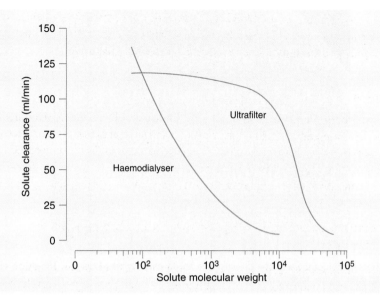

Fig. 5 Clearance vs solute molecular weight profiles for a haemodialyser (diffusive transfer) and an ultrafilter (convective transfer), The human kidney possesses a similar profile to that of the ultrafilter.

the dialyser dose should be, but there is evidence that higher values (>1.2) reduce both morbidity and mortality in patients. Improved membranes and haemodialyser designs which produce high values of K mean that the duration of dialysis can be reduced, with advantages both for those providing the dialysis and for the patient whose life is less disrupted. Nevertheless, such short, high flux dialysis may be associated with increased morbidity and mortality [5].

☐ THE FUTURE

Development of materials

Materials' development, which has driven progress and also dialysis and ultrafiltration performance, will continue. Reducing the blood response to the materials is an important aim, but the complexity of the blood-material interaction often means that improvement in one aspect of the response is accompanied by reduced performance in others. For example, surface modification by applying biomimetic coatings to polymer surfaces is unlikely to be applicable to dialyser membranes because of the resulting degradation of transfer characteristics.

Improved transfer properties

The utilisation of the improved transfer properties of membranes and hollow fibres may be limited by the concentration gradients they produce in the blood. This has already occurred in hollow fibre blood oxygenators where transfer of oxygen and carbon dioxide is limited by the concentration gradients within the blood. It has led to design changes to mix the blood to disrupt the concentration gradients. In the longer term, similar problems will arise in dialysers, and it is likely that novel designs, analogous to those of blood oxygenators, will be required.

Adsorption

The most important and exciting area of progress will be the development of adsorption as a method of blood purification. Activated charcoal and ion exchange resins have been used to treat blood (usually in cases of acute poisoning) and ultrafiltrate, but they absorb a wide range of solutes. Selective adsorbents bind several, generally related, plasma components, mostly by utilising chemical interactions:

☐ dextran sulphate binds to negatively charged molecules including lipoprotein

☐ the amino acids, tryptophan and phenylalanine, bind immunoglobulins (Igs) and circulating immunocomplexes by non-specific, non-covalent hydrophobic interactions

☐ staphylococcal protein-A binds Ig subclasses 1, 2 and 4, and has been used to remove immune complexes.

Specific adsorbents are based on antibodies or antigens bound to a membrane surface. Antibodies against specific Igs, low density lipoproteins and β2-microglobulin have been developed.

Adsorbents are generally used to treat plasma, which requires an initial plasma separation, but methods are being developed which allow the treatment of whole blood. The development of increasingly selective and specific adsorbents which can be used to treat whole blood offers the possibility of new therapies, particularly for autoimmune disease, but the aims and applications must be clinically led.

REFERENCES

1 Vanholder R, De Smet R, Hsu C, *et al.* Uraemic toxicity; the middle molecule hypothesis revisited. *Semin Nephrol* 1994; 14: 205–18.

2 Courtney JM, Sundaram S, Lamba NMK, *et al.* Monitoring of the blood response in blood purification. *Artif Organs* 1993; 17: 260–6.

3 Kolff WJ, Berk HTJ. The artificial kidney: a dialyser with a great area. *Acta Med Scand* 1944; 117: 121–34.

4 Hoenich NA, Woffindin C, Ronco C. Haemodialysis and associated devices. In: Jacobs C, Kjellstrand CM, Koch KM, Winchester JF (eds). *Replacement of renal function by dialysis.* Dordrecht: Kluwer Academic Publishers, 1996: 188–230.

5 Barth RH. Pros and cons of short, high efficiency, and high flux dialysis. In: Jacobs C, Kjellstrand CM, Koch KM, Winchester JF (eds). *Replacement of renal function by dialysis.* Dordrecht: Kluwer Academic Publishers, 1996: 418–453.

FURTHER READING

Jacobs C, Kjellstrand CM, Koch KM, Winchester JF (eds). *Replacement of renal function by dialysis.* Dordrecht: Kluwer Academic Publishers, 1996.
This is an extremely useful volume which contains review chapters and additional references. Chapters of interest other than those listed above, are:

1   Quellhorst EA. Ultrafiltration/hemofiltration practice, pp 380–9.
2   Gurland H, Samtleben W, Lysaght MJ, *et al.* Extracorporeal blood purification techniques: plasmapheresis and haemoperfusion, pp 472–500.
3   Vanholder R, de Smet R, Vogeleere P, *et al.* The uraemic syndrome, pp 1–33.
4   Sargent JA, Gotch FA. Principles and biophysics of dialysis, pp 34–102.
5   Colton CK, Lysaght MJ. Membranes for haemodialysis, pp 103–13.
6   Henderson LW. Biophysics of ultrafiltration and hemofiltration, pp 114–45.

☐ SELF ASSESSMENT QUESTIONS

1   The most important driving force in dialysis is:
   (a) Solute concentration
   (b) Pressure
   (c) Osmosis
   (d) Membrane thickness
   (e) Adsorption

2   The most important resistance to transport in dialysis is:
   (a) Solute concentration
   (b) Pressure
   (c) Osmosis
   (d) Membrane thickness
   (e) Adsorption

3   The most important driving force in ultrafiltration is:
   (a) Solute concentration
   (b) Pressure
   (c) Osmosis
   (d) Membrane thickness
   (e) Adsorption

4   The most important resistance to transport in ultrafiltration is:
   (a) Solute concentration
   (b) Pressure
   (c) Osmosis
   (d) Membrane thickness
   (e) Adsorption

5   Dialysis membranes:
   (a) Separate the filtrate and dialysate
   (b) Separate the blood and dialysate

(c) Select the solute which is dialysed

(d) Transport high molecular weight solutes but not low molecular weight solutes

(e) Transport low molecular weight solutes but not high molecular weight solutes

6   Blood interacts with dialysis membranes, and the first event on contact is:

(a) Protein coating of the membrane

(b) Haemolysis of red cells

(c) Endotoxin generation

(d) Fibrinolysis

ANSWERS

| 1a | 2d | 3b | 4d | 5b, e | 6a |